Better Food
for Pregnancy

The Hospital for Sick Children

Better Food for Pregnancy

Nutrition Guide plus more
than 125 Recipes for Healthy
Pregnancy and Breastfeeding

Daina Kalnins, MSc, RD, and Joanne Saab, RD

The Hospital for Sick Children

The publisher acknowledges the financial support of the Government of Canada through the Book Publishing Industry Development Program.

Canadian Cataloguing in Publication Data
Kalnins, Daina
        Better food for pregnancy : nutrition guide plus more than 125 recipes for healthy pregnancy and breastfeeding / Daina Kalnins, Joanne Saab.

Includes index.
ISBN-13: 978-0-7788-0136-8
ISBN-10: 0-7788-0136-5

1. Pregnancy—Nutritional aspects. I. Saab, Joanne II. Title.

RG559.K34 2006   618.2'42   C2005-906120-0

Editors: Bob Hilderley, Senior Editor, Health; and Sue Sumeraj
Copyeditor and proofreader: Sheila Wawanash
Index: Gillian Watts
Design and page composition: PageWave Graphics Inc.
Illustrations: Kveta
Cover photo: Jerzyworks/Masterfile

Published by Robert Rose Inc.
120 Eglinton Ave. E., Suite 800, Toronto, Ontario Canada M4P 1E2
Tel: (416) 322-6552 Fax: (416) 322-6936.

Printed and bound in Canada
1 2 3 4 5 6 7 8 9 CPL 14 13 12 11 10 09 08 07 06

Contents

Preface. 6

Top 20 Frequently Asked
  Questions about Nutrition
  and Pregnancy 7

PART 1
**Better Nutrition for
Pregnancy**

1. Food Nutrition Basics 14
2. Food Safety 32
3. Pre-Pregnancy Nutrition . . . 48
4. Early Pregnancy Nutrition
   (First Trimester). 70
5. Mid-Pregnancy Nutrition
   (Second Trimester) 82
6. Late Pregnancy Nutrition
   (Third Trimester). 92
7. Post-Partum Nutrition
   and Breastfeeding 98
8. Good Nutrition for Life . . . 130

PART 2
Better Recipes for Pregnancy
Healthy Meal Plans 132
Best Recipes for
  Vital Nutrients 135

*Recipes with
Nutritional Analyses*
  Breakfasts. 141
  Appetizers and Snacks 155
  Soups 165
  Salads. 177
  Poultry 199
  Fish and Seafood 215
  Meat 231
  Vegetarian 247
  Sides 265
  Pasta. 271
  Desserts 281

Nutritional Analysis 296
Contributing Authors. 297
Resources 298
References. 300
Acknowledgments 310
Index 311

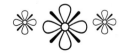

Preface

WHAT BETTER TIME TO LEARN about good nutrition than during the planning and earliest stages of a pregnancy? The nutritional status of a mother prior to conception and throughout pregnancy influences the nutritional status of the newborn baby and the future health of the child. Optimal nutrition provided to an unborn baby during the developing stages may prevent chronic disease in adulthood.

This is not just a question of eating well for two; it means eating smarter. Not only are calorie needs increased during pregnancy, but specific nutrients (such as iron and folic acid) are in higher demand, even before pregnancy! A balanced diet with these required nutrients needs to be supplied to the baby.

In this book, we provide the basics of a better diet for pregnancy that includes optimum intake of macronutrients — proteins, carbohydrates and fats — and required micronutrients, such as vitamins and minerals. We also identify foods that may help with morning sickness and foods that are not safe to eat during pregnancy. While this is not a "diet" book for losing weight, we do present information on appropriate weight gain during pregnancy and getting back into shape after pregnancy with good food selection. The need to eat better goes beyond the stages of pregnancy to breastfeeding your baby and establishing better eating habits for your kids. For each stage in your pregnancy, from conception to breastfeeding, we present not only nutritional advice, but also healthy recipes and meal plans for the two of you.

As co-authors of the best-selling books *Better Baby Food* and *Better Food for Kids*, we were inspired to write this book to provide mothers with the information they need to prepare for pregnancy and to provide optimal nutrition for themselves and for their babies. Our careful selection of recipes offers a wide variety of foods to enjoy, making food preparation a pleasure to savor, not a task to suffer. Understanding the principles of good nutrition and knowing how to prepare good food — that's what you will find in *Better Food for Pregnancy*.

Top 20 Frequently Asked Questions about Nutrition and Pregnancy

Women who are planning a pregnancy or who are pregnant often question the nutritional value and the safety of certain foods, as well as risks their lifestyle may present to the fetus. Here are the most frequently asked questions and their answers. Fuller answers are provided later in the book, but these short answers should serve as a quick reference to nutrition and lifestyle in pregnancy.

1. **Q.** I am very nauseated and worried that I am not getting enough to eat. How can I know if I am eating enough?

A. Mild to moderate nausea and vomiting do not generally result in poor nutritional status for the expectant mother or the fetus. Usually symptoms of nausea subside by 18 weeks of gestation. If you continue to experience nausea and vomiting throughout your pregnancy, you should speak with your health-care provider. For more information on nausea and vomiting, see page 79.

2. **Q.** I am having intense cravings for certain foods. Is this normal?

A. Cravings or aversions to certain foods are quite common during pregnancy. The cause of these intense cravings is unknown. Provided that the food is not harmful, you can give in to these cravings now and then. For more information on food cravings, see page 78.

3. **Q.** Do I need to take a multivitamin during pregnancy?

A. You do not need to take a multivitamin if you eat a well-balanced diet during pregnancy. Following the United States Department of Agriculture (USDA) MyPyramid or Canada's Food Guide to Healthy Eating will provide you with the nutrients you need. Nevertheless, if you are planning a pregnancy or become pregnant, you should take an additional folic acid supplement containing at least 400 mcg (0.4 mg). There is strong evidence that folic acid supplementation can help prevent neural tube defects. Additional iron may also be recommended by your doctor. If your diet is less than perfect, a multivitamin can help to provide some additional vitamins and minerals. For more on multivitamins, see pages 64 and 76–77.

4. **Q.** How much folic acid do I need? I am worried about my baby developing spina bifida.

A. The Recommended Dietary Allowance (RDA) of folic acid for pregnant women is 600 mcg, or 0.6 mg, per day. This should come from a combination of a supplement containing at least 400 mcg (0.4 mg) of folic acid and from dietary sources, including enriched grains, fruits and vegetables. For more information on folic acid, see pages 25–27 and 58–59.

5. **Q.** Is it safe to drink herbal teas during pregnancy?

A. Some herbal teas are safe to drink during pregnancy and some are not. For example, chamomile tea, commonly used for relaxation, is not safe to use during pregnancy, while citrus peel, ginger, lemon balm, orange peel and rose hip teas are safe. For more information on herbal teas, see pages 41 and 44.

6.

Q. My gums are bleeding when I brush my teeth. Is this normal?

A. This is a fairly common occurrence during pregnancy because of increased blood flow to the gums. To help minimize the bleeding of gums, be sure to brush three times a day, floss daily and see your dentist regularly. For more information on dental health, see page 90.

7.

Q. Is it safe to drink diet soda pop?

A. Occasionally consuming diet colas containing aspartame, acesulfame potassium (ace K) or sucralose is considered safe during pregnancy. Beverages sweetened with saccharin or cyclamates should be avoided during pregnancy. For more information on the safety of artificial sweeteners, see page 42.

8.

Q. I have heard about listeria in cheese. What cheeses can I eat?

A. Hard cheeses, such as Cheddar and Parmesan, as well as soft pasteurized milk products, such as cottage cheese, cream cheese and yogurt, are safe to eat. Unpasteurized cheese, such as Brie, Camembert and feta cheese, should be avoided. For more information on listeria, see page 32.

9.

Q. Should I avoid eating peanuts to prevent my baby from developing food allergies?

A. This is a very controversial topic in the scientific community. Avoiding peanuts during pregnancy may or may not prevent your child from developing an allergy. However, the American Academy of Pediatrics (AAP) suggests that in families where there is a high risk of having a baby with an allergy (sibling or parent also has an allergy or asthma), a pregnant woman may wish to eliminate peanuts from her diet during her pregnancy. For more information on allergies, see pages 77 and 122–26.

10. **Q.** What can I do to help with constipation?

A. Try increasing your fiber intake through the consumption of high-fiber foods, such as whole grains, fruits, vegetables and lentils. Exercise regularly when possible, and take in 12 cups (3 L) of fluid daily, including milk, water, soup and juices. For more information on constipation, see page 88.

11. **Q.** What can I do to treat my hemorrhoids?

A. The best way to treat hemorrhoids is to prevent constipation by drinking plenty of fluid (12 cups/3 L) each day and getting enough fiber in your diet from fruits, vegetables and whole grains. Regular exercise is also important. If hemorrhoids continue to be a problem, speak with your health-care provider, who can recommend an ointment to help with the pain associated with hemorrhoids. For more information on hemorrhoids, see page 89.

12. **Q.** Can I eat something to help prevent stretch marks?

A. There is no evidence that suggests anything you eat will prevent the development of stretch marks. Stretch marks are colored changes to the skin that happen when the skin is stretched beyond its natural limits during pregnancy. For more information on stretch marks, see page 97.

13. **Q.** Can I drink protein shakes or eat protein bars during pregnancy?

A. It is not recommended that pregnant women consume protein shakes and bars. These foods contain a large amount of protein. One protein bar can contain as much as 35 grams of protein, which is about half of your day's protein needs in one snack. Protein bars and shakes can also contain herbs that may not be safe to use during pregnancy. For more information on protein, see pages 21 and 67.

14. **Q.** Which herbs are not safe to use during my pregnancy?

A. The safety of many herbal remedies or herbs has not been adequately studied. At this time, the following herbs have been determined by the Motherisk program at The Hospital for Sick Children to be unsafe to consume during pregnancy: aloe vera, black cohosh, burdock, calendula, chamomile, chaste tree, dong quai, feverfew, goldenseal, hops, juniper, licorice, ma huang, passionflower, peppermint and slippery elm. Unsafe means there is evidence to show that the herb might cause harm to the fetus. It does not mean that this will happen in each case, but avoidance is strongly recommended. Please note that if a herb is not listed here, that does not mean it is safe to use during pregnancy. For more information on herbs, see pages 41 and 44.

15. **Q.** I have cravings for Chinese food. Should I ask for no MSG to be added to my food?

A. At this time, there is no evidence that monosodium glutamate (MSG) is harmful during pregnancy. MSG is often used as a flavor enhancer. Some research with mice does show that MSG crosses the placental barrier, but studies do not indicate that this is true in humans. MSG is high in sodium, however, so for women who are required to lower their sodium intake, limiting MSG intake would be recommended. It would be prudent for women to ask for foods that are MSG-free during pregnancy in order to decrease their salt intake. For more information on MSG intake, see page 121.

16. **Q.** Is it safe to use a microwave oven when I am pregnant?

A. Current studies indicate that it is safe to use a microwave oven. For more information on microwave exposure, see page 39.

17.

Q. Is it safe to drink tap water while I am pregnant, or should I be buying bottled water?

A. It is safe and considerably less expensive to use municipal tap water rather than bottled water. If you have concerns about your local water supply, contact your water supply company, usually listed on your municipal tax bill or water bill. For more information on water safety, see pages 45–47.

18.

Q. I am 9 months pregnant and like to jog. When should I quit exercising?

A. Active women can continue to exercise as long as they are able. Jogging in the last trimester may not be recommended due to lower-abdominal discomfort because of the weight of the fetus. Check with your physician for advice on your individual pregnancy — a lot will depend on your general health and the progression of your pregnancy. Any discomfort felt during exercise should be seen as an indicator to stop. For more information on exercise, see pages 63, 75, 89–90 and 128.

19.

Q. How long will it take to lose the weight I gained during pregnancy?

A. This depends on how much was gained during the pregnancy, your activity level after pregnancy and your general diet. It would not be unreasonable to expect to be back to your pregnancy weight about 6 to 7 months after the birth of your baby. For more information on weight loss, see pages 126–27.

20.

Q. Can I drink coffee every day during my pregnancy?

A. One cup of coffee per day should be okay. For more information on coffee and caffeine guidelines, see page 39–40.

PART 1

Better Nutrition for Pregnancy

CHAPTER 1

Food Nutrition Basics

FOOD PROVIDES US WITH ENERGY needed for all bodily functions. When we walk, talk, breathe or think, we need energy from food. Without this food energy, we could not survive.

Our primary sources of food energy are macronutrients — carbohydrates, proteins and fats. These macronutrients are converted into energy in the body by the action of micronutrients — minerals, vitamins, amino acids, essential fatty acids and enzymes. Some of these micronutrients are manufactured in our bodies, but others are found only in our food.

Let's look at the energy requirements for pregnant women before exploring the role macronutrients and micronutrients play in pregnancy nutrition.

Did You Know ...

Calorie Requirements

Intake of calories needs to increase over the course of the 40 weeks of pregnancy to support changes in the mother and fetus.

- Growth of maternal tissues, including the uterus, placenta and mammary tissues
- Expanding blood supply to these tissues
- Growth and activity of the fetus
- Loss of maternal tissues at birth
- Preparation for breastfeeding

Energy

Energy Needs

Food energy is commonly measured in calories. Current recommendations suggest that women of normal weight and average activity level need about 2,000 to 2,400 calories daily. Pregnant women need about an additional 100 calories a day in the first trimester and 300 extra calories per day in the second and third trimester. This means that most adult pregnant women need about 2,100 to 2,700 calories of energy a day, depending on the stage of pregnancy. However, some micronutrient requirements during pregnancy, such as iron and folate, increase as much as 50%. These nutrient requirements are affected by a woman's basal metabolic rate, pre-pregnancy weight, age, rate of weight gain and activity level. Obese women should not gain much weight during pregnancy. Every woman is different; energy needs are very individualized.

 What is metabolism?

Metabolism is the breaking down and the building of substances in the body in order to maintain life, including the way nutrients are handled in the body. Basal metabolic rate (BMR) refers to the energy requirements of the body at rest.

❀ What is a calorie?

A calorie is the standard unit for measuring the amount of energy available in the food we eat and the amount of energy we use in physical activity. Technically, 1 calorie is the amount of energy needed to raise the temperature of 1 gram of water by 1 degree Celsius. Because calories are small units of measure, they are usually expressed as kilocalories (kcal) or Calories (with a capital C) to indicate 1,000 calories. In this book, we have chosen to use the kcal nomenclature when making specific energy measurements and simply "calories" when we are discussing energy needs.

Women carrying multiples, such as twins, triplets or quads, need more calories than women carrying a single baby. Twin pregnancies require approximately 150 additional calories a day, so about 450 calories more each day over pre-pregnancy needs in the second and third trimesters, while triplets and quads need even more calories. Women expecting multiple babies should speak with a dietitian to ensure that all their nutritional needs are being met.

In North America, where overweight and obesity are prevalent, too much weight gain during pregnancy can be an issue. Women need to focus on eating nutrient-rich foods that are high in vitamins and minerals, not just calorically dense foods.

Weight Management

To suggest that pregnant women need to eat more calories raises the question of weight management during pregnancy. Eating too many calories without expending this added energy can result in weight gain. Pregnant women need to choose their foods wisely to ensure nutrient-dense foods are chosen while avoiding putting on excess weight. Following the United Sates Department of Agriculture MyPyramid eating guide or Canada's Food Guide to Healthy Eating, maintaining an active lifestyle and letting your appetite guide what you eat are all terrific ways to ensure that you eat enough for both you and your baby without overdoing it.

Did You Know ...

Fetal Calories

Near the end of pregnancy, the fetus will need about 125 calories of energy a day.

How much food makes up 300 calories?

In your second and third trimester, you will need to add 300 calories a day to your diet. You'd be surprised to find how very little food is needed to meet this requirement. Some examples of food choices that are equal to about 300 calories include:

- skim milk: 2$\frac{1}{2}$ cups (625 mL)
- ice cream: 1 cup (250 mL)
- bagel ($\frac{1}{2}$) with Cheddar cheese and tomato
- tuna sandwich with cucumber

Dietitians recommend that these 300 calories be spread out over the course of the day among three meals and one to two snacks, rather than trying to consume an additional 300 calories at any one time.

Macronutrients

Macronutrients comprise carbohydrates, proteins and fats.

Carbohydrates

Carbohydrates provide the largest percentage of calories in the North American diet, usually between 40% and 55% of total daily calories. The acceptable range, according to the Dietary Reference Intakes (DRIs), is 45% to 65% of total caloric intake. Carbohydrates include cereals and grains, such as wheat, rice, oats and barley. Fruits, vegetables and honey are also sources of carbohydrates. Milk and dairy products contain carbohydrates, but to a lesser extent than cereals, fruits and vegetables. The brain and red blood cells use carbohydrates as an important source of energy. If carbohydrates are not available, the body adapts by using protein or fat as a source of energy.

Kinds of Carbohydrates
Carbohydrates are also known as sugars and classified according to their "length" as short-chain or simple sugars and long-chain or complex sugars.

Simple Sugars

The simple "single" sugars are glucose, fructose and galactose. These are also known as monosaccharides. The disaccharides (two sugars connected together) are sucrose, lactose and maltose.

Sucrose is made up of glucose and fructose. This carbohydrate is commonly found in fruits and vegetables. It is the type found in table sugar. Lactose, made up of glucose and galactose, is found in milk and dairy products. Maltose, made from two glucose units, is found in cereals, such as wheat or barley.

Complex Sugars

Long-chain carbohydrates are called polysaccharides and include starches and modified starches. They are made up mainly of glucose found in plant foods. Non-starch polysaccharides are more commonly known as dietary fiber.

 What is lactose intolerance?

Individuals who are intolerant to milk are usually lactose intolerant. The enzyme lactase, found on the wall of the small intestine, is required to break down lactose. Lactose intolerance is not caused by a milk allergy, but by an inability to break down lactose due to a lack of or limited amount of the enzyme lactase. The undigested lactose accumulates in the gastrointestinal tract and becomes food for bacteria living in our digestive system. These bacteria produce the gas that causes the symptoms of lactose intolerance, including flatulence, bloating and abdominal cramps, as well as diarrhea.

The occurrence of lactose intolerance differs among races. Most Caucasian North Americans of European descent maintain their lactase activity. For other races, such as African Americans, Native Americans, Asians and Mediterraneans, lactose intolerance affects as many as 70% to 90% of women. Although almost all females are born with high amounts of lactase and are able to digest milk and milk products, many of us lose lactase and by adulthood are considered lactose intolerant.

People who suffer from lactose intolerance are not able to eat many dairy products with lactose, but may be able to consume fermented dairy products, such as some cheeses and yogurt. This is because the lactose in these dairy products has already been converted to lactic acid during the fermentation process. The good news is that, over time, many people with lactose intolerance do gradually build up a tolerance to lactose and are able to consume increasing amounts of dairy products. Enzyme tablets containing lactase are available to help women digest lactose and can be used during pregnancy.

What does dietary recommended intake mean?

The Dietary Reference Intakes (DRIs) are nutrient recommendations based on the most recently available scientific information. The DRIs actually include four reference values: the Recommended Dietary Allowance (RDA), the Estimated Average Requirement (EAR), Adequate Intake (AI) and the Tolerable Upper Intake Level (UL). The RDA, EAR and AI are used to determine the amount of a macronutrient or micronutrient required. The amount of energy required in individuals is labeled the Estimated Energy Requirement (EER). The difference between these values (RDA, EAR and AI) lies in the amount of evidence available to support the daily required recommendation for that nutrient. In any case, the RDA, EAR or AI are the recommended daily amounts for individuals. The UL sets the maximum safe level to consume on a daily basis.

 ## Dietary Recommended Intake of Carbohydrates

A minimum amount of carbohydrates during pregnancy has been determined to be 175 grams a day. If not enough carbohydrate is available for normal body functions and non-carbohydrate sources are used for energy, this can be potentially harmful to the fetus.

Glycemic Index

The glycemic index of foods is used to describe the effect that certain carbohydrates have on blood sugar, providing a guide to how fast a certain food raises blood sugar levels. The longer it takes to raise the blood sugar level, the better that food is in keeping blood sugar levels more stable. This becomes important in those with diabetes, as certain foods may help control glucose levels better than others.

Generally, a food that has a lower glycemic index is preferable to one that has a higher glycemic index. For example, an oat bran cereal or chickpeas would have a lower glycemic index than plain white bread or potatoes. In situations where a quick increase in blood sugar is required, the foods that are higher on the glycemic index would be recommended.

Low Glycemic Index Foods

Skim milk, plain yogurt, sweet potato, oat bran bread, oatmeal, lentils, kidney beans, chickpeas

Medium Glycemic Index Foods

Banana, raisins, split pea soup, brown rice, couscous, whole wheat bread, rye bread

High Glycemic Index Foods

Dried dates, instant mashed potatoes, baked white potatoes, instant rice, white plain bagel, soda crackers, french fries, ice cream, table sugar

Good Sources of Dietary Carbohydrates

- Whole-grain breads and cereals
- Lentils
- Fruits and vegetables
- Milk

Fiber

Fiber is a carbohydrate that escapes digestion in the stomach and small intestine but can be used as energy by microorganisms in the large intestine, or colon. Fiber is needed to prevent constipation and increase the bulk of stools. Dietary fiber is found in many foods, including fruits, vegetables, legumes, whole grains such as oats, rye and barley, and wheat bran.

Significantly, our bodies do not have the enzyme needed to break down fiber into small enough pieces to be absorbed, and so fiber passes through your digestive tract without being digested. This allows fiber to do a couple of things.

First, it helps to slow down the speed at which food passes through the small intestine, which increases the amount of nutrients that are absorbed from food. It also helps to lower blood cholesterol levels, mainly "bad" low-density lipoprotein (LDL) cholesterol. Fiber also helps to absorb water and increase stool bulk. Certain types of dietary fiber help to increase the speed at which food moves through the gastrointestinal tract, especially the colon, or large intestine. This prevents excess water from being absorbed in the colon and helps to keep the stool soft and moving through your body. Basically, it helps keep you regular. Fiber helps to maintain good blood sugar control. A diet high in fiber may also reduce the risk of diverticulitis and colon cancer, which is the second leading cause of cancer death in North America.

 ## Dietary Recommended Intake of Fiber

Most North Americans do not get enough fiber in their diet. Current AI recommendations suggest that adults should aim for an intake of 21 to 38 grams of fiber a day to maximize its beneficial effects while minimizing any negative effects associated with too much fiber. The AI for women who are pregnant is 28 grams of fiber a day.

This can be obtained by eating approximately 5 servings of fruits and vegetables a day and 6 servings of breads and cereals daily, choosing whole grains instead of refined white bread products and whole fruits with their skins when possible.

Be sure to drink lots of fluid when increasing the amount of fiber you eat (at least 12 cups/3 L a day of all fluids). When you eat more fiber without drinking more water, it can make constipation worse by increasing the volume of stool you produce without extra water to keep it moving through your colon. Any increases in fiber intake should be done slowly. Increasing fiber intake quickly can initially cause an increase in gas production, or flatulence.

Eating too much fiber, although rare, can also be problematic, reducing the absorption of certain minerals, such as calcium, iron, magnesium and zinc.

Did You Know ...

Amino Acid Needs

During the first 20 weeks of pregnancy, all the amino acids your baby needs to make protein must be provided from your diet. After 20 weeks of pregnancy, your baby's liver is able to make some non-essential amino acids on its own.

Good Sources of Dietary Fiber

Oatmeal, 1 cup (250 mL) cooked	4.0 g
Whole wheat toast, 2 slices	3.8 g
Raisin bran cereal, 1 cup (250 mL)	8.2 g
Apple, raw with skin	3.7 g
Blueberries, ½ cup (125 mL)	2.0 g
Broccoli, steamed, ½ cup (125 mL)	2.3 g
Kidney beans, ½ cup (125 mL) boiled	6.5 g
Dry-roasted almonds, 1 oz (30 g)	3.9 g

Proteins

Proteins are the building blocks for all the tissues in the body. During pregnancy, protein is needed for the development of the baby's organs and tissues. Your baby uses some of the protein supplied by you as an energy source. It is also needed to help support the growth of a mother's uterus, placenta and mammary glands.

Proteins are made up of amino acids. Amino acids are considered to be "non-essential" if the body can make enough of them on its own, and "essential" when the body cannot make them in sufficient quantities and we need to obtain them from our diet.

Dietary Recommended Intake of Protein

During pregnancy, the requirements for protein are higher than they were before pregnancy. Protein needs increase over the course of pregnancy, and it is suggested that an extra 25 grams of protein daily are needed, for a total of 71 grams of protein each day. These protein requirements for pregnancy are based on what is considered to be the normal needs of a non-pregnant woman plus extra added for the growth of fetal and maternal tissues.

Most women in North America eat more than the recommended amount of protein every day. The average woman does not need to increase her protein intake consciously during pregnancy.

Fats

The fat in food is an essential element of our diet, storing an important source of concentrated energy for use when required, providing us with essential fatty acids and transporting important fat-soluble micronutrients — vitamins A, D, E and K. Triglycerides and phospholipids, for example, are combinations of fatty acids involved in fat storage, cell structure and transportation of fat in the bloodstream. The DRI fat intake range is 20% to 35% of total energy intake.

Saturated vs. Unsaturated Fats

Fats can be saturated or unsaturated, depending on their chemical structure. Saturated fats do not contain chemical double bonds, whereas unsaturated fats do. Monounsaturated fatty acids have one double bond, while polyunsaturated fatty

Did You Know ...
Protein Levels

If your diet does not contain enough protein, then the amount of protein stored by your body will be reduced to ensure that the fetus receives the protein it needs. However, significantly reduced protein intake can influence birth length, and a baby may not reach its full height potential. Too much protein may also retard fetal growth and contribute to premature birth.

Did You Know ...

Fat Choices

Choosing fats that are monounsaturated or polyunsaturated while limiting, but not eliminating, saturated fatty acids is often recommended for a healthy diet.

Did You Know ...

Limited Fats

The DRI recommendations for foods high in saturated fats and trans fatty acids state that they should be limited during pregnancy. There is no defined upper level that is considered to be safe. Saturated fats can raise "bad" cholesterol (low-density lipoprotein, or LDL) levels and total blood cholesterol. Trans fatty acids also raise cholesterol levels in a similar way as saturated fats. They also lower "good" cholesterol (high-density lipoproteins, or HDL) levels, so are potentially more damaging.

acids have more than one double bond. The location of this bond determines if it is a "cis" or a "trans" fat. Fat with the cis conformation occurs more often in nature, while the trans fats are more often manufactured or altered.

Limit use of saturated fats, such as butter and coconut oil, as well as commercial products that contain saturated fats, such as sweets and pastries. Saturated fats are found in animal products, so choose the less fatty cuts of meat and lower-fat varieties of dairy products.

Trans Fatty Acids

Trans fatty acids are found in small amounts naturally in meat and in dairy products. They are also manufactured by decreasing the number of double bonds by adding hydrogen to make unsaturated fats more solid at room temperature. Because this process increases the shelf life of oils, trans fatty acids are often added to processed foods, such as crackers, cookies and other snack foods, to provide a desired crispy texture.

However, because of the negative association between trans fatty acids and coronary heart disease, food manufacturers have started eliminating these fats from food production. While other factors influence the risk of heart disease, such as decreased levels of activity and decreased intake of fruits and vegetables, a decrease in trans fats, with an increased emphasis on omega 3 fatty acids, is desirable.

Trans fatty acids are found in many commercially baked products, such as potato chips, crackers, cookies and other sweet foods. Trans fatty acids are also found in products that

Good Sources of Monounsaturated Fats

- Margarine spreads with canola oil or olive oil base
- Olive oil, canola oil, peanut oil
- Avocados
- Peanuts, hazelnuts, cashews, almonds

Good Sources of Polyunsaturated Fats

- Safflower oil, sunflower oil, corn oil, soy oil
- Fish oils and seafood
- Polyunsaturated margarines
- Walnuts, brazil nuts, seeds

contain hydrogenated or partially hydrogenated vegetable shortenings. The U.S. Food and Drug Administration and Health Canada require that manufacturers disclose the amount of trans fatty acids in the product on food labels.

Omega 3 and Omega 6 Essential Fatty Acids

Essential fatty acids are required for human development and must be taken in as part of the diet. These essential polyunsaturated fatty acids have many structural and metabolic functions. They are important components of cell membranes. The central nervous system contains a high amount of fatty acids. Visual function depends on an adequate supply of essential fatty acids.

 What is the ideal ratio of omega 3 to omega 6 fatty acids?

While these fats are found together in many other foods, the North American diet is overweighted with omega 6 fatty acids, at a ratio of more than 10:1, resulting in an excessive amount of omega 6 fatty acids compared to omega 3 fatty acids. Our health is influenced by the ratio of omega 6 to omega 3 fatty acids in our diet. A very high consumption of omega 6 fatty acids in relation to omega 3 fatty acids may decrease our natural defense against certain disease states, such as heart disease, asthma and arthritis. A recommended healthy ratio of omega 6 to omega 3 fatty acids is about 4:1.

The DRI (AI) for omega 6 fatty acids during pregnancy is 13 grams per day, or 5% to 10% of total calories. The AI for omega 3 fatty acids is 1.4 grams per day, or 0.6% to 1.2% of total calories.

The essential fatty acids include omega 3 (double bond at the third carbon) and omega 6 (double bond at the sixth carbon) fatty acids. Omega 3 and omega 6 fatty acids are called essential because the body is not able to form them, so these fatty acids must be derived from dietary fat.

Omega 3 fatty acids help to regulate inflammation and the inflammation process. They can reduce the risk of cardiac disease or coronary heart disease and may help in the prevention of high blood pressure. Omega 6 fatty acids play an important role in lowering cholesterol levels and are involved in the inflammation process.

Omega 3 and omega 6 fatty acids are essential for the normal development of the fetus. During its metabolism, the

Omega 3 Supplements

The use of omega 3 fatty acid supplements is becoming increasingly popular. However, the dietary form of these fatty acids is recommended because it is likely that other components of the foods containing omega 3 fatty acids are important as well.

omega 3 fatty acid known as linolenic acid is converted to docosahexaenoic acid (DHA) and eicosapentaenoic acid (EPA). The omega 6 fatty acid known as linoleic acid is converted to arachidonic acids (AA), which are structural fatty acids in the brain. DHA and AA are important for brain and retina (visual) development in the fetus. Some studies suggest that the fetus may not be able to adequately make the conversion of linolenic acid to DHA in the first few months of life, thus requiring a direct supply of DHA. DHA is found, already formed, in breast milk and is added to some infant formulas.

The fetus not only depends on the mother's dietary intake of essential fatty acids, but also on the function of the placenta and fat stores of the mother. Because of the interaction of each of these components on the availability of essential fatty acid supply to the fetus, women should consume a diet balanced with essential fatty acids prior to pregnancy so that the body can have them available to the growing fetus in the future.

Good Sources of Omega 3 Fatty Acids

- Flax seeds and flax seed oil
- Canola oil and soy oil
- Fatty fish (salmon or trout)
- Eggs containing omega 3 fatty acids

Good Sources of Omega 6 Fatty Acids

- Corn oil, sunflower oil, safflower oil, peanut oil
- Egg yolks
- Lean meats

Cholesterol

Cholesterol is another fat important to cell membranes. Cholesterol is also a component of hormones. The body makes it own cholesterol in the liver and in other cells of the body. Regulation of its level in the blood is determined by internal mechanisms and, to a lesser extent, by dietary intake, primarily from animal sources of food (meat, poultry, eggs, dairy products, seafood, butter and lard).

There are two types of cholesterol in the blood: low-density lipoprotein (LDL) cholesterol and high-density lipoprotein (HDL) cholesterol. LDL is often referred to as the "bad" cholesterol because it contributes to the narrowing of arteries, which can lead to heart disease and stroke. Saturated fats tend to raise LDL levels in the blood. HDL is often referred to as the "good" cholesterol because it helps to clean out arteries and to clear the blood of LDL.

It is the ratio of HDL to LDL that is important when talking about blood cholesterol levels. A higher amount of HDL compared to LDL is desirable. Monounsaturated and polyunsaturated fats tend to lower blood cholesterol levels. Regular physical activity and exercise and a high-fiber diet may also help reduce cholesterol levels in the blood.

Dietary Recommended Intake of Fat

Keep the contribution of fat to your diet to 20% to 35% of total energy intake during pregnancy. Remember, fats are an important part of a healthy diet, so there is no need to restrict them too much.

Micronutrients

Several micronutrients are vital to the health of the mother and the fetus during pregnancy, including folic acid, calcium, vitamin D, iron and zinc.

Folate (Folic Acid)

Folate is a B vitamin needed for the normal growth and division of all cells — not just human cells, but all animal, plant and microbial cells. It is involved in the making of our genetic material, DNA (deoxyribonucleic acid) and RNA (ribonucleic acid). It is also required for the growth and development of our red blood cells.

During pregnancy, a time when so much cell division and growth are occurring, the need for folate increases. Pregnant women specifically need more folate to support their expanding blood volume, as well as the growth of maternal and fetal tissues. Later in pregnancy, folate helps to promote normal fetal growth and prevents some forms of anemia of pregnancy. It also offers protection against other complications of pregnancy, including detachment of the placenta, hemorrhage and low birth weight. In its supplemental form, folate is termed folic acid.

Among all neural tube defects, 90% to 95% occur in pregnancies where there is no family history of other neural tube defects. Neural tube defects often develop before a woman even realizes she is pregnant. Current research suggests that taking a folic acid supplement of 400 mcg (0.4 mg) daily, before becoming pregnant and until the end of the first trimester, may help to reduce the risk of these defects by up to 50%.

Neural Tube Defects

Providing your body with adequate folate before and during early pregnancy helps to prevent neural tube defects. Neural tube defects include spina bifida, as well as lesser-known defects such as anencephaly and encephalocele. Neural tube defects happen because of the improper development and closure of the neural tube (which eventually becomes part of the spine and brain) by 25 days after conception. Pregnancies affected by a neural tube defect may result in miscarriage or stillbirth. Children may also be born with a mild to severe disability.

The good news is that once folate is transferred from mother to fetus, it cannot be returned to the mother. This is to help ensure that your baby's folate stores will not be depleted to meet your folate needs later in pregnancy. During pregnancy, folate is not as well absorbed as it was before pregnancy, and the amount that is removed through the urinary tract system increases. This is an important factor in making folate deficiency a global pregnancy issue.

 Who should be concerned about neural tube defects?

All women who do not consume adequate folic acid are at risk of having a baby with a neural tube defect. Some women may be more at risk if other factors are present:

- They have a family history of NTDs or a previous pregnancy involving an NTD.
- They have diabetes.
- They take anticonvulsant drugs (e.g., women with epilepsy).

If you have an increased risk of having a baby with a neural tube defect, speak with your doctor. She may advise you to take higher amounts of folic acid.

 Dietary Recommended Intake of Folate

The current DRI (RDA) for folate is 600 mcg (0.6 mg) a day for pregnant women from both dietary and supplement sources of folic acid. This is 50% more than the DRI for non-pregnant women of 400 mcg (0.4 mg) daily. This increase helps to meet the demands of tissue growth during pregnancy. However, current data suggests that the average Canadian female consumes only about 200 mcg (0.2 mg) of folate a day.

Good Sources of Folate

Food: While folate is present in most foods, wheat germ is a very concentrated source, containing 178 mcg (0.18 mg) of folate per 100 grams. Other excellent sources include organ meats, such as liver and kidney. These foods are not consumed very often or in large quantities, however. Fruits and vegetables provide the most significant source of folate in most diets. Yet another reason to eat up your fruits and veggies!

Enriched foods: For many women, consuming 600 mcg (0.6 mg) per day of folate by food sources alone is difficult. Folate is susceptible to destruction by heat, UV light and oxidation. During cooking, some foods lose between 50% and 90% of their original folate content. To solve this problem, the American and Canadian governments in 1998 required that white flour and pasta products labeled "enriched" also include added folic acid. It is estimated that this enrichment adds about 100 mcg (0.1 mg) to the average woman's diet every day.

Vitamin supplements: Many prenatal multivitamin and mineral supplements contain more than 400 mcg (0.4 mg) of folic acid in each tablet. Be careful not to overdo it. There is a tolerable upper limit (UL) set for folic acid of 1,000 mcg (1.0 mg) daily from supplemental sources. Although there have been no reported adverse effects of taking too much folic acid, this does not mean that none exist. However, there is no risk of toxicity from folic acid through dietary sources.

Calcium

Calcium is an important mineral required for keeping our bones and teeth strong and for normal functioning of the heart, nerves and muscles. Calcium is also required for the development of the fetal skeleton.

During pregnancy, the absorption of calcium increases as the demand for this mineral increases, ensuring that the fetus receives an adequate supply of calcium. Not only is it essential that the dietary intake of calcium is adequate during pregnancy, but the efficiency of calcium absorption also needs to be enhanced. Other minerals and vitamins, such as phosphorous and vitamin D, are required for normal calcium metabolism.

Calcium is found in milk and dairy products, tofu, some vegetables (such as broccoli) and fish bones (such as canned salmon and sardines). Most of the calcium in our bodies (99%) is found in the bones.

Dietary Recommended Intake of Calcium

The DRI (AI) for calcium is 1,000 mg per day during pregnancy, which is the same requirement as pre-pregnancy. Teenage girls, however, do need more if they are pregnant: 1,300 mg per day both before and during pregnancy. The maximum safe level of calcium intake per day (UL) is 2, 500 mg per day, before and during pregnancy.

Good Sources of Dietary Calcium

- Milk
- Cheese
- Tofu
- Certain vegetables (for example, broccoli)
- Bones of fish (for example, sardines and salmon)

Vitamin D

Vitamin D, or calciferol, plays an important role in calcium absorption and, therefore, in bone formation and maintenance. It can be produced by the action of the sun on the skin, where a precursor of vitamin D is located. If sunlight is available, there is a limited dietary requirement for vitamin D. Not all individuals are exposed to adequate sunlight throughout the year (such as those residing in the Northern Hemisphere), however, and cultural reasons (such as dress) prevent adequate exposure for others. Then, the dietary form of vitamin D is required.

Dietary Recommended Intake of Vitamin D

The DRI (AI) for vitamin D is 200 IU per day, both before and during pregnancy. The safest highest level (UL) is considered to be 2,000 IU per day. However, some experts believe that the DRI (AI) for vitamin D is much too low. Because of the use of sunscreens, which significantly reduce the formation of vitamin D in our bodies from the sun, and limited exposure to the sun in general, as is recommended to reduce the incidence of skin cancer, we are not getting the amount of vitamin D we need. Check with your doctor to sure you are getting enough vitamin D.

Vitamin D conversion and regulation are dependent on the amount of calcium and phosphorous found in the blood, as well as on the level of vitamin D circulating in the blood. The kidneys play an important role in converting vitamin D to an active form. The kidneys also regulate the amount of vitamin D in the blood by increasing its production when blood levels are low, and by decreasing production when levels are high.

Good Sources of Vitamin D

- Fortified milk
- Fortified margarines
- Fish oils
- Fortified cereals
- Liver

Iron

Iron is a mineral involved in many metabolic processes. It is found in animal foods (heme iron) and plants (non-heme iron). The absorption of heme iron in the body is much greater than non-heme iron absorption. By consuming foods that contain vitamin C, non-heme iron absorption is increased.

Iron is stored in the body. Men have about 4 grams of iron in their body, while women have about 2.5 grams. When iron and blood levels of hemoglobin (a protein in the blood that carries iron) are low in the body, anemia may develop. Because oxygen is carried on the hemoglobin molecule, anemia can result in a decrease in oxygen being supplied to maternal and fetal tissues during pregnancy. Anemia can also occur when there is not enough circulating iron for metabolic processes that involve this mineral, even if stores of iron are adequate. Iron deficiency is the most common nutrient deficiency in both developing and developed countries.

Dietary Recommended Intake of Iron

The DRI (RDA) for iron during pregnancy is 27 mg per day. Pre-pregnancy it is 18 mg per day. The upper safe limit (UL) is 45 mg per day.

Good Sources of Dietary Iron

- Meat and poultry
- Firm tofu
- Beans and lentils
- Dried fruit
- Fortified cereals

Vitamin B-12

It is critical that pregnant or breastfeeding women on a vegetarian diet, especially a vegan diet, receive a regular source of vitamin B-12 every day if their diet is not supplemented. This is also true for infants of breastfeeding vegetarian mothers who do not take a vitamin B-12 supplement. Infants who do not receive an adequate source of vitamin B-12 are at particularly high risk for deficiency. Studies indicate that a mother's intake and absorption of vitamin B-12 during pregnancy may be more important than what her actual vitamin B-12 stores are.

With prolonged iron deficiency anemia, vitamin B-12 deficiency can occur regardless of vitamin B-12 intake. This is because iron deficiency anemia damages the lining in the stomach and can lessen the production of gastric acid, an intrinsic factor important for the absorption of vitamin B-12.

In North America, vitamin B-12 fortification is permitted. Common foods that are fortified with vitamin B-12 include tofu burgers, soy milk, breakfast cereals and nutritional yeasts. Read all the labels to ensure that an adequate amount of vitamin B-12 is being consumed.

 ## Dietary Recommended Intake of Vitamin B-12

The Recommended Dietary Allowance (RDA) for vitamin B-12 is 2.6 mcg per day. The upper limit for vitamin B-12 intake during pregnancy has not been determined.

Good Sources of Vitamin B-12

- Beef
- Salmon
- Dairy products
- Eggs
- Pork
- Clams and oysters, cooked

Zinc

Zinc is an essential trace element involved in growth and metabolism. Deficiency of zinc compromises the immune system. Zinc is found in organs and tissues in the body, but it must be supplied by the diet. As is the case with calcium and iron, absorption of zinc increases when there is a low supply or a zinc deficiency.

High intakes of phytate (found in whole grains and cereals), as well as calcium and iron, may interfere with zinc absorption. Women who smoke during pregnancy also decrease the amount of zinc available to the fetus. Strenuous exercise and infections may decrease the amount of zinc transferred to the fetus.

Did You Know ...

Inadequate Fetal Zinc

During pregnancy, zinc is deposited in the fetus and in the uterine muscle. One of the factors that cause low birth weight may be the result of inadequate fetal zinc supply.

Dietary Recommended Intake of Zinc

The DRI (RDA) for zinc is 11 mg per day during pregnancy, and 8 mg per day pre-pregnancy. The safe upper limit (UL) is 40 mg per day

Good Sources of Dietary Zinc

- Meat and poultry
- Dairy products
- Breakfast cereals
- Pecans and cashews
- Baked beans
- Fish

CHAPTER 2

Food Safety

YOU NEED TO BE AWARE of the foods you eat during pregnancy more than at other times during your life. Aim to eat foods that are good for you, but also avoid foods that may not be so good for you and your unborn baby. It is always important to practice safe food-handling techniques, but this is particularly true during pregnancy, when your growing baby is especially sensitive to food-borne illness. Safe food-handling practices are useful for preventing the spread of germs and infections caused by listeria, Toxoplasma gondii, *salmonella and E. coli.*

Did You Know ...

In the United States, the Centers for Disease Control estimates that about 2,500 people become seriously ill with listeriosis each year and almost 30% of those cases are pregnant women.

Food-Borne Illnesses

There are two food-borne illnesses — listeriosis and toxoplasmosis — that are of particular concern for pregnant women in North America because of their potential risk to the fetus. Two other food-borne infections — salmonellosis and E. coli — can affect the health of the mother.

Listeriosis

Listeriosis is caused by the bacterium *Listeria monocytogenes*. This disease is rare but significant because it can be very serious in pregnant women and the fetus.

Listeria is found in unpasteurized dairy products and uncooked (raw) meat, poultry and fish, as well as vegetables with contaminated soil adhering. It may be found in ready-to-eat foods, such as deli meat and hot dogs, where contamination may occur after processing.

Food contaminated with listeria may not look, smell or taste different than uncontaminated food. Listeria can survive cold temperatures and can even grow on refrigerated foods. Listeria is killed by heat, including pasteurization and cooking foods well.

Symptoms of listeriosis include mild flu-like nausea, vomiting, headache, fever and achy muscles. Symptoms occur between 2 and 30 days after eating an infected food.

If the infection becomes severe, it can cause disorientation, stiff neck and even convulsions.

Infection from listeria can happen at anytime during pregnancy. Early in pregnancy, listeriosis can cause miscarriage. Later in pregnancy, it can cause premature birth, stillbirth or an acute infection in the newborn. It is possible for the mother to become infected with listeria without necessarily passing the infection on to the fetus. Early diagnosis and treatment are critical for the well-being of the baby. Listeriosis can be treated with antibiotics, which in most cases will prevent the infection from spreading from mother to fetus.

 How to Avoid Listeriosis

The most important thing you can do to avoid listeria bacteria is to practice safe food-handling techniques and to avoid food that may be contaminated with listeria.

1. Avoid soft, unpasteurized cheeses such as Brie, Camembert, blue-veined cheeses, feta and Mexican-style cheese, such as queso fresco, queso blanco and panela. However, these cheeses can be found in pasteurized forms. Read labels carefully to be sure they are safe to eat. If a label does not state the food is pasteurized, assume the cheese has not been. Hard cheeses such as Cheddar and mozzarella are safe to eat. Dairy products that have been pasteurized, such as cheese slices, cottage cheese, cream cheese and yogurt, are also safe.

2. Avoid hot dogs and deli meats, unless they are properly reheated until steaming or reach a minimum internal temperature of 160°F (71°C).

3. Avoid cold pâtés and meat spreads, such as liverwurst.

4. Avoid refrigerated smoked seafood, such as salmon, unless it has been fully cooked, in a casserole, for example.

Toxoplasmosis

Toxoplasmosis is a relatively rare infection caused by a single-celled parasite known as *Toxoplasma gondii*. Symptoms are often mild, or there may be no symptoms at all. In fact, only 10% of affected women appear to have symptoms. Toxoplasmosis is often mistaken for the stomach flu. Fetal infection is less common when the mother is infected in the first or second trimester. Early diagnosis can reduce the severity of fetal infection.

It is estimated that in the United States between 400 and 6,000 young children are affected each year by *Toxoplasma gondii*.

Cat Feces

Toxoplasma gondii is carried in cat feces. Women who are pregnant and have cats should avoid changing the litter box and being exposed to feces that may contain toxoplasma. Have your husband or partner change the litter. If no one else is able to change the litter box, make sure you wear rubber gloves and wash your hands really well after changing the litter box. Also avoid garden soil or children's sandboxes that may have been in contact with cat feces.

In infants, toxoplasmosis can cause mental retardation, seizures, hearing loss and other problems. Luckily, when the mother is infected, less than 50% of cases infect the fetus.

Toxoplasma has been found in pigs and sheep, where it can infect the meat we may eat. Almost all food-borne toxoplasmosis cases come from raw or undercooked meat, primarily pork and lamb rather than beef or poultry. Fruits and vegetables can also become contaminated from infected manure, so be sure to wash fruits and vegetables well before eating.

Salmonellosis

Salmonella poisoning happens when food has been infected by the salmonella bacteria. This bacteria is commonly found in raw poultry, eggs and unpasteurized milk, as well as contaminated meats and water. Salmonella can also be carried by pets, such as turtles and birds. Symptoms of salmonella poisoning include diarrhea, headaches, stomach cramps,

 Safe Food-Handling Practices

Safe food-handling practices should always be used, especially during pregnancy, to prevent the spread of germs and infections caused by listeria, *Toxoplasma gondii*, salmonella and E. coli.

1. Always wash hands well before handling foods. Keep work surfaces clean and disinfect surfaces when dealing with raw foods.
2. Wash all fruits and vegetables well to remove soil that may be contaminated.
3. Avoid cross contamination between raw and cooked foods. Do not handle raw meats and raw fruits and vegetables at the same time. Be sure to sanitize any cutting boards or utensils after handling raw meats and before using for other foods.
4. Cook foods until they are at the proper internal temperature. Check with a food thermometer. Adequate cooking and reheating of foods will destroy any microorganisms that may infect foods.
5. Always keep hot foods hot (> 140°F/60°C) and cold foods cold (< 39°F/4°C).
6. Reheat leftovers and ready-to-eat meats, such as hot dogs or deli meats, until they are steaming or at least 165°F (73°C).
7. Do not eat raw meats, including uncooked hot dogs, raw fish or sushi, poultry, raw eggs or unpasteurized milk products.
8. Defrost foods overnight in the refrigerator and not on the counter.

nausea and vomiting, fever and possibly blood in the stool. Mild salmonella cases generally clear up on their own within four to seven days, but sometimes severe cases require treatment with antibiotics.

E. coli

Escherichia coli, more commonly known as E. coli, refers to a group of bacteria normally found in human and animal intestines. Certain virulent strains of E. coli can cause severe bloody diarrhea, abdominal cramping, kidney failure and even death. You can become sick from E. coli by eating contaminated ground beef, alfalfa or bean sprouts, lettuce, salami and undercooked red meat, as well as unpasteurized milk, apple juice, cider and untreated water.

Safe Food Preparation Temperature Chart
INTERNAL FOOD TEMPERATURES

Beef:	Ground beef	160°–165°F	71°–73°C
	Medium	160°F	71°C
	Well done	170°F	76°C
Pork		160°–170°F	71°–76°C
Poultry		165°–180°F	74°–82°C
Fish		165°F	74°C
Egg dishes		160°F	71°C

Food-Borne Contaminants

Women need to be cautious in avoiding not only food-borne illnesses, but also food-borne contaminants from environmental and chemical hazards. The contaminant that has drawn the greatest attention is mercury levels in fish. Is it safe to eat fresh or canned tuna? Is any fish safe to eat? How much fish can I eat? These are some of the questions you may have.

Mercury

Mercury is a naturally occurring element in the environment; however, it is also a byproduct of some industries that is released into the air as a pollutant. When mercury pollution falls from the air and enters our waterways, including rivers, lakes and oceans, it turns into methylmercury. Methylmercury can be harmful to the fetus and young children.

Fish absorb methylmercury as they feed in polluted waters. Levels of methylmercury accumulate in these fish. Fish that swim and eat at the bottom of the ocean are heavier in weight and accumulate more mercury than other types of fish. These fish should be avoided by pregnant and nursing women, as well as by young children. Intake of these fish should also be limited in the general population.

Foods to Avoid during Pregnancy

Soft Cheeses

Soft cheeses contain the bacteria *Listeria monocytogenes*. All pregnant women should avoid unpasteurized soft cheeses, including Brie, Camembert, blue-veined cheeses (e.g., Roquefort), feta cheese and soft Mexican cheeses, such as queso blanco, queso fresco, quesa de hoja and queso de crema. These cheeses may be available in pasteurized forms, so be sure to read all labels carefully. If the label does not state the cheese has been pasteurized, then it must be assumed that the cheese is unpasteurized. Cream cheese and cottage cheese, as well as yogurts, are all pasteurized and safe to eat during pregnancy.

Fish Consumption Guidelines

FDA AND EPA STATEMENT

In the United States, the Food and Drug Administration (FDA), in conjunction with the Environmental Protection Agency (EPA), announced a joint statement on methylmercury in fish in March 2004. They recommend that women who are planning to become pregnant, are pregnant or are breastfeeding, as well as young children, should "reduce their exposure to the harmful effects of mercury" by following these guidelines:

1. Avoid shark, swordfish, king mackerel and tilefish, which all contain high levels of mercury.

2. Eat up to 12 oz (375 g) per week (two average meals) of fish and shellfish that are low in mercury to receive the beneficial health effects of fish. Examples of fish low in mercury include canned light tuna, salmon, pollock, sole, shrimp, haddock, catfish and mahi mahi.

3. Limit intake of canned albacore tuna to one meal or 6 oz (175 g) per week because canned white, or albacore, tuna has higher levels of mercury than canned light tuna. Eat fish lower in mercury for the balance of the week.

4. Check your local authorities about the safety of fish caught in local waters. This includes fish caught by friends and family in local rivers and lakes. If no information is available, the FDA and EPA suggest consuming a maximum of 6 oz (175 g) of the fish in question and then not consuming any more fish that week.

HEALTH CANADA RECOMMENDATIONS

The current Canadian guidelines suggest that 0.5 ppm of mercury in fish is considered safe for the general population, including women of childbearing age, pregnant and nursing women and young children. Health Canada suggests that women of childbearing age, pregnant women and young children should eat a maximum of one meal per month of top-predator fish that may contain higher levels of mercury, including shark, swordfish and fresh or frozen tuna.

DIETITIANS' RECOMMENDATIONS

Both the Dietitians of Canada and the American Dietetic Association believe that fish contribute to a well-balanced diet. We should not forget all the benefits of eating fish when we are talking about the concerns of mercury in fish. Fish contains omega 3 fatty acids, which contribute to heart health. Research also suggests that omega 3 fatty acids improve visual and neural acuity in unborn babies. Fish is an excellent high-quality protein and low in saturated fat that can increase blood cholesterol. Fish has other essential nutrients, such as zinc and iron, which can contribute to a healthy diet.

Raw Meats and Raw Fish

Raw meats and fish can contain salmonella, *Toxoplasma gondii*, or E. coli microorganisms. Be sure to avoid any foods containing raw meats, such as meat pâtés, liverwurst, steak tartare or beef cooked rare or medium rare. Meat should be cooked to a minimum of 155°F to 165°F (71°C to 73°C). Do not eat poultry that is still pink inside. Also avoid all raw fish, shellfish and seafood, including mussels, clams, oysters and sushi. Some fish found in sushi may also contain high levels of mercury that should be avoided during pregnancy. Fish should be cooked until it flakes easily with a fork and is no longer pink inside.

Fish with High Levels of Mercury

Avoid fish with known mercury contamination. This includes shark, tilefish, king mackerel and fresh or frozen tuna. Canned light tuna can be eaten, up to 12 oz (375 g), or about 2 cans, per week.

 ## Are soy foods safe to eat during pregnancy?

Soybeans contain phytoestrogens, which are naturally occurring compounds with estrogen-like activity. Phytoestrogens have been shown to produce mild hormonal action in the body. It has been suggested that these compounds may affect the development of an infant's hormonal system or the reproductive organs in a male fetus. This is a very controversial topic in the scientific community, and the findings have not been conclusive. Populations that typically consume large amounts of soy have not exhibited any unusual increase in birth defects related to the male genitalia. As always, we recommend eating a well-balanced diet that can include soy-based foods, such as soy breads, soy milk and tofu.

Deli Meats and Hot Dogs

These meat products should not be eaten raw, to prevent infection from listeria. These foods may be eaten when well heated and cooked until steaming (at least 165°F/74°C). This includes cured meats, such as salami.

Raw Eggs

Egg-based or egg-added foods, such as Caesar salad, some homemade mayonnaises, ice creams, custards and hollandaise sauces, may contain raw eggs. They should be avoided. At holiday time, unpasteurized eggnog is also a concern and should be avoided. Raw eggs may have been exposed to salmonella.

Unwashed Fruits and Vegetables

Eat all kinds of fruits and vegetables during pregnancy, including raw, uncooked veggies, but be sure to wash all fruits and vegetables thoroughly, because any soil they were grown in may potentially be contaminated with *Toxoplasma gondii*.

Unpasteurized Milk and Dairy Products

Avoid these foods during pregnancy because they may contain the bacterium *Listeria monocytogenes*.

Caffeine

Caffeine is a well-known stimulant that affects the central nervous system, increasing heart rate and alertness. Caffeine is also known as a diuretic, which means it can increase the elimination of fluids from the body by increasing urination. Caffeine is found in coffee, tea, chocolate, some soft drinks and other foods. It is also a component of certain medications.

 How much caffeine can I drink during pregnancy?

According to Health Canada, caffeine intake prior to and during pregnancy from all sources should be limited to about 300 mg per day, or approximately 2 to 2½ cups of brewed coffee. However, the Motherisk program at The Hospital for Sick Children recommends 150 mg a day, while the National Women's Health Information Center, US Department of Health and Human Services, recommends avoiding caffeine altogether during pregnancy. Consult with your doctor on an acceptable amount of caffeine.

Sources of Caffeine

On average, where 1 cup = 250 mL, 300 mg of caffeine would be contained in:

- less than $2\frac{1}{2}$ cups of percolated or filter drip coffee
- 4 to $4\frac{1}{2}$ cups instant coffee
- less than $3\frac{1}{2}$ cups of strong tea
- 7 to 16 cans of cola beverages
- 16 cups of hot cocoa from mix
- 10 regular dark chocolate bars

(**Source:** Nutrition for a Healthy Pregnancy, National Guidelines for the Childbearing Years, Health Canada, Oct., 2002. Reprinted with the permission of the Minister of Public Works and Government Services Canada, 2005.)

Did You Know ...

Curtail Caffeine

Because caffeine can have negative effects on reproduction and fetal development, its consumption, from all sources, should be curtailed prior to conception and during pregnancy.

Measuring Caffeine Intake

Because caffeine content varies depending on the type of product (coffee, tea, cola, for example), it is best to check with the manufacturer to determine the exact amount of caffeine. Also be sure to measure the volume of fluid in a take-out container. One "cup" of coffee may actually be 2 cups (500 mL) or more.

Caffeine Withdrawal

If intake is above 300 mg per day, then it is wise to decrease intake gradually to the acceptable level before becoming pregnant. When caffeine is removed from the diet, many individuals claim that they get withdrawal symptoms, including headache, irritability and drowsiness. However, studies have shown that the expectation of caffeine withdrawal leads to the symptoms; caffeine does not have a pharmacological withdrawal effect. In any case, it is wise to limit caffeine intake before becoming pregnant by decreasing intake slowly to an acceptable level of 150 to 300 mg or less per day. One suggestion for coffee lovers would be to prepare a mixture of decaffeinated and regular coffee, or to make the change to decaffeinated coffee. Some decaffeinated coffees do contain a small amount of caffeine.

Alcohol

Alcohol consumption is not recommended while trying to become pregnant or during pregnancy. Although moderate consumption before pregnancy is not likely to put the fetus at risk later on, federal health agencies (the American Pregnancy Association and Health Canada's National Guidelines for the Childbearing Years) recommend that alcohol consumption should be avoided. It is not known what a safe level of alcohol before or during pregnancy might be. Because of the detrimental effects of alcohol on a fetus, no amount of alcohol can be safely recommended. Alcohol may also displace foods that contain important nutrients, so this is an important consideration.

Herbal Products

Herbal products are used by many women for their possible medicinal benefits. These products are considered to be foods by the United States Federal Drug Administration (FDA) and the Natural Health Products Directorate (NHDP) of Canada. They are not subject to the same evaluation procedures as prescription drugs. Recently, testing for safety and effectiveness has begun on these herbal products, but information about their safety during pregnancy is scarce. Women who continue to take herbal products before and during pregnancy should do so with caution. Check with your doctor for advice on the safety of these products. If the safety of a product is unknown, it would be prudent not to take it before or during pregnancy.

As with herbal remedies, not all herbal teas can be recommended during pregnancy, as the contents and their effects on pregnancy are unknown. According to the National Guidelines for the Childbearing Years in Canada, a maximum of 2 to 3 cups (500 to 750 mL) of herbal tea is recommended as a limit. Ingredients that are considered safe include citrus peel, ginger, lemon balm and rose hip. Chamomile teas have been reported to have negative effects on the uterus and, therefore, are not recommended during pregnancy. Limit drinking herbal teas to those defined as safe.

Did You Know ...

No-Calorie Caution

Although pregnant women can safely use all approved sweeteners throughout their pregnancy, sweeteners do not provide additional energy or calories that may be needed to support pregnancy and breastfeeding.

Artificial Sweeteners

Artificial sweeteners are also known as non-nutritive sweeteners. They do not provide calories or energy to the diet and do not influence blood sugar levels. Artificial sweeteners can be used by pregnant women who have diabetes or who need to watch their caloric intake. Some pregnant women simply enjoy the taste of foods sweetened with non-nutritive sweeteners.

In Canada, all sweeteners must go through extensive testing before Health Canada will approve them for use.

 Approved Tabletop Sweeteners

Aspartame (NutraSweet®/Equal®), ace K, or acesulfame potassium (Sunett®), sucralose (Splenda®) and neotame are considered safe to use during pregnancy and lactation. However, saccharin (Hermesetas®) can cross the placenta into fetal tissues. Health Canada suggests that saccharin and cyclamates (Sugar Twin®/Weight Watchers®) be used during pregnancy and lactation only under the advice of a physician. Choose one of the other available sweeteners as an alternative.

Aspartame: Sold as NutraSweet® for use in foods, such as breakfast cereals, desserts, candy and soft drinks, and as Equal® for use as a tabletop sweetener. Aspartame is made up of two amino acids, aspartic acid and phenylalanine. It is digested like any other protein, but is used in such small amounts that it does not contribute calories to the diet. It is 200 times sweeter than sugar. Aspartame has been extensively studied. The FDA and the American Academy of Pediatrics, as well as Health Canada, consider it safe for pregnant women and the fetus. The exception to this is mothers who have a rare genetic disease known as phenylketonuria (PKU). Women with PKU must limit the amount of phenylalanine in their diets; other artificial sweeteners would be considered better choices.

Ace K (acesulfame potassium): Sold under the brand name of Sunett®. This is the latest non-nutritive sweetener approved for use in Canada. Ace K is found in a variety of desserts, beverages, candies and gum and is also used as a tabletop sweetener. Ace K is not metabolized in the body and is excreted unchanged by the kidneys. Animal studies have shown no toxic effects of ace K, and it is considered safe for use by pregnant and breastfeeding women. You should speak with your doctor before using ace K if you are on a potassium-restricted diet or have allergies to sulfa-based drugs.

Once approved, they are considered safe for use by all Canadians, including pregnant and lactating mothers, as well as young children. In the United States, approved sweeteners are classified as generally recognized as safe (GRAS) by the FDA and are considered acceptable for use during pregnancy. Each sweetener has an acceptable daily intake (ADI) set for it, suggesting how much is safe to consume on a daily basis. These ADIs are for individuals, based on body weight. It is generally accepted that the "normal use" of sweeteners does not pose a health risk.

Sweeteners can be a part of a well-balanced diet, but caution should be used to ensure that nutrient needs are being met and that sweeteners are not replacing other nutrient-dense food choices.

Sucralose: Made from real sugar and sold as Splenda®. It is 400 to 800 times sweeter than sugar and is stable in extreme hot and cold temperatures, which makes it ideal for use in many different hot and cold beverages, baked goods and canned or frozen fruits and vegetables. Sucralose is not well absorbed by the body and is basically excreted unchanged. It is considered safe for use by pregnant and lactating women.

Neotame: The most recently approved non-nutritive sweetener in the United States. It is rapidly metabolized and then eliminated completely by the body. It is considered safe for use by women who are pregnant or breastfeeding.

Cyclamate: Known as Sucaryl® and used in Sugar Twin® and Weight Watchers®. In Canada, it is available only as a tabletop sweetener. Cyclamate is heat stable and can be used in hot or cold foods without losing its sweet flavor. It is about 30 times sweeter than sugar and has no aftertaste. Health Canada suggests that pregnant and lactating women use cyclamate only on the advice of their physician.

Saccharin: Sold under the brand name of Hermesetas®. It is the oldest artificial sweetener on the market and is 300 times sweeter than sugar. Saccharin has received negative media attention because of its alleged relationship with cancer. However, studies have not been able to prove a link between saccharin and cancer, and the US Department of Health and Human Services does not consider saccharin to be a known carcinogen. Saccharin is not metabolized and passes unchanged through the body. Saccharin can cross the placenta and may stay in the fetal tissues, but there is no evidence that it is harmful to a growing baby. For this reason, however, the American Dietetic Association suggests that pregnant women may want to limit their saccharin intake and choose alternative sweeteners for consumption. Health Canada has approved the use of saccharin only as a tabletop sweetener and suggests that pregnant and lactating women only use saccharin on the advice of their physician.

❋ Quick Guide to Food Safety

Food	Safe/Avoid	Reason/Microorganism
CHEESE		
Unpasteurized soft cheeses, including Brie, Camembert, blue-veined cheeses, soft Mexican cheeses	Avoid	May contain Listeria monocytogenes
Cottage cheese	Safe	
Cream cheese	Safe	
Hard cheeses, such as Cheddar or mozzarella	Safe	
DAIRY PRODUCTS		
Yogurt	Safe	
MEAT		
Raw meat, including beef, pork and lamb	Avoid	May contain E. coli, salmonella or T. gondii
Deli meats	Okay if cooked until steaming	May contain Listeria monocytogenes
Hot dogs	Okay if cooked until steaming	May contain Listeria monocytogenes
Pâtés or liverwurst	Avoid	May contain Listeria monocytogenes
FISH		
Raw fish, including oysters, mussels, clams and sushi	Avoid	May contain salmonella, Clostridium botulinum or Listeria monocytogenes
Tuna, fresh or frozen	Avoid	May contain high levels of mercury
Tuna, canned light	Limit to 12 oz (360 g) a week	
Tuna, canned albacore	Limit to 6 oz (180 g) a week	May contain higher levels of mercury
Salmon, canned or fresh	Safe	
CAFFEINE		
Caffeine in coffee and tea	150–300 mg a day = < 1–2½ cups (< 250–625 mL) brewed coffee or < 2–3½ cups (< 500–875 mL) of strong tea	Higher levels may cause low birth weight
HERBAL PRODUCTS		
Herbal teas	2–3 cups a day (500–750 mL) of citrus peel, ginger, lemon balm, orange peel or rose hip tea Avoid chamomile tea	Unknown safety of some herbal teas during pregnancy Chamomile may have negative effects on the uterus
ARTIFICIAL SWEETENERS		
Saccharin (Hermesetas®) and cyclamate (SugarTwin® and Weight Watchers®)	Avoid unless under advice of physician	Health Canada suggests pregnant and lactating women avoid saccharin and cyclamate unless advised by a physician

Organic Foods

More and more women are choosing to eat organic food when planning their pregnancy or during their pregnancy, trusting this food will provide the best nutritional environment for the growth of their baby. However, whether organic foods are more beneficial to overall health than foods that are not grown organically is a hotly debated topic.

Both non-organic and organic food production are regulated by federal agencies. Some research has shown that organic food is usually higher in vitamin C. Iron and magnesium levels may sometimes be higher, but B vitamins and vitamin A are generally the same. Nitrate content is usually less in organic foods. Nitrates are also used to preserve cured meats (hot dogs, deli meats) and prevent growth of harmful bacteria. Try to limit intake of nitrates, as high dietary intake may be associated with certain forms of cancer.

 ## Is tap water safe to drink during pregnancy?

In North America, the municipal water supply is considered to be safe. The safety of local tap water depends on the disinfection process, which usually involves chlorination of the water. Disinfection is necessary to kill the microorganisms and viruses that cause serious illnesses or even death. Information on the safety of individual municipal or tap water is available from your local water supplier (which can be found on your water bill or at your local tax office). You can also check with the Environmental Protection Agency in the United States for your local water supply information. For contact information, see the Resources section in this book. Well water should be tested at regular intervals. Contact your local public health office for more information on testing procedures and services. For anyone using water from lakes, streams or rivers, be sure to treat the water completely before consumption.

According to Health Canada's Nutrition for a Healthy Pregnancy, National Guidelines for the Childbearing Years, women who are planning pregnancy or who are pregnant should let tap water run freely in the morning to prevent excess intake of lead or copper that may have accumulated in the pipes overnight. This is true for both older and newer homes. Water from the hot water tap should not be consumed because it may contain higher amounts of lead or copper than that from the cold water tap. Again, these precautions should be taken even before a pregnancy, so that it is already a habit by the time a woman is pregnant. Lead or copper can interfere with the health and well-being of the fetus.

Water Requirements and Safety

Water is an important element of the diet and should be consumed instead of sweetened beverages to quench thirst. The recommended amount of fluid is 12 cups (3 L) daily from food and beverages (water, milk, juice, soups). Women who are pregnant need extra water to support the increase in blood volume that occurs during pregnancy and to prevent dehydration. Adequate hydration may also help relieve the symptoms of constipation. Women who have nausea and vomiting associated with early pregnancy may only be able to take small amounts of water between meals instead of during meals to decrease the feeling of fullness that may worsen their nausea.

However, many women have concerns about the safety of tap water and bottled water, which, if not answered, may lead them to substitute other beverages for water in their diet.

Water Filters

Various forms of water filters are available, ranging from complex municipal water treatment plants to tap filters. Filters are used not only to clean contaminants from the water, but also to improve the taste. Check with the manufacturer of your household filter to see what components it is designed to remove (e.g., if fluoride is removed, you may need a supplement).

 What are trihalomethanes?

Chlorine is commonly used to help disinfect and treat drinking water. When chlorine reacts with certain elements in the water, a byproduct is trihalomethanes (THMs). The level of THMs is an indicator of the safety of the water. High levels of THMs may have an adverse effect on health. Water treatment facilities ensure that THM levels stay within a safe range. Bottled water, in general, may have lower levels of THMs, but this will vary depending on the manufacturer. Water filters may be used to decrease the level of THM exposure, but they won't completely eliminate them. Be sure to maintain filter devices; otherwise, they may become a source of bacterial contamination.

Is bottled water better?

Many consumers today rely on bottled water for their intake of fluid, believing that bottled water is safer than tap water. Prepackaged water is subject to government regulations in the United States and Canada. The Word Health Organization (WHO) has international standards for bottled drinking water as well.

Bottled water that claims to be from a spring or mineral source must come from an underground source. Bottled water may not contain any fluoride, unless indicated on the bottle. If bottled water is the sole source of water intake, fluoride may be lacking in the diet (this is especially important for young children). Inform your physician if this is the case, and supplementation may be required (most prenatal vitamin supplements do not contain fluoride). Other bottled water may come from a public water supply, which is treated to remove or decrease some of the minerals. Especially when traveling to remote areas, caution should be taken when consuming bottled water because there have been reports of regular local water being used. Bottle seals should be checked carefully.

Bottled water should be refrigerated after opening. Health Canada recommends storing sealed bottled water in the refrigerator. Bottled water normally contains small amounts of harmless bacteria, but storing in a warm place will increase their content. Bottled water usually has a two-year shelf life.

For more information on bottled water, refer to the Health Canada website, Health Products and Food Branch, Questions and Answers on Bottled Water (www.hc-sc.gc.ca/food) or the Environmental Protection Agency in the United States (www.epa.gov/epahome).

Safe Water Consumption Guidelines

- Drink plenty of water before and during pregnancy, about 3 quarts or liters a day from all liquid and food sources.
- Use water as a thirst quencher instead of juices or sweetened drinks.
- If you are unsure of the safety of tap water, consult your local water supplier and your doctor.
- Bottled water is not sterile, although it may contain lower amounts of byproducts of disinfection.
- Check with your national health organization for the latest information on drinking-water safety.

CHAPTER 3

Pre-Pregnancy Nutrition

"WOMEN TODAY MAY HAVE COMPROMISED HEALTH *due to a busy lifestyle, with limited time to focus on healthy eating and living," according to a joint paper released recently by the Dietitians of Canada and the American Dietetic Association. Women may not be preparing healthy meals, relying instead on fast foods or convenience foods, and may not be exercising regularly, leading them to become overweight or obese.*

In fact, Canadian statistics revealed that 21% of women are obese and 3% to 5% of women aged 18 to 44 years have iron deficiency anemia. Statistics Canada reports that 57% of women do not meet the recommended requirement of five or more servings of fruits and vegetables a day. Clearly, this is not the ideal lifestyle when preparing for a healthy pregnancy.

However, pre-pregnancy can be the ideal time to start making changes to lifestyle, especially diet, so that both the mother and the fetus are healthy. More and more research is being presented that proves the association between prenatal nutrition and postnatal health. Researchers are suggesting that the nutrients provided during pregnancy affect the fetus into adulthood. An adequate intake of energy and nutrients is essential for a healthy pregnancy. Research supports the need for a healthy diet before, during and after pregnancy.

Food Guides

One of the best ways to ensure a healthy diet before pregnancy is to follow the nutritional advice in the United States Department of Agriculture (USDA) MyPyramid guidelines or Canada's Food Guide to Healthy Eating. Each guide separates food into different food groups with similar nutrients. A healthy diet should consist of appropriate serving sizes of foods from the following food groups: milk and milk products, bread and cereals, meat and alternatives, and fruits and vegetables. If you are meeting your recommended daily intake of the different food groups, then you are likely in nutritional balance and receiving the appropriate nutrient needs. In pregnancy, these needs change, but not dramatically.

Quick Tips for Healthy Eating

- Enjoy a variety of foods.
- Eat an adequate amount of cereals, breads and other grain products.
- Eat plenty of fruits and vegetables.
- Eat lower-fat dairy products and leaner meats, fish and poultry.
- Limit salt and caffeine.
- Avoid alcohol intake during pregnancy.
- Along with these good eating habits, remember to participate in regular physical activity.

(Based on Canada's Food Guide to Healthy Eating)

Energy Needs

During pre-pregnancy, energy requirements are not increased above normal, unless the woman is underweight or overweight. You need to achieve an energy balance, so that the energy or calories going into your body equal the energy going out, including energy used for day-to-day activities and exercise. If you are overweight, you need to decrease your total energy or calorie intake and increase physical activity. If you are underweight, you likely require an increased energy intake, ideally from all food groups. For example, increasing energy intake by eating more fat alone would not be recommended, unless your diet was already very low in fat.

Risks with Being Overweight

Results from the 1996–1997 National Population Health Survey revealed that approximately 20% of Canadian women who are in their childbearing years had a BMI that was greater than 27. Women with this BMI are considered to be overweight and are at greater risk of health-related problems. They are putting their babies at risk as well.

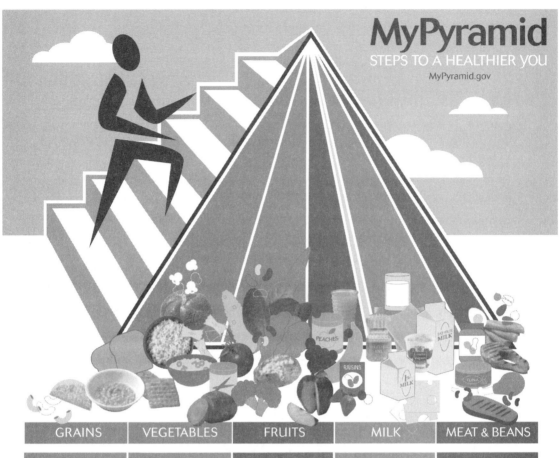

MyPyramid
STEPS TO A HEALTHIER YOU
MyPyramid.gov

GRAINS	VEGETABLES	FRUITS	MILK	MEAT & BEANS
GRAINS Make half your grains whole	**VEGETABLES** Vary your veggies	**FRUITS** Focus on fruits	**MILK** Get your calcium-rich foods	**MEAT & BEANS** Go lean with protein
Eat at least 3 oz. of whole-grain cereals, breads, crackers, rice, or pasta every day 1 oz. is about 1 slice of bread, about 1 cup of breakfast cereal, or ½ cup of cooked rice, cereal, or pasta	Eat more dark-green veggies like broccoli, spinach, and other dark leafy greens Eat more orange vegetables like carrots and sweetpotatoes Eat more dry beans and peas like pinto beans, kidney beans, and lentils	Eat a variety of fruit Choose fresh, frozen, canned, or dried fruit Go easy on fruit juices	Go low-fat or fat-free when you choose milk, yogurt, and other milk products If you don't or can't consume milk, choose lactose-free products or other calcium sources such as fortified foods and beverages	Choose low-fat or lean meats and poultry Bake it, broil it, or grill it Vary your protein routine — choose more fish, beans, peas, nuts, and seeds

For a 2,000-calorie diet, you need the amounts below from each food group. To find the amounts that are right for you, go to MyPyramid.gov.

Eat 6 oz. every day	Eat 2½ cups every day	Eat 2 cups every day	Get 3 cups every day; for kids aged 2 to 8, it's 2	Eat 5½ oz. every day

Find your balance between food and physical activity
- Be sure to stay within your daily calorie needs.
- Be physically active for at least 30 minutes most days of the week.
- About 60 minutes a day of physical activity may be needed to prevent weight gain.
- For sustaining weight loss, at least 60 to 90 minutes a day of physical activity may be required.
- Children and teenagers should be physically active for 60 minutes every day, or most days.

Know the limits on fats, sugars, and salt (sodium)
- Make most of your fat sources from fish, nuts, and vegetable oils.
- Limit solid fats like butter, stick margarine, shortening, and lard, as well as foods that contain these.
- Check the Nutrition Facts label to keep saturated fats, trans fats, and sodium low.
- Choose food and beverages low in added sugars. Added sugars contribute calories with few, if any, nutrients.

MyPyramid.gov
STEPS TO A HEALTHIER YOU

U.S. Department of Agriculture
Center for Nutrition Policy and Promotion
April 2005
CNPP-15

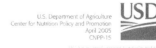

USDA

Strategies to reduce weight and achieve a lower BMI should be encouraged. In most cases, an increase in activity, along with changes in diet patterns and choices of food, would be recommended to achieve a healthy body weight.

Health Risks if Overweight

- Type 2 diabetes
- High blood pressure
- Heart disease
- Sleep disorders
- Infertility
- Larger than normal babies, or in some cases a baby who is a lower than normal weight at birth
- Children who are overweight later on in life

Risks with Being Underweight

A mother who is underweight before pregnancy also carries some greater health risks than someone with a normal BMI.

Some studies suggest that women with a low BMI prior to becoming pregnant who gain weight normally during pregnancy still have an increased risk of having a low-birth-weight infant. The reasons for this include a lower blood plasma volume in the mother, with decreased cardiac output, which would lead to a diminished nutrient supply to the fetus, resulting in poorer growth of that fetus.

Health Risks if Underweight

- Associated infertility issues
- Lower birth weight
- Increased risk of diabetes later in life
- Minimal nutritional reserve and therefore an increased risk of having a preterm infant or an infant with intrauterine growth retardation (IUGR)

Did You Know ...

Macronutrient Distribution

The distribution of the macronutrient energy sources in a typical North American diet is typically about 55% carbohydrates, 10% proteins and 35% fats. The DRI acceptable range of energy intake (as a percent of total daily calories) for carbohydrate is 45% to 65%, for protein 10% to 35% and for fat 20% to 35%. Some people have proposed that a change in this distribution — for example by reducing carbohydrates and increasing proteins (low-carb, high-protein diet) — might promote weight loss. But none of the studies have proven that one way of shifting the nutrients is better than the other for achieving a healthy body weight over the long term.

Did You Know ...

Weight Risks

There are risks with being overweight and with being underweight, particularly for women who are planning a pregnancy.

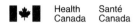

Health   Santé
Canada   Canada

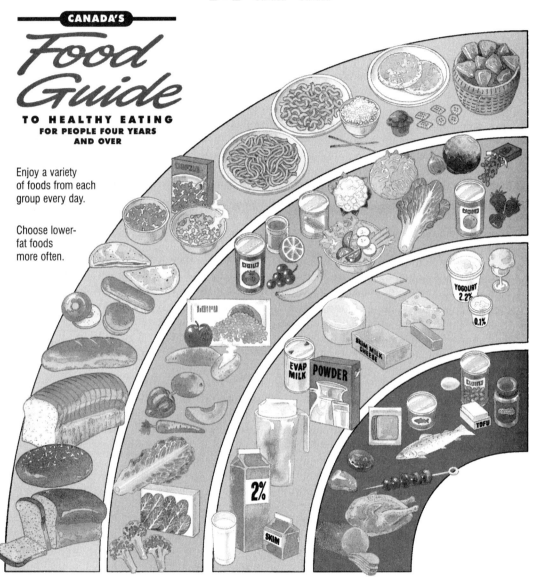

CANADA'S

Food Guide

TO HEALTHY EATING
FOR PEOPLE FOUR YEARS
AND OVER

Enjoy a variety
of foods from each
group every day.

Choose lower-
fat foods
more often.

Grain Products
Choose whole grain
and enriched
products more often.

Vegetables and Fruit
Choose dark green and
orange vegetables and
orange fruit more often.

Milk Products
Choose lower-fat milk
products more often.

Meat and Alternatives
Choose leaner meats,
poultry and fish, as well
as dried peas, beans
and lentils more often.

Canada

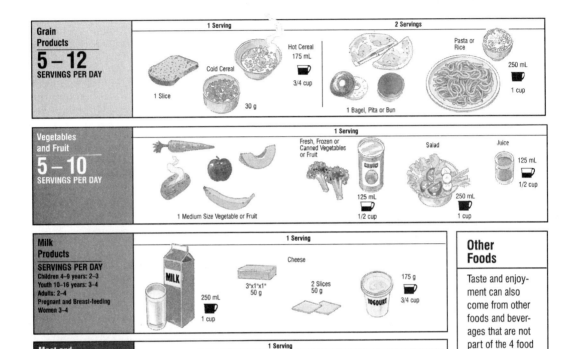

Grain Products
5 – 12
SERVINGS PER DAY

1 Serving
Cold Cereal
1 Slice
Hot Cereal 175 mL
3/4 cup
30 g

2 Servings
Pasta or Rice
1 Bagel, Pita or Bun
250 mL
1 cup

Vegetables and Fruit
5 – 10
SERVINGS PER DAY

1 Serving
1 Medium Size Vegetable or Fruit
Fresh, Frozen or Canned Vegetables or Fruit
125 mL
1/2 cup
Salad
250 mL
1 cup
Juice
125 mL
1/2 cup

Milk Products
SERVINGS PER DAY
Children 4–9 years: 2–3
Youth 10–16 years: 3–4
Adults: 2–4
Pregnant and Breast-feeding Women 3–4

1 Serving
MILK
250 mL
1 cup
Cheese
3"x1"x1"
50 g
2 Slices
50 g
175 g
3/4 cup

Meat and Alternatives
2 – 3
SERVINGS PER DAY

1 Serving
Fish
Meat, Poultry or Fish
50–100 g
1/3–2/3 Can
50–100 g
1-2 Eggs
Beans
125–250 mL
TOFU
100 g
1/3 cup
Peanut Butter
30 mL 2 tbsp

Other Foods

Taste and enjoyment can also come from other foods and beverages that are not part of the 4 food groups. Some of these foods are higher in fat or Calories, so use these foods in moderation.

Different People Need Different Amounts of Food

The amount of food you need every day from the 4 food groups and other foods depends on your age, body size, activity level, whether you are male or female and if you are pregnant or breastfeeding. That's why the Food Guide gives a lower and higher number of servings for each food group. For example, young children can choose the lower number of servings, while male teenagers can go to the higher number. Most other people can choose servings somewhere in between.

Consult *Canada's Physical Activity Guide to Healthy Active Living* to help you build physical activity into your daily life.

Enjoy eating well, being active and feeling good about yourself. That's VITALIT®

Source: Canada's Food Guide to Healthy Eating, Health Canada, 1997. Reprinted with the permission of the Minister of Public Works and Government Services Canada, 2005.

What is a healthy body weight?

Determining whether a weight is appropriate for height and therefore healthy can be determined by using the body mass index (BMI).

To calculate the BMI, you divide your weight in kilograms by your height in meters squared — or your weight in pounds is multiplied by 700 and then divided by your height in inches squared.

Take, for example, a woman who is 5 feet, 5 inches (65 inches) tall, or 165 cm (1.65 meters), and weighs 145 lbs, or 65.9 kg.

CALCULATION OF BMI
Imperial: 145 lbs x 700 ÷ 65 x 65 = 24
Metric: 65.9 kg ÷ 1.65 x 1.65 = 24

WEIGHT RANGES
Normal = BMI 20–25   Overweight = BMI > 25–29
Underweight = BMI < 19   Obese = BMI > 30

For example, a woman who is 5 feet 6 inches (168 cm), weighing between 124 and 149 lbs (56 to 68 kg) is normal weight, weighing 161 lbs (73 kg) is overweight, and weighing 192 lbs (87 kg) is obese. Someone who has a BMI under 19 is considered to be underweight. This range of BMI may not apply to someone with an increased muscle mass — for example, a bodybuilder, as muscle weighs more than fat and a higher BMI for that individual would not mean they are overweight. An accurate use of the BMI, therefore, needs to include level of physical activity, growth and muscle mass.

By calculating your BMI, you can determine if you are in the range of a healthy body weight. It would be prudent for you to calculate your BMI prior to pregnancy and discuss this with a dietitian or physician to determine if it is appropriate. This will allow you to know if you are at an appropriate weight or if you should try to increase or decrease weight prior to becoming pregnant and give you an easier way to determine if weight gain is appropriate during the pregnancy.

Body Image

Some women perceive that they are overweight when they are, in fact, at an appropriate weight for their height and have a normal BMI. Health Canada reports that over half of women in their childbearing years think that they should lose weight when they are at a healthy weight. An unhealthy and unrealistic body image is prevalent in North American society, and a large proportion of women who are contemplating a pregnancy are at risk of undereating because of societal pressures to be thin. Women who continue to have a desire to lose weight despite being at an appropriate BMI should be counseled on healthy eating and a healthy lifestyle that includes exercise.

 ## Are low-carb diets effective for weight loss and management?

Low-carbohydrate diets have been popular because of the belief that they will promote weight loss while allowing consumption of generous amounts of fats and proteins. However, research has not consistently proven that these low-carbohydrate diets are any more beneficial for weight loss than the usual diet that includes approximately 40% to 55% of energy as carbohydrates. In fact, many researchers suggest that limiting fruits, vegetables and cereals to accommodate the diet can actually be harmful. Low-carbohydrate diets can contribute to iron and folate deficiency due to insufficient intake of grains and cereals.

An effective program for weight loss includes a combination of total calorie reduction, along with exercise, without limiting any one food group. Simply balancing all types of foods can allow for a reasonable total daily calorie intake. Understanding the role of carbohydrates in the diet and having an appreciation of the different forms of carbohydrates can allow an individual to select a diet that is both sensible and healthy.

Eating Disorders

Women with eating disorders often have a distorted body image, causing them to think they are constantly overweight when in fact they are very thin, often below a BMI of 19. Anorexia nervosa, bulimia nervosa and binge-eating disorders can result in undernutrition, creating significant negative health effects on a fetus and baby. If adequate nutrition is not provided by the mother to the fetus during pregnancy, such as when a woman purposely restricts caloric intake, then the risk of having a low-birth-weight baby is very high. The infant may suffer lifelong consequences. Women with an eating disorder who abuse diuretics may have a higher risk of having a child with a neural tube defect.

Support for women with an eating disorder is essential before and during a pregnancy. Women who suffer from an eating disorder will be challenged by the normal weight gain of pregnancy and require counseling to encourage a healthy, non-restricted diet during pregnancy.

Teenage Pregnancy

Teenage pregnancy poses a greater risk of delivering a baby prematurely (born before 37 weeks) or having a baby with a low birth weight. Reasons for this may include inadequate nutrient intake due to the extra energy demands for growth in the adolescent's own body, along with the energy needs of the fetus. Adolescents may not be aware of the extra nutritional needs for calories, protein, fiber, vitamins and minerals. Teen girls are more likely to have poor diet habits along with nutritional deficiencies. They may require educational, emotional and professional health-care support to ensure that energy and nutrient needs are met during pregnancy. This is especially true if they have financial restrictions and are eating on the run because of school or employment obligations. More frequent visits to a health-care team may be required to monitor the growth of the baby and their own weight gain.

Older Women (over 35 years of age)

There are some special risks for women planning pregnancy who are more than 35 years of age. These include increased risk of diabetes and high blood pressure for the mother, as well as a placental problem called placenta previa, where the placenta may cover some or all of the opening of the cervix. One study found that older women were 20% more likely to have a premature baby, and 20% to 40% of these women were more likely to have a low-birth-weight baby. A higher percentage of older women also have a higher BMI and, therefore, have the risks associated with being overweight. However, with proper monitoring and attention to their health, women more than 35 years of age can and do have healthy, thriving babies.

Nutrient Needs

With more attention being given to nutrition these days, more women are becoming better informed about healthy eating when they are planning a pregnancy. However, some women are overweight or underweight before conception, and some women may be low in calcium, vitamin D, folic acid, iron, zinc and essential fatty acids.

Calcium

Calcium is essential for the growth of the fetus and, therefore, should be adequately supplied before becoming pregnant to establish a healthy intake at the time of conception and during the pregnancy. Fortunately, if the body is in short supply of calcium, calcium absorption will be enhanced, but if intake is really low, then this improvement in absorption will not be enough to compensate for a low dietary intake.

Foods that are high in calcium include milk and milk products, some kinds of tofu, certain vegetables (e.g., broccoli) and fish with bones (e.g., canned sardines and salmon with bones). Certain foods may interfere with the absorption of calcium, including legumes, such as beans and lentils, spinach and sweet potatoes. These plant foods contain oxalates and phytates, which decrease the absorption of calcium.

Did You Know ...

Calcium Deficiency

The US Third Natural Health Examination Survey indicated that 75% of women between 20 and 50 years of age were not receiving an adequate intake of calcium prior to pregnancy.

Dietary Sources of Calcium

Dietary sources of nutrients can be ranked as Excellent, Good and Source.
(Based on usual serving size.)

EXCELLENT SOURCE of Calcium (275 mg or more)

- Milk: all types
- Swiss cheese
- Tofu set with calcium sulphate
- Plain yogurt
- Sesame seeds, whole
- Fortified plant-based beverages

SOURCE of Calcium (55 mg or more)

- Cheese: creamed cottage or ricotta cheese
- Legumes: beans (most kinds), cooked or canned
- Greens: cooked bok choy, kale, turnip, mustard greens, broccoli
- Oranges
- Scallops, cooked
- Oysters, cooked
- Nuts: almonds, dried sunflower seeds

GOOD SOURCE of Calcium (165 mg or more)

- Cheeses: mozzarella, Edam, brick, Parmesan, Gouda, feta
- Processed cheese spread and slices
- Yogurt, flavored
- Sardines, small canned
- Salmon, canned with bones

Note: Spinach, chard, beet greens, sweet potatoes and rhubarb are not good sources of calcium because these foods also contain oxalate or phytate, which inhibit calcium absorption.

Note: There may be new products coming on the market that have added milk solids. Orange juice may also be fortified with calcium. Some may be Sources, Good Sources, or Excellent Sources of calcium. Read labels to find out what amounts of calcium are added.

(Based on Nutrition for a Healthy Pregnancy, National Guidelines for the Childbearing Years, Health Canada, Oct., 2002. Reprinted with the permission of the Minister of Public Works and Government Services Canada, 2005.)

Dietary Recommended Intake of Calcium

Based on the DRI, a woman's daily calcium requirement is 1,000 mg a day (AI) prior to pregnancy. An intake of 2 cups (500 mL) of milk, ¾ cup (175 mL) of yogurt and 3 oz (90 g) of canned salmon with bones would be enough to provide this requirement. The AI for calcium does not change during pregnancy.

Did You Know ...

Vitamin D Deficiency

Recent evidence suggests that vitamin D deficiency may affect the infant's immune system later in life, not just bone and skeletal development. Some researchers suggest that vitamin D deficiency during pregnancy may lead to Type 1 diabetes later in life. Sunscreens eliminate the formation of Vitamin D in the skin by the sun, so this source cannot be counted on for Vitamin D. Make sure your diet contains an adequate supply of Vitamin D and try to get some sunlight exposure.

Vitamin D

Ensuring that an adequate supply of vitamin D is present before becoming pregnant leads to an increased chance of adequate intake during pregnancy and the birth of a healthy child.

Vitamin D is made available to the body through the action of sunlight on the skin, as well as through the diet. Moderate exposure to sunlight is recommended for this important source of vitamin D. Women who are at risk of vitamin D deficiency before conception include those who are not exposed to sunlight for climate or for cultural reasons. Malnutrition in general may also be associated with low levels of vitamin D.

Foods that are high in vitamin D include milk, fortified soy beverages, powdered and evaporated milk, margarine and fatty fish, such as salmon.

Dietary Recommended Intake of Vitamin D

The DRI (AI) for vitamin D for women of childbearing age is 200 IU per day.

Folic Acid

Women of childbearing age should take a folic acid supplement of 400 mcg (0.4 mg) daily before becoming pregnant and until the end of the first trimester to reduce the risk of neural tube defects, such as spina bifida.

Dietary Sources of Folate

Dietary sources of nutrients can be ranked as Excellent, Good and Source. (Based on usual serving size.)

EXCELLENT SOURCE of Folate
- Chickpeas, lentils
- Spinach, asparagus, cooked
- Romaine lettuce
- Orange juice, canned pineapple juice
- Sunflower seeds

SOURCE of Folate
- Beans (fava, kidney, pinto, romano, soy, white beans), cooked
- Lima beans, cooked
- Corn, bean sprouts, cooked broccoli, green peas, Brussels sprouts, beets
- Oranges
- Melon: honeydew
- Raspberries, blackberries
- Avocado
- Roasted peanuts
- Wheat germ

GOOD SOURCE of Folate
- Carrots, beet greens, sweet potato, snow peas, summer or winter squash, rutabaga, cabbage, green beans, cooked
- Cashews, roasted peanuts, walnuts
- Eggs
- Strawberries, bananas, grapefruit, cantaloupe
- Whole wheat or white bread
- Pork kidney
- Breakfast cereals
- Milk: all types

Note: Addition of folic acid to white flour and pasta products labeled "enriched" became mandatory as of November 1998. This mandatory fortification will add approximately 100 mcg (0.1 mg) of folic acid to the average woman's diet every day.

(**Source:** Nutrition for a Healthy Pregnancy, National Guidelines for the Childbearing Years, Health Canada, Oct., 2002. Reprinted with the permission of the Minister of Public Works and Government Services Canada, 2005.)

Iron

In pre-pregnancy, an adequate supply of iron can prepare the body with sufficient stores for the higher demands during pregnancy. By adjusting a diet that may be deficient in iron before pregnancy occurs, a woman will be more likely to maintain an adequate intake during and after pregnancy. With enough iron on board, a woman should have the energy required for normal daily activities.

If iron is low, then energy levels decrease, possibly leading to a less active lifestyle due to decreased muscle function, which would affect general health and well-being.

Did You Know ...

Iron Stores

Iron stores may also be depleted around the time of delivery, so adequate iron intake/supplementation before and after birth is essential.

Dietary Recommended Intake of Iron

The DRI (RDA) for iron for women during their childbearing years is 18 mg per day. During pregnancy, this increases to 27 mg per day. The maximum safe level (UL) is 45 mg per day.

Did You Know ...

Iron Deficiency

Canadian studies have shown that many women in their childbearing years do not meet their daily requirements for iron. Studies from Australia indicate that between 13% and 18% of both vegetarian and non-vegetarian women of childbearing age may have low iron stores. This is also true for adolescent girls, where increased iron requirements along with decreased caloric intake would result in iron deficiency. This combination could affect the growth of the adolescent, as well as the growth of the future fetus.

Again, the better the health of a woman before pregnancy, the more likely the chances that a healthy lifestyle will be maintained during pregnancy. Iron deficiency can also lower immunity, increasing risk of infection and decreasing resistance to illness.

Risk Factors for Poor Iron Status

- Diet low in meat, fish, poultry
- Diet low in vitamin C
- Frequent consumption of tea or coffee close to mealtime
- Regular acetylsalicylic acid (ASA) use
- Menorrhagia (excessive menstrual loss)
- Three or more annual blood donations
- Pregnancy
- Multiple gestations
- Parity of three or more (more than three pregnancies)

(**Source:** Nutrition for a Healthy Pregnancy, National Guidelines for the Childbearing Years, Health Canada, Oct., 2002. Reprinted with the permission of the Minister of Public Works and Government Services Canada, 2005.)

Zinc

Did You Know ...

Zinc Needs

For pregnancy, 100 mg of zinc are required. Of this 100 mg, approximately 7% is required by the mother, 50% by the fetus and 25% by the uterus.

When planning your pregnancy, you should monitor your dietary intake of zinc because it is important in maintaining healthy metabolic and immune systems. Inadequate intake of zinc may affect the growth of the fetus, possibly leading to intrauterine growth retardation. Alcohol intake and smoking (which should be avoided before and during pregnancy) can also decrease the placental transfer of zinc to the fetus. Women who have problems with their digestive system may require supplemental zinc. Their physician would be their best guide on whether or not they require zinc supplementation.

Dietary Sources of Heme and Non-Heme Iron

Dietary sources of nutrients can be ranked as Excellent, Good and Source.
(Based on usual serving size.)

SOURCES OF HEME IRON

**EXCELLENT SOURCE of Heme Iron
(3.5 mg or more)**
- N/A.

**GOOD SOURCE of Heme Iron
(2.1 mg or more)**
- Beef, ground or steak, cooked
- Blood pudding

**SOURCE of Heme Iron
(0.7 mg or more)**
- Chicken, ham, lamb, pork, veal
- Halibut, haddock, perch, salmon, canned or fresh
- Shrimp, cooked
- Sardines and tuna, canned
- Eggs

Note: Dietary iron has two forms: heme iron and non-heme iron. Generally, heme iron is more easily absorbed than non-heme iron.

(**Source:** Nutrition for a Healthy Pregnancy, National Guidelines for the Childbearing Years, Health Canada, Oct., 2002. Reprinted with the permission of the Minister of Public Works and Government Services Canada, 2005.)

SOURCES OF NON-HEME IRON

**EXCELLENT SOURCE of Non-Heme
Iron (3.5 mg or more)**
- Beans (white beans, soybeans, lentils, chickpeas), cooked
- Clams and oysters, cooked
- Seeds: pumpkin, sesame, squash, sunflower
- Breakfast cereals enriched with iron
- Tofu

**GOOD SOURCE of Non-Heme Iron
(2.1 mg or more)**
- Beans (lima, red kidney beans, chickpeas, split peas), cooked

**SOURCE of Non-Heme Iron
(0.7 mg or more)**
- Nuts: peanuts, pecans, walnuts, pistachios, roasted almonds, roasted cashews
- Cooked pasta, egg noodles
- Bread
- Pumpernickel bagel
- Bran muffin
- Oatmeal, cooked
- Wheat germ
- Beets, canned, drained
- Pumpkin, canned or cooked
- Dried fruit: seedless raisins, peaches, prunes, apricots

Zinc is found in many foods, including meat and dairy products. However, certain foods may also interfere with the absorption of zinc. These include foods that are high in dietary phytate (such as legumes like soybeans), fiber or calcium. Consumption of these foods will not lead to a deficiency if there is adequate consumption of zinc.

Dietary Recommended Intake of Zinc

In the United States, women receive about 10 mg per day of zinc, while the recommended daily amount is 8 mg per day. During pregnancy, extra zinc demands are required for the fetus as well as the mother. The DRI (RDA) for zinc during pregnancy is 11 mg per day. If there is an inadequate supply of dietary zinc, then the body will try to adapt by increasing the absorption of this mineral; however, this will not compensate for a lack of dietary zinc.

Essential Fatty Acids

According to the National Guidelines for the Childbearing Years, "Essential fatty acid intake may be low if the major sources of fat in the diet are higher-fat commercial bakery products or fried foods prepared with partially hydrogenated vegetable oils or vegetable oil shortening." Prior to pregnancy, a woman should ensure that the supply of omega 3 and omega 6 fatty acids is adequate, by consuming a diet containing fatty fish, lean meat and eggs (egg yolk).

Common vegetable oils, such as canola and soy, also contain large amounts of essential fatty acids, especially omega 3 fatty acids. Margarines and salad dressings made from these oils are good sources of these fatty acids. Sunflower, peanut and corn oils, as well as nuts and peanuts, are good sources of omega 6 fatty acids, but not the omega 3 fatty acids.

Therefore, a variety of these foods is recommended so that a balance of the omega 3 and omega 6 fatty acids is provided by the diet. The typical North American diet is composed of foods that are relatively higher in proportion of energy from omega 6 fatty acids compared to omega 3 fatty acids. It would be prudent to increase intake of foods that are high in omega 3 fatty acids.

Dietary Recommended Intake of Fatty Acids

The DRI (AI) for omega 6 fatty acids is 13 grams per day, or 5% to 10 % of total calories, while the DRI (AI) for omega 3 fatty acids is 1.4 grams per day, or 0.6% to 1.2% of total calories. The DRI (AI) during lactation is 13 grams per day for omega 6 fatty acids and 1.3 grams per day for omega 3 fatty acids.

Lifestyle Choices

Exercise

Exercise is an important part of a healthy lifestyle and should be encouraged before pregnancy. Following a daily exercise routine will have a very positive impact on the health and well-being of the mother and the fetus. By having an established exercise regimen prior to becoming pregnant, a woman will find it easier to incorporate exercise during pregnancy.

Benefits of Exercise

- Increased daily energy levels
- Increased muscle strength
- Limited or controlled weight gain and limited fat retention
- Improved attitude
- Improved body-image satisfaction
- Improved overall well-being

Smoking

Smoking is associated with many well-known health risks to the smoker, including heart disease and high blood pressure, and to the fetus. Smoking during pregnancy or the exposure of a mother to secondhand smoke (defined as passive smoking) increases the risk of preterm birth, increases the risk of low birth weight, decreases head circumference at birth and increases the incidence of sudden infant death syndrome (SIDS).

Exposure of the fetus to smoke can also lead to decreased lung function and an increased risk of infections. Smoking and secondhand smoke have also been associated with behavioral disorders in the child, such as attention deficit/hyperactivity disorder (ADHD), and increased risk of heart disease and hypertension later in life. A mother who smokes during pregnancy may increase her child's risk of having airway disease or wheezing illnesses because the function of the airways is dependent on a healthy fetal development. One study found that adult men whose mothers smoked during their pregnancy had a lower sperm concentration and a higher risk of low sperm count, which was dose dependent.

Did You Know …

Daily Exercise

According to Canada's Physical Activity Guide to Healthy Active Living, at least 30 to 60 minutes of daily exercise, such as walking, running, swimming and bicycling, are recommended. Some studies suggest that a healthy level of exercise throughout pregnancy will lead to a quicker recovery after delivery and possibly less complicated labor. The level of exercise should be discussed with your doctor.

Activities that pose a risk of falling, such as downhill skiing, or that involve bodily contact, such as soccer or field hockey, should be avoided during pregnancy.

Did You Know ...

Drug Risks

Risks of recreational drug use include a premature delivery, delays in fetal brain development and increases in maternal blood pressure. Drug use before and during pregnancy must be brought to the attention of primary health-care providers so they can assist in discontinuing their use.

Did You Know ...

Folic Acid Needs

In addition to eating a well-balanced diet, the Office of Nutrition Policy and Promotion at Health Canada recommends that women contemplating a pregnancy should take a supplement of 400 mcg (0.4 mg) of folic acid every day, beginning at least one month before pregnancy, to reduce the risk of having a child born with a neural tube defect or spina bifida.

For many health reasons, it is recommended that smoking or being exposed to smoking be discontinued prior to becoming pregnant so that the mother and fetus have decreased risk of developing these conditions.

Recreational Drugs

Recreational drug use should be discontinued prior to and during pregnancy. The risks to the fetus can be lifelong. Women who use recreational drugs such as cocaine, marijuana or ecstasy may also take less care of their own health, putting their unborn child at risk as well. Drug-dependent women may be undernourished, which also affects the fetus.

Vitamin Supplements

A diet that includes foods from the four major food groups from Canada's Food Guide or is based on the USDA MyPyramid will provide women with the essential nutrients for themselves and to support a pregnancy. The exception is folic acid, which needs to be supplemented if dietary intake is inadequate. Iron supplements may also be required. Prenatal multivitamins often contain adequate folate and iron.

Women who must restrict their intake of some foods or food groups (for example, vegetarians) may require supplementation with certain vitamins or minerals. This should be discussed with a physician.

Medications

Before taking any medications, including over-the-counter remedies for a common headache, women contemplating pregnancy or who are pregnant should check with their physician to ensure that the medication is safe. An excellent resource for understanding the risk of taking medications before and during pregnancy is *The Complete Guide to Everyday Risks in Pregnancy and Breastfeeding*, prepared by the Motherisk Program at The Hospital for Sick Children.

Special Diets

Vegetarianism

Well-planned vegetarian diets, including strict vegan diets, can be appropriate for women during pregnancy and lactation. The American Dietetic Association and Dietitians of Canada state that the nutritional benefits of vegetarian diets include lower intakes of saturated fat and dietary cholesterol. They also include higher intakes of carbohydrates, including fiber, as well as other vitamins and minerals, such as magnesium, potassium, folate and antioxidants, particularly vitamin C and vitamin E. Studies have shown that babies born to vegetarian mothers have similar birth weights to babies born to mothers who eat meat.

New products are continually being developed for vegetarian diets. There is an extensive choice of fortified foods, including soy milks, meat alternatives, fruit juices and breakfast cereals, which allow the well-informed consumer to obtain sufficient amounts of all nutrients needed for a well-balanced diet. If you are on a vegetarian diet, speak with your doctor about any concerns you may have. Your physician may connect you with a dietitian for a further nutrition consultation if warranted.

Vegetarian Diet Benefits Can Include

- Lower body mass index (BMI)
- Lower blood cholesterol levels
- Less death from heart disease
- Lower rates of blood pressure and hypertension
- Lower rates of other lifestyle diseases, such as diabetes and colon cancer

Kinds of Vegetarian Diets

There are many different types of vegetarian diets. Lacto-ovo vegetarians do not eat meat, fish or poultry, but choose to include both eggs and dairy as a part of their diet. Vegans are stricter vegetarians who choose not to include animal products of any kind. Vegans represent a small proportion of all vegetarians. Semi-vegetarians do not eat red meat, but do include occasional poultry and fish in their diets. For pregnant women consuming a vegetarian diet, both lacto-ovo and vegan diets can be a healthy alternative to a mixed diet.

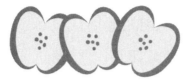

Vegetarian food guide rainbow

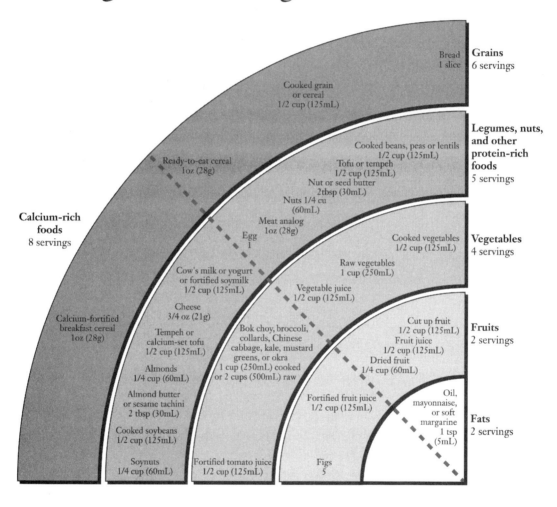

Grains
6 servings
Bread 1 slice

Cooked grain
or cereal
1/2 cup (125mL)

Legumes, nuts, and other protein-rich foods
5 servings

Ready-to-eat cereal
1oz (28g)

Cooked beans, peas or lentils
1/2 cup (125mL)

Tofu or tempeh
1/2 cup (125mL)

Nut or seed butter
2tbsp (30mL)

Nuts 1/4 cu
(60mL)

Meat analog
1oz (28g)

Egg
1

Calcium-rich foods
8 servings

Cooked vegetables
1/2 cup (125mL)

Vegetables
4 servings

Cow's milk or yogurt
or fortified soymilk
1/2 cup (125mL)

Raw vegetables
1 cup (250mL)

Cheese
3/4 oz (21g)

Vegetable juice
1/2 cup (125mL)

Calcium-fortified
breakfast cereal
1oz (28g)

Tempeh or
calcium-set tofu
1/2 cup (125mL)

Bok choy, broccoli,
collards, Chinese
cabbage, kale, mustard
greens, or okra
1 cup (250mL) cooked
or 2 cups (500mL) raw

Cut up fruit
1/2 cup (125mL)

Fruit juice
1/2 cup (125mL)

Dried fruit
1/4 cup (60mL)

Fruits
2 servings

Almonds
1/4 cup (60mL)

Almond butter
or sesame tachini
2 tbsp (30mL)

Fortified fruit juice
1/2 cup (125mL)

Oil,
mayonnaise,
or soft
margarine
1 tsp
(5mL)

Fats
2 servings

Cooked soybeans
1/2 cup (125mL)

Soynuts
1/4 cup (60mL)

Fortified tomato juice
1/2 cup (125mL)

Figs
5

Special Nutrient Needs

However, vegetarian diets can pose some risks if not adequately supplemented with specific nutrients. It is especially important for pregnant women to make sure their vegetarian diet is well planned to ensure energy and nutrient needs are being met. Follow the Vegetarian Food Guide Rainbow provided by the Dietitians of Canada.

Energy: Caloric intake is typically lower in vegetarians than in non-vegetarians; nevertheless, vegetarians usually consume adequate calories. Many vegetarians have a BMI less than 20, so they need to eat enough to gain appropriate weight during pregnancy.

Protein: Vegetarians can receive adequate protein from plant sources when a variety of plant foods are eaten and caloric intake is adequate. The protein needs of vegetarians may be higher than the protein needs of non-vegetarians because some plant proteins are not as usable as protein from animal sources. Lacto-ovo vegetarians typically meet and exceed protein requirements, similar to non-vegetarian diets.

Iron: The American Dietetic Association and Dietitians of Canada suggest that the iron needs of vegetarians may be almost twice the recommended levels for non-vegetarians because of the low availability of plant-based, or non-heme, iron. Non-heme iron tends to be more sensitive than heme iron to both inhibitors and enhancers of iron absorption.

Many compounds interfere with the absorption of iron, most notably high intakes of phytates, which is particularly problematic because many plant foods that are high in iron are also high in phytates. Other inhibitors of iron absorption include calcium, fiber, coffee and tannins found in tea.

However, vegetarian diets are typically higher in vitamin C and other organic acids found in fruits and vegetables that help with the absorption of plant-sourced iron in the body. Vitamin C can help to improve iron absorption and can also help to lessen the negative effect that phytates have on iron absorption. However, even well-planned lacto-ovo vegetarian diets may require additional iron supplementation during the second and third trimesters.

Did You Know ...

Complementary Proteins

Some health-care professionals used to suggest that vegetarians eat "complementary proteins" containing different essential amino acids at each meal. Current thinking suggests that assorted plant foods consumed over the course of the day can provide all the essential amino acids that your body needs.

Did You Know ...

Iron Supplements

Researchers have found that although iron stores may be lower in vegetarians than in omnivores, who also eat meat, the risk of iron deficiency anemia is similar. Iron deficiency anemia is a common problem in pregnancy regardless of diet type. An iron supplement may be suggested to prevent or treat iron deficiency anemia.

Calcium: There is no evidence to suggest that vegetarians have poor calcium intake, especially for lacto-ovo vegetarians who drink milk. Vegans are at a higher risk of not consuming enough calcium and need to choose a wide variety of non-dairy foods that contain calcium. High-calcium plant foods that are also low in oxalates are better absorbed because oxalates inhibit calcium absorption. Good examples include bok choy and broccoli. During pregnancy, however, it may be difficult to obtain enough calcium through vegetable sources only. Fortified milk alternatives, such as soy milk or rice milk, will help to provide additional calcium in the diet.

Vitamin D: Vitamin D tends not to be a concern for vegetarians who eat dairy products and for vegans who have adequate exposure to sunlight daily, because the body is capable of producing its own vitamin D when skin is exposed to the sun. This becomes more of a concern in the winter months, when sunlight exposure is less frequent, and with extensive sunscreen use, which is nevertheless important to prevent skin cancer and premature aging.

Vitamin B-12: Vegans are at risk for vitamin B-12 deficiency because this vitamin is only found in significant amounts in foods derived from animal sources. Lacto-ovo vegetarians may also be at risk for vitamin B-12 deficiency during pregnancy and should consider supplementary sources of vitamin B-12.

 Dietary Recommended Intake of Vitamin B-12 for Vegans

Vegans should consume a vitamin B-12 supplement of at least 1 mcg (0.74 mmol) or the equivalent found in fortified foods, such as meat analogues, every day.

Zinc: Vegetarians generally do not have a problem obtaining adequate zinc in their diets, although high intakes of fiber, calcium, oxalates and phytates, as well as supplemental iron, can interfere with zinc absorption. Good vegetarian sources of zinc include nuts, legumes, whole grains, milk and egg yolks.

What is DHA?

DHA (docosahexaenoic acid) is an omega 3 fatty acid that has been shown to play a role in the development of a baby's brain and eyes. Babies born to vegetarian mothers have been shown to have lower spinal cord and blood levels of DHA than babies born to mothers who eat meat. The DHA levels in the breast milk of vegan mothers also tend to be lower than that of lacto-ovo vegetarian and non-vegetarian mothers.

While the importance of these low levels is not yet known, it is recommended that women on a vegetarian diet include a source of linolenic acid (a precursor of DHA) in their diet before conception, during pregnancy and while lactating. Some sources of linolenic acid include flax seeds, flax seed oil, canola oil and soy oil.

Folate: Vegetarians tend to have higher intakes of folate than non-vegetarians; nevertheless, women on a vegetarian diet are advised to take a folic acid supplement of 400 mcg (0.4 mg) daily before and during pregnancy until the end of the first trimester. This supplement should be taken by all women of childbearing age before getting pregnant because neural tube defects develop in the early weeks of pregnancy, often before a women realizes that she is pregnant. Ask your health-care provider for guidance about your own individual situation.

Lactose-Free Diets

For those pregnant women who are lactose intolerant and want to consume dairy products during their pregnancy, lactase tablets containing the enzyme purified from yeasts and molds can be used. For mothers who choose to continue to avoid dairy products, other sources of calcium and vitamin D, such as fortified milk alternatives like soy milk, should be chosen and a supplement containing these nutrients should be considered.

CHAPTER 4

Early Pregnancy Nutrition (First Trimester)

THE FIRST TRIMESTER OF GESTATION is extremely important in determining the eventual health of your baby. The first trimester begins with the first day of your last menstrual period and continues until the end of week 12. However, trimesters are arbitrary in nature. There is nothing that makes the last day of week 12 more significant than the first day of week 13. Trimesters are simply general guides in dividing a pregnancy into stages.

The first trimester is a time of rapid growth and cell division. All organ systems are formed in the first trimester and continue to grow and develop throughout the course of pregnancy. Most malformations also begin during the critical embryonic period between week 6 and week 10.

During the first trimester, you should aim to maintain a healthy weight, take care of several special nutrient needs to support growth and development of the fetus, and avoid foods that put mother and fetus at risk.

Healthy Body Mass Index

In the first trimester of pregnancy, some weight gain can be expected. During the first 3 months of pregnancy, for a woman with a normal or healthy BMI, average weight gain may only be about 2 to 8 lb (1 to 3.5 kg). A healthy BMI range is still about 20 to 25 in the early days of pregnancy. In women with a BMI over 27, very little weight gain should occur in the first trimester — about 1 to 2 lbs (0.5 to 1.0 kg). Pregnant women with a BMI under 19 should achieve a slightly higher weight gain during pregnancy to improve their own nutritional status and to support the growth of the fetus.

The rate of weight gain in the first trimester will also depend on the health of the mother, including nausea and/or vomiting, which may result in less weight gain at the start, with catch-up weight gain at the end of the trimester.

First Trimester Growth and Development

- During the first trimester, limb buds appear and then grow. By the end of the first trimester, fingers and toes are formed.
- The central nervous system forms. By day 25 after conception, the neural tube, which forms the brain and spinal cord, closes.
- Muscle and bone formation begins to take place and the skeleton begins to form.
- The heart develops and divides into four chambers. By week 13, the heart begins to beat about 140 times a minute.
- The lungs are formed and the fetus begins to "breathe" amniotic fluid.
- The fetus begins to practice sucking by pursing lips, turning its head and swallowing amniotic fluid.
- The kidneys begin to function and begin to pass urine from around week 10.
- The small intestine is able to contract and relax by week 11.
- The eyes, ears and nose are also developing.
- The eyelids fuse shut and will remain that way until about week 27.
- By the end of the first trimester, the sex of the baby will be apparent to the naked eye (although still too early to see on ultrasound) and the baby will move freely within the uterus; however, it is still too early to be felt by the mother. By the end of the first trimester, the fetus will be about 3.5 inches (9 cm) long and weigh about 1.7 oz (48 g), about the size of a peach.

Recommended Rate of Weight Gain

Rates of weight gain for the duration of the pregnancy for normal weight, underweight and overweight women have been suggested by the Institute of Medicine's Food and Nutrition Board (1990) and the March of Dimes.

If you are normal weight before pregnancy: Gain 25 to 35 lbs (11 to 16 kg) during pregnancy.

If you are overweight before pregnancy: Gain 15 to 25 lbs (7 to 11 kg) during pregnancy.

If you are underweight before pregnancy: Gain 28 to 40 lbs (13 to 18 kg) during pregnancy (depending on your pre-pregnancy weight).

If you have a multiple pregnancy (twins, triplets or more): Gain 35 to 45 lbs (16 to 20 kg). You will need to gain more weight during pregnancy depending on the number of babies you are carrying. See your health-care provider for guidance.

(**Source:** Reprinted by permission from March of Dimes, 2005)

Some women gain very little weight in the first trimester, due to feeling unwell. This should be monitored by a physician. Referral to a registered dietitian may be recommended. A dietitian can assist in selecting appropriate nutrient-rich foods that would help with weight gain. Fortunately, the additional energy needs of the fetus are not as great during the first trimester as they are in the second and third trimesters.

Approximate Weight Breakdown of 30 lbs (14 kg) Gained

Blood	3.0 lbs (1.4 kg)
Breasts	3.0 lbs (1.4 kg)
Womb	2.0 lbs (0.9 kg)
Fetus	7.5 lbs (3.4 kg)
Placenta	1.5 lbs (0.7 kg)
Amniotic fluid	2.0 lbs (0.9 kg)
Fat, protein, other nutrients	7.0 lbs (3.2 kg)
Water retained	4.0 lbs (1.8 kg)

Nutritional Needs

Energy

Energy needs increase by about 100 kcal per day in the first 10 to 12 weeks of pregnancy, from a regular diet of approximately 2,000 to 2,400 kcal. This is good news for those not feeling well, because there is less pressure to take in more food. Despite the old wives' tale, you don't have to eat for two; it would be unhealthy to do so because too much weight would be gained.

Protein

Increased protein intake is needed for the developing fetus, for supporting the uterus and mammary glands, and for increasing blood volume and skeletal muscle. Recommended protein foods include lean meat, chicken, fish, eggs and low-fat milk or other dairy products. Tofu, lentils and nuts

How much food makes up 100 kcal?

It is quite easy to increase energy intake by an extra 100 kcal per day. Here are some examples of foods that contain 100 kcal:

- Milk, 1% M.F.: 1 cup (250 mL)
- Vanilla yogurt, 1.9% M.F.: $\frac{1}{3}$–$\frac{1}{2}$ cup (75–125 mL)
- Cottage cheese, 2% M.F.: $\frac{1}{2}$ cup (125 mL)
- Egg, fried with 1 tsp (5 mL) butter or margarine: 1
- Salmon, baked: $1\frac{1}{2}$–2 oz (45–60 g)
- Chicken thigh, roasted: 2 oz (60 g)
- Plums: 3
- Blueberries, fresh: $1\frac{1}{4}$ cup (300 mL)
- Banana: 1 medium
- Apple: 1 large
- Tomatoes: 4 medium
- Carrots: 3 medium

Recommended Recipes

100-CALORIE FOOD ITEMS

In the Better Recipes for Pregnancy section of this book, you will find a number of recipes that contain approximately the 100 calories you need to add to your diet during the first trimester of pregnancy. (Based on 1 serving or as otherwise indicated.)

Rapini with Balsamic Vinegar	Mango-Cucumber Salad
Strawberry Sorbet	Couscous
Lemony Biscotti	Cauliflower Popcorn Snack
Borscht	(1 cup/250 mL)
Thai-Style Beef Salad	Green Beans and Tomato
Sweet Green Pea Soup	Grandma's Rolled Oat Cookies
Mango, Strawberry and Cucumber Salad	Lentil Dip (2 tbsp/25 mL)
Asian Cucumber Salad	Fiber-full Bran Pancakes (1)

and seeds are also good choices. Higher-fat choices, such as regular cuts of meat and chicken with skin, are recommended for those who are trying to gain weight, while the leaner varieties of meat are recommended for those of normal weight or for those with a higher BMI.

Dietary Recommended Intake of Protein

The DRI (RDA) for protein for women during the three trimesters of pregnancy is 71 g per day. The percentage of calories in your diet from protein should be 10% to 35% of total daily calories.

Did You Know ...

Multiple Pregnancy Weight Gain

Weight gain, particularly the rate of weight gain in the initial 28 weeks of a multiple pregnancy, will have an effect on the birth weight of the babies. The Institute of Medicine recommends a total weight gain of 35 to 45 lbs (16 to 21 kg) for a twin pregnancy. Underweight women should gain at the higher range, while overweight women should gain at the lower range of this scale.

Did You Know ...

Multiple Vitamins

The Institute of Medicine (1990) recommends a multivitamin with minerals and an iron supplement of 30 mg per day for women with multiple pregnancies. This supplement should also include 15 mg of zinc, 2 mg of copper, 250 mg of calcium, 2 mg of vitamin B-6, 400 mcg of folate, 50 mg of vitamin C, and 5 mcg (200 IU) of vitamin D.

Fat

Women often decrease their intake of calories from fat when watching their weight, but may be at risk of being deficient in the essential fatty acids, such as the omega 3 and omega 6 fatty acids. These fatty acids are important for the fetus as well as the mother. Fat intake should represent about 20% to 35% of the total daily energy intake.

Multiple Pregnancy

A healthy multiple pregnancy outcome can be assisted with the appropriate nutritional advice and with close monitoring of the growth of the babies. By receiving counseling on an appropriate diet, the weight gain of the mother can be improved and a healthier birth weight of the multiples can be expected. Better fetal growth has been shown to improve the health outcome for the babies as well as that of the mother. There is a higher risk of having babies with low birth weight than when having only one baby. Again, this is why it is so important to have the proper nutritional counseling and monitoring when multiples are expected.

Multiple Pregnancy Diet

The American Dietetic Association suggests that women with a multiple pregnancy increase their servings from the various food groups to the following levels:

> 3 servings of milk and milk products

> 3 servings of meat or alternatives

> 3 servings of vegetables

> 2 servings of fruit

> 6 servings of breads or cereals

It has been suggested that a weight gain of about 1.5 lbs (0.7 kg) per week after the first trimester is adequate for a twin pregnancy. For triplets, the same weight gain of 1.5 lbs (0.7 kg) per week is recommended, but beginning in the earlier stages of pregnancy, for a total weight gain of 50 lbs (23 kg).

Early Pregnancy Exercise

It is never too late to start an exercise program. For someone who is normally not very active, an exercise program that is mild in the beginning can be started at the early stages of pregnancy. Your physician will be able to guide you on the amount and type of exercise that is safe. Brisk walking, bicycling, swimming and some floor exercises are usually recommended.

For women who are already active, especially if you are involved in strenuous activities, such as running, lifting weights and endurance-type sports, your level of activity during early pregnancy should also be discussed with your doctor.

Liquids should be consumed at the beginning, during and after activity to maintain good hydration. Increased activity also requires increased energy intake.

Benefits of Exercise in Early Pregnancy

- Decreased feeling of nausea associated with early pregnancy
- Improved cardiac function
- Improved mental state of the mother
- Easier and less complicated labor
- Quicker recovery after giving birth
- Control of weight gained during pregnancy
- Limited accumulation of fat after delivery
- Overall improved health
- Studies also suggest the benefits to the fetus include leaner bodies at 5 years of age and better developmental outcomes

Did You Know ...

Vigorous Activity

According to Health Canada, vigorous or strenuous activity should be avoided in the first trimester because of the possibility of overheating the fetus when at its critical development stage. Scuba diving is contraindicated at any stage of pregnancy because gas bubbles may form in the circulatory system of the fetus. Contact sports and any exercise that increases risk of falling are not recommended.

Did You Know ...

Exercise Recommendations

The executive and council of the Society of Obstetricians and Gynaecologists of Canada recommends that all women without contraindications should be encouraged to participate in aerobic and strength-conditioning exercises as part of a healthy lifestyle during their pregnancy. Health Canada recommends that women include 15 to 30 minutes, 3 to 5 days a week, of physical activity in their daily lives. The American College of Obstetricians and Gynecologists recommends at least 30 minutes on most, if not all, days.

Lifestyle

Alcohol

Did You Know ...

Fetal Alcohol Syndrome

Fetal alcohol syndrome (FAS), caused by a mother's alcohol intake during pregnancy, is a lifelong condition affecting people in many ways. Children with FAS have physical and mental disabilities, including problems with memory, learning, attention span, communication and hearing that persist into adulthood. FAS is entirely preventable by avoiding alcohol during pregnancy. The lifelong consequences are not worth the risk.

The use of alcohol is not recommended in early pregnancy because alcohol passes from the mother's bloodstream across the placenta into the fetus and is associated with several serious conditions:

- Decreased birth weight
- Interference with hormones that promote growth of the fetal brain as well as the body
- Interference with the hormones of the mother, leading to an altered hormonal environment that may also influence the growth and well-being of the fetus
- Fetal alcohol syndrome

Studies of children exposed to alcohol during pregnancy show difficulty with processing information and with activities that involved working memory, such as arithmetic.

There is no known amount of alcohol considered or proven in studies to be safe. Abstain from alcohol before and during pregnancy.

Vitamin Supplements

Physicians often recommend vitamin supplements in early pregnancy. Results of North American surveys reveal that many women in their childbearing years are deficient in the intake of iron (11% to 13% of women), calcium (up to 75% of women), and fruits and vegetables (up to 57% do not receive 5 or more servings), while intake of high-energy, low-nutrient foods has increased. In the United States, these low-nutrient foods make up more than 31% of total daily energy intake.

Iron is of particular concern because of the extra demands placed on the woman for this mineral during pregnancy and the risk of anemia and its negative effects on the fetus. Folic acid supplements are recommended for all women of childbearing age. Vitamin B-12 may be recommended for women who are following vegetarian diets. Reports have revealed irreversible neurological consequences of this deficiency in infants born to women with vitamin B-12 deficiency.

Should I take a multivitamin throughout my pregnancy?

Generally speaking, it should be possible for almost all pregnant women to meet their needs for most nutrients through a well-balanced diet alone. Most experts agree, however, that taking a multivitamin throughout the course of your pregnancy is an easy way to ensure adequate intakes of many vitamins and minerals — a nutritional safety net for times when your diet may not be 100% perfect.

A good prenatal vitamin should include 400 mcg (0.4 mg) of folic acid, as well as calcium and zinc. The folic acid is required until the end of the first trimester. An iron supplement with 30 mg of iron may be recommended. Although most prenatal vitamins contain iron, this may not be enough for some women with anemia. Certain groups of women, such as vegans, young mothers, women who do not drink milk and women who follow very restrictive diets, may require additional supplementation. If you are concerned, speak with your doctor, who may refer you to a dietitian.

Safe Levels

Safe vitamin levels for pregnancy are based on the Dietary Reference Intakes (DRIs), which show acceptable upper limits. Vitamin supplements should not contain an excess amount of any one nutrient, unless prescribed by the physician. There are certain vitamins that may be harmful in elevated amounts to the fetus; for example, vitamin A. Always check the amount of vitamin A in the chosen supplement and ensure that is does not exceed the DRI. A vitamin A supplement should not exceed 3,000 mcg (10,000 IU) per day. Use of any vitamin supplements should always be discussed with your physician.

Food Allergies

Approximately 4% to 6% of children have some type of food allergy. The prevalence of food allergies and the sensitization to allergenic foods has increased in the past decade. The most common foods to trigger an allergic reaction in North America include cow's milk and all other dairy products, eggs, peanuts, nuts, fish, wheat and soy. It is common to grow out of an allergy to cow's milk, egg and soy by early childhood. In fact, most children grow out of their milk allergy by age 5. Allergies to nuts, peanuts and fish tend to persist into adulthood. The question of whether food allergies can be prevented in early infancy through avoidance or by exclusive breastfeeding remains a controversial subject that is hotly debated among scientists.

Did You Know ...

Vitamin Risks

There are certain vitamins that may be harmful to the fetus in increased amounts. Vitamin A, for example, can be harmful in excess doses. Always check that your supplement does not exceed the UL, or upper safe limit, as described by the DRI. The RDA is 700 mcg (2,300 IU) per day pre-pregnancy and during pregnancy. The UL is 3,000 mcg (10,000 IU) per day.

Should I avoid certain foods during pregnancy to prevent my child from developing food allergies after birth?

The short answer to this question is no. Studies have not been able to demonstrate that avoiding specific foods, such as cow's milk or eggs, during pregnancy can prevent food allergies from developing in the child. However, studies have shown that mothers who choose to avoid milk and egg products during pregnancy compromise their weight gain, which can be potentially more dangerous to the fetus than the risk of sensitizing the baby to certain food allergens.

The American Academy of Pediatrics (AAP), as well as scientific committees in Europe and Australia, do not recommend an avoidance diet that excludes essential foods during pregnancy. The only food that may be an exception to this rule is peanuts. The AAP suggests that avoiding peanuts during pregnancy for mothers of children who are at high risk of developing an allergy will not lead to a nutritional deficiency because peanuts are not an essential food during pregnancy. High-risk infants include those babies who have at least one parent or sibling with a documented food allergy. This avoidance during pregnancy may also help mothers prepare to eliminate peanuts from their diets while breastfeeding.

Food Cravings and Aversions

Some pregnant women experience a mild to intense desire or distaste for certain foods during pregnancy. It has been speculated that these cravings are the result of a woman's body trying to compensate for certain nutritional deficiencies, but current scientific research does not support this theory.

Some common foods that pregnant women crave include chocolate, pickles, citrus fruit, potato chips and ice cream. Common foods that some pregnant women seem to avoid include coffee, tea, spicy foods, meat and eggs. Generally speaking, there is no harm in giving in to these cravings. It can be a source of concern, however, when your cravings are for high-calorie foods that may contribute to an increase in calories and potentially add extra, unwanted weight gain. The opposite can be true for certain aversions — for example, to meat — which can lead to a reduced intake of calories and less weight being gained.

Use some common sense. Don't force yourself to eat something that makes you feel ill. Eat a well-balanced diet and give in to your cravings every now and then.

Nausea and Vomiting

Nausea and vomiting (often called morning sickness) are probably the most common symptoms of early pregnancy. Although the term "morning sickness" is used to describe the symptoms, nausea and vomiting occur at any time of the day in about 80% of women. These symptoms usually occur between weeks 10 and 18 of pregnancy, but may begin as early as weeks 6 to 8. Nausea is reported in between 70% and 85% of women, while vomiting is reported in about 50% of women.

There is no difference in the birth weight of infants with mothers who experience nausea and vomiting compared to those without these symptoms. However, in women with severe nausea and vomiting, the infant's birth weight may be lower.

Possible Causes

The exact cause of nausea and vomiting during early pregnancy is unknown, but may be due to the change in hormones, such as progesterone, estrogen and HCG, during pregnancy. Other hormones may be involved as well. Increased stress levels during pregnancy may be considered a cause of nausea and vomiting. Often, in these women, the psychological response to the persistent nausea and vomiting may exacerbate the condition.

For most women, the symptoms only last for a few weeks, but for about 15% to 20%, the symptoms persist longer, even until delivery. In severe cases of nausea and vomiting (hyperemesis gravidarum), women experience persistent vomiting, with weight loss and ketonuria (the spilling of ketones in the urine). When there is not enough food intake, the body uses fat for its source of energy. The end products of the breakdown of fat is ketones. These severe cases are reported to occur among three in every 1,000 women or up to one in every 200 women.

Common Treatments

Often, women are able to assess on their own which strategies alleviate the symptoms the best. Some of these include simply getting adequate rest, not getting overtired and avoiding stuffy, hot rooms. A well-ventilated, cool environment is better tolerated than a humid, warmer one. Although exercise has not been studied, regular activity may also help reduce the symptoms of nausea while providing the health benefits of regular exercise and activity.

Did You Know ...

Nutritional Status

Despite the perceived negative effect on dietary intake, mild to moderate cases of nausea and vomiting during pregnancy do not result in a poorer nutritional status of the mother. Usually, most women are able to a catch up in weight gain once symptoms subside.

Did You Know ...

Treatment Strategies

In most instances, the symptoms of nausea and vomiting can be controlled by diet or other strategies, but in severe cases, such as with hyperemesis gravidarum, medication or hospitalization may be required.

Acupuncture and hypnosis have been reported to be helpful in relieving the nausea and vomiting in early pregnancy, but these were found to be mainly successful in those with anxiety-associated issues. Medications are occasionally prescribed by a physician.

Nutritional Strategies for Preventing and Relieving Morning Sickness

- Eat small amounts of foods, commonly cereals (crackers, dry cereal), as snacks.
- Avoid certain foods that induce the symptoms, such as coffee, certain meats and high-fat foods.
- Eat small, frequent meals.
- Don't allow yourself to get hungry.
- Eat a small amount of crackers or other dry food before getting out of bed when the body has been fasting.
- Try high-protein snacks to help decrease symptoms.
- Drink cold fluids that are carbonated or slightly sour between meals.
- Try some crunchy, fresh foods, such as celery sticks or fresh cucumber slices.

Fatigue

Many woman experience increased fatigue in the first few weeks of pregnancy and then again in the last trimester. There are several possible causes of fatigue that are nutrition-related.

Causes

Increased progesterone: One of the reasons for the increase in fatigue in early pregnancy may include the increased level of the hormone progesterone, which helps to support the growing fetus and tissue surrounding it. Progesterone is produced by the placenta for this purpose.

Increased blood volume: The volume of a woman's blood, needed to carry nutrients to the fetus, also increases substantially during pregnancy, leading the heart and other organs to consume more energy than before pregnancy. This may also result in the woman feeling short of breath more easily.

Increased emotional stress: The anxiety that may accompany pregnancy can be caused by nausea and vomiting and the decreased amount of sleep due to these symptoms.

Anemia (lack of iron): Anemia is common during pregnancy and may be a cause of fatigue. Iron is deposited into the fetal and placental tissue during pregnancy. The iron needs of the fetus will override those of the mother, but a woman with iron deficiency anemia will increase the chance of having an infant born prematurely or at a low birth weight.

Treatments

Sleep: If possible, frequent, short naps (15 minutes) during the day may help you to cope with the increased fatigue. Ensuring adequate sleep every night is also important. You might consider going to bed at an earlier time.

Diet: Without a doubt, eating a balanced diet with the additional 100 calories required in early pregnancy (first 10 weeks) for the growing fetus will provide the energy needed for the pregnancy, as well as for the well-being of the mother. Eat fruits and vegetables as snacks, as well as whole grains, lean meats and dairy products. Foods that are high in fat and sugar may actually decrease energy levels. Adequate intake of fluids is also recommended. These include water, milk, lightly sweetened carbonated beverages and limited caffeine and tea.

Iron: Women in the United States receive only about 15 mg of iron daily, while the DRI (RDA) for iron during pregnancy is 27 mg a day. During pregnancy, women need to consume foods that are high in iron, ensuring that plant sources of iron (non-heme iron) are taken with vitamin C–containing foods (such as tomatoes, oranges, orange juice, mangoes, strawberries) to enhance their absorption of this important mineral. An iron supplement may be indicated in some women, under the guidance of their physician.

Exercise: Exercise of some sort is recommended every day, even when a woman feels extremely fatigued (unless this is against the physician's recommendations). Establishing a daily exercise routine by walking short distances and stretching will actually make you feel better. Exercise will help increase metabolism and muscle strength, making it even easier to support the pregnancy as the fetus grows.

Did You Know ...

Ginger Extracts and Vitamin B-6

Some studies have shown that ginger extracts and vitamin B-6 (pyridoxine) can alleviate the nausea experienced by women in early pregnancy. The exact amounts of ginger or vitamin B-6 used in the studies varies, however. The DRI (UL) for pyridoxine during pregnancy is 100 mg per day. It is believed that the active oils found in ginger provide the medicinal effects of this spice. These oils may help to empty the stomach, simulating digestion and relieving nausea. The safety of ginger supplementation has not been proven during pregnancy, so ginger should not be used long-term during pregnancy. Before trying either ginger or pyridoxine (or any alternative treatment), their use should first be discussed with your doctor. Vitamin B-6 is available by prescription from your doctor.

CHAPTER 5

Mid-Pregnancy Nutrition
(Second Trimester)

THE SECOND TRIMESTER lasts from week 13 to week 26. The fetus begins to look like a baby now. The eyes and ears, which were on the side of the head, now start to move into their normal position on the face. The fetus is moving freely, and the mother may begin to feel this movement around week 18, although there is great variability here and the mother may not begin to feel the fetus move until the end of the second trimester. This is called "quickening." The fetus is also able to respond to sound now.

The placenta gradually begins to take over most of the hormone production in this trimester, and as hormone levels even out, you may begin to feel normal again. The nausea that may have plagued you in the first trimester will likely begin to subside.

During the second trimester, you should aim to get the extra daily calories you need by eating nutrient-rich foods. Also make time for leisure or social activities that you can enjoy during your pregnancy and will continue to enjoy once your baby is born. Take precautions against complications of pregnancy — iron deficiency anemia, gestational diabetes, constipation, heartburn and hemorrhoids. Now is also a good time to take care of your dental health. Don't neglect your exercise program. Keeping fit will serve you well as you head into the third trimester and prepare for giving birth to your baby.

Energy Needs

An extra 300 calories of energy is required in the second trimester of pregnancy to develop maternal and fetal tissues. Extra energy is also needed for regular physical activity (with the extra weight of the fetus, more energy is required by the body for usual activities). It is not too difficult to add 300 calories to your diet, but be careful not to eat too much extra food, as excessive weight gain is not desirable. Some women think they can eat all they want during pregnancy, but this is simply not true — and not healthy for the mother or the fetus.

Second Trimester Growth and Development

- The second trimester is a time of rapid skeletal development and the organ systems are now functioning on a basic level, all requiring energy and nutrients.
- By the end of the second trimester, the fetus will weigh between 1½ and 2 lbs (700 and 900 g) and the crown to rump length will be about 9.2 inches (23 cm). Fat begins to form on the fetus around 17 weeks and continues to help the fetus gain weight until birth.
- During the second trimester, fingernails grow to full length and the fetus may begin to suck its thumb. Fine "lanugo" hair insulates the body and a hairline may be visible on the head. The umbilical cord is now thick and strong. Between week 20 and week 24, the fetus has regular periods of sleep and activity.
- Around week 20 of pregnancy, a thick white paste called vernix begins to be secreted through the glands of the skin. Vernix helps to protect the skin from amniotic fluid, and some may still be present at birth.
- By week 21 of pregnancy, the digestive system will allow the fetus to swallow the amniotic fluid and reabsorb the water in it. The amniotic sac contains a large quantity of fluid, which includes nutrients needed for growth, as well as the urine that has been passed. The unused portion of the amniotic fluid now passes into the large bowel and will become meconium (the baby's first stool).
- Around week 22, the organ systems, such as the liver and pancreas, are becoming specialized for their own specific functions.
- Around week 26, the eyelids, which were previously fused shut, now open and close freely.
- By the end of the second trimester, survival of the baby may be expected if the baby is born prematurely.

Iron Deficiency Anemia

Pregnant women may be prone to iron deficiency anemia. By attending to your diet, you can help to prevent this condition. Although many women have healthy nutrient stores during their pregnancy, some become iron deficient during pregnancy. During weeks 12 to 25 of pregnancy, more iron is used by the mother for increasing her blood cell volume. Blood markers of iron status usually fall at this time. In women who have normal iron stores in pre-pregnancy, iron deficiency can still occur, especially in the later stages of pregnancy due to the increased demands of the fetus at about week 30 of gestation.

If the mother is iron deficient, the placenta may not be able to provide sufficient iron to the growing fetus. If the mother's intake of iron is low, the placenta nevertheless continues to provide the fetus with its needed supply. The placenta plays a very important role in regulating the iron transfer from mother to fetus. Fortunately, the absorption of iron from the diet increases as well so that iron supply is sufficient, provided the diet is sufficient too.

Iron Supplementation

In women who are iron deficient, iron supplementation will improve iron status. About 12% of women have anemia before becoming pregnant; in these women, there should be an increased emphasis on ensuring adequate iron intake during pregnancy.

Since many iron supplements are reported to irritate the stomach, it would be prudent to attempt to increase dietary iron intake. Foods high in iron include beef, pork, chicken and tofu. Tofu or any other vegetable (non-meat or non-animal) sources of iron should be taken with foods high in vitamin C to enhance its absorption.

 What is pica?

Pica is defined as the intake of non-food items. During pregnancy, pica may be associated with anemia or iron deficiency, although the items may contain no iron. Women may have cravings for items that include clay, chalk, coffee grounds, paint chips and plaster. It is definitely recommended to avoid eating these materials because intake may result in intestinal blockage or severe illness. Intake of paint, for example, may result in lead poisoning.

Gestational Diabetes

Gestational diabetes is a complication in pregnancy that occurs in about 2% to 5% of women. The cause of elevated blood sugar in gestational diabetes is not due to the lack of insulin secretion, as in Type 1 diabetes, but to insulin resistance. Insulin resistance is mediated by the hormones produced by the placenta. This means that the insulin is secreted in response to increasing amounts of sugar, or glucose, in the blood, but the insulin cannot perform its normal function of allowing glucose to enter cells because insulin cannot get into the cell (known as insulin resistance) to perform this function.

Risk Factors for Gestational Diabetes

- Overweight or obese before pregnancy
- Advanced maternal age
- Birth weight of an infant from previous pregnancy more than 9 lbs
- Gestational diabetes in a previous pregnancy
- Multiple gestation
- African or Hispanic ancestry
- Recurrent infections

Blood glucose levels measured in week 24 to week 28 week of gestation should be used to define gestational diabetes. However, women with multiple risk factors are tested in the first trimester and again in the second and third trimester, even if the first test was negative. An oral glucose tolerance test (OGTT) is performed. Blood is taken and then you are asked to drink a sweetened beverage with a specific amount of sugar. About 1 to 2 hours after drinking the beverage, another sample of blood is taken. These levels are then compared to normal ranges to determine the diagnosis.

Symptoms of Gestational Diabetes

- Increased thirst and urination
- Fatigue
- Weight loss despite increased appetite
- Blurred vision
- Nausea and vomiting
- Frequent infections (bladder, vagina and skin)

Some of these symptoms (fatigue, nausea and vomiting, increased urination) are usual symptoms of pregnancy, so women should seek the advice of their physician if they are concerned about gestational diabetes. Many women have no symptoms, so it is important to test for gestational diabetes routinely during a pregnancy.

Did You Know ...

Ketosis

If energy intake is restricted too much, then the body will use fat for energy, resulting in ketosis (end products of fat metabolism), which can be harmful to the fetus. Studies have shown that sensible calorie restriction in obese women has decreased the incidence of high-birth-weight infants.

Did You Know ...

At Risk

Women with gestational diabetes have a greater chance of developing it again in future pregnancies and developing Type 2 diabetes later in life.

Prevention and Treatment

Often, preventative measures, such as attention to diet, exercise and weight loss, can help improve the symptoms and keep blood sugar levels under control. Insulin is not necessarily needed with gestational diabetes. It may be used if reduction in blood sugar levels does not reach recommended levels within 2 weeks of lifestyle changes.

Dietary

Dietary measures include restricting daily energy intake, with the assistance of a registered dietitian, for those who are overweight or obese. The energy distribution that is often recommended includes 45% to 65% from carbohydrates (spread over three meals and three snacks), 20% to 35% from fat and 10% to 35% from protein. With a lower percentage of energy from carbohydrates, there is less hyperglycemia, or elevated blood sugar levels.

The amount of calorie restriction in overweight or obese women is based on individual needs and should be done with caution.

Exercise

Exercise or physical activity may also decrease insulin resistance and may help improve blood glucose levels in women with gestational diabetes. The health state of the mother should be considered before any exercise routines are started, and these should be discussed with the physician. Excessive exercise should be avoided.

Medical Monitoring

Some studies suggest that women with a BMI over 25 or those with impaired glucose tolerance (higher than normal blood sugars following a glucose challenge drink but not in the diabetic range) are more likely to develop diabetes later on in life. Following pregnancy, women with gestational diabetes should be encouraged to adopt a healthy lifestyle that includes daily exercise, following the USDA MyPyramid food guide or Canada's Food Guide to Healthy Eating. Women who have had gestational diabetes should be screened regularly for diabetes within 6 months of giving birth.

Heartburn

At some point during pregnancy, it is estimated that 30% to 50% of women will experience heartburn. Although most common in the third trimester, some women experience heartburn throughout their pregnancy. Some women find heartburn to be a minor nuisance, but for others, it becomes a major complaint throughout pregnancy.

As the uterus expands during pregnancy, it presses up on your stomach, forcing stomach contents and gastric acid up into the lower esophagus. This is made worse by hormones that help relax the valve that keeps the esophagus and stomach separated, making it easier for acid to move up into the food pipe.

Tips for Managing Heartburn

Heartburn is most common after meals, so some simple dietary and lifestyle strategies may help reduce side effects during pregnancy.

- Eat small, frequent meals to reduce the amount of food in your stomach. Try to limit fatty foods because fat can slow the transit time of food out of the stomach, which can exacerbate the problem because the esophageal sphincter is already relaxed from pregnancy hormones.
- Eat slowly and chew your food well.
- Drink fluids between meals when possible to limit how full you become at mealtimes.
- Avoid spicy, greasy foods and foods that contain caffeine because these foods are known to irritate heartburn.
- Try to sit upright and not lie down for at least 1 hour after meals. This prevents food from slipping back up the food pipe and allows more time for food to pass from your stomach into the small intestine.
- When it is time to lay down, raise the head of your bed with extra pillows.
- Avoid eating or drinking anything other than water before going to bed.
- Wear loose-fitting clothing that does not constrict or add additional pressure on your stomach.
- Try to avoid stress whenever possible.
- Talk to your doctor if heartburn becomes problematic or begins to interfere with your dietary intake.

(**Source:** Nutrition for a Healthy Pregnancy, Nutritional Guidelines for the Childbearing Years, Health Canada, Oct., 2002. Reprinted with the permission of the Minister of Public Works and Government Services Canada, 2005.)

Be sure to speak with your doctor before starting any over-the-counter medications to help with your heartburn. Your doctor may recommend safe antacids and be able to prescribe something if heartburn is severe or interfering with your nutritional intake.

Constipation

Constipation is another common complaint during pregnancy. It is estimated that somewhere between 11% and 38% of all pregnant women experience problems with constipation at some point during pregnancy. This may also be true for women who never experienced any problems with constipation before becoming pregnant.

During pregnancy, constipation may be caused by hormone changes that relax the digestive tract and slow gastric motility. This slowed motility increases the amount of time that food spends in the digestive system, particularly in the colon. The longer digested food spends in the colon, the more water is absorbed from the stool (and back into the body), making it dryer and harder and more difficult to pass.

The growing uterus also puts additional pressure on the bowels, making stool harder to pass, and finally, lifestyle habits, such as bed rest, inadequate physical activity and iron supplements that prevent anemia, can all contribute to constipation. Iron supplements may also cause your stool to change color, turning it black. It is important to note that the iron in foods does not cause constipation.

Tips for Managing Constipation

Simple dietary and lifestyle changes can help to manage the constipation experienced during pregnancy.

- Try to take in about 12 cups (3 L) of fluid every day. This includes water, milk, soups and fruit juices (and water found in fruit and vegetables). Drinking lots of fluid may help to keep stool soft and easy to pass. Caffeine-free warm or hot liquids may also help to stimulate the bowels.

- Exercise. If you're not already regularly exercising, try to make small changes, such as going for a walk on your lunch break or taking the dog for a stroll around the block. You do not need to be running a marathon to take advantage of the benefits of physical activity. Exercise helps to keep your bowels moving and your stool pattern regular.

- Increase your fiber intake. Aim for between 25 and 35 grams of fiber daily. Fiber helps increase stool bulk and keeps food moving through the gastrointestinal tract. Fruits, vegetables, lentils and whole grains are all great sources of dietary fiber.

- Speak with your physician if constipation becomes problematic. Your doctor may be able to prescribe a stool softener or bulk-forming agent to help. You should not take an over-the-counter medication or laxative while pregnant before speaking with your doctor because some of these medications may not be safe to take.

Tips for Managing Hemorrhoids

PREVENTION

The best way to treat hemorrhoids is to prevent constipation:

- Consume adequate fluid, including milk, water, soup and fruit juices. Aim to get about 12 cups (3 L) of fluid every day.
- Get adequate fiber in your diet. Eat lots of whole grains, fruits and vegetables.
- Exercise. Even moderate amounts of activity, like walking, can help.

TREATMENT

If hemorrhoids are already a problem for you, try these remedies:

- Continue to try to eliminate constipation.
- Try getting enough rest to relieve the pressure on the lower intestines during the latter part of your pregnancy.
- Speak with your doctor, who may be able to suggest an ointment to help shrink hemorrhoids and relieve the pain and itching they cause.

Hemorrhoids

Hemorrhoids are varicose veins (enlarged veins) in the rectum that occasionally protrude through the anal sphincter. They are a common complaint during pregnancy, especially toward the end, when the additional pressure from the growing baby and uterus put stress on the veins in the rectum.

Hemorrhoids are extremely uncomfortable and may itch and burn. If you strain to have a bowel movement because stool is hard and difficult to pass, you may cause hemorrhoids to become worse. They may push out around the anal opening, and there may also be bright red blood associated with hemorrhoids.

Exercise during Mid-Pregnancy

If you have been feeling poorly because of nausea and vomiting, you will likely begin to feel better during mid-pregnancy and may be ready to resume or start an exercise program, if this isn't already part of your daily routine. Symptoms of fatigue may also be decreased by this time.

Did You Know ...

Safe Exercise Levels

The executive and council of Obstetricians and Gynaecologists of Canada recommends 15 minutes, three times a week, of continuous exercise, working up to 30 minutes about four times a week. These exercise levels have been reported to be safe to the mother and fetus. Nevertheless, you should seek advice from your physician to determine safe levels of exercise during your individual pregnancy, especially if you plan to exercise at higher levels of activity or for athletic training. Referral to a physiotherapist or exercise physiologist may be recommended.

Exercise Cautions

- Maintaining your balance becomes an issue at this stage of pregnancy, so any activity that causes loss of balance, such as bicycling or downhill skiing, should be avoided or done with caution.

- Stretching and yoga exercises have not been properly studied in pregnant women; however, they do not necessarily have to be discouraged.

- Scuba diving is contraindicated at any stage of pregnancy.

- After 16 weeks of pregnancy, exercises that involve the supine position (lying on your back) may have to be avoided because the pressure of the fetus on the vena cava (a large vein in the back of the uterus) may cause symptoms of hypotension (low blood pressure).

- Chest pain, increased shortness of breath, painful uterine contractions and other discomfiting symptoms should be reported to your doctor.

Dental Health

Nutritional intake during pregnancy affects fetal tooth development. Fetal teeth develop between month 3 and month 6, so it is important to have a sufficient intake of many nutrients at this stage, especially protein, calcium, phosphorous and vitamins A, C and D — all of which play a role in healthy tooth formation.

Mothers also need to take care of their dental health during pregnancy because increasing hormone levels may increase the susceptibility to gingivitis. Studies have shown that women with severe gum disease may be at risk for preterm labor, yet another reason to maintain good oral hygiene during pregnancy.

Dental Conditions

Gingivitis

Gingivitis is a common problem during pregnancy. Rising levels of the hormone progesterone during pregnancy cause increased blood flow to the gums and may cause gums to become red, tender or puffy. Gums may also have a tendency to bleed when you brush your teeth. This sensitivity is an exaggerated response to plaque caused by high progesterone levels.

Pregnancy Tumors

Occasionally, gums that are sensitive due to gingivitis may develop an overgrowth of tissue called pregnancy tumors.

These are small growths usually found between teeth and may be related to excess plaque. Pregnancy tumors tend to bleed easily and have a raw-looking surface. These growths usually resolve on their own without dental intervention. If the tumor causes difficulty swallowing or speaking, you should see your dentist for an evaluation. Sometimes these tumors must be surgically removed after the baby is born.

Tips for Dental Health

SNACK FOOD CHOICES

Many pregnant women tend to snack between meals. This helps ensure adequate intake of nutrients over the course of the day and helps reduce the feelings of morning sickness. However, choose your snacks wisely. Sometimes food cravings or the idea that we are "eating for two" cause us to overindulge in foods that are not necessarily good for our teeth. Snacks that are high in sugars and carbohydrates may encourage tooth decay. Choose snacks that are good for maternal and fetal teeth:

- Raw carrot and celery sticks with a low-fat sour cream dip
- Fresh fruit slices
- Low-fat yogurt

ORAL HYGIENE

Follow these guidelines to maintain good oral hygiene during pregnancy:

- Brush teeth after each meal, at least three times a day, with a toothpaste containing fluoride. If brushing your teeth triggers morning sickness, try brushing after eating, when your stomach is more settled. If brushing causes severe nausea, a fluoride mouthwash may help instead of brushing; however, this should not be a substitute for regular brushing and flossing. Sometimes even a change in the flavor of toothpaste may help.
- Floss daily.
- See your dentist regularly. This will help reduce the plaque levels that contribute to gingivitis during pregnancy.

 Is calcium leached from the mother's teeth during pregnancy?

This is a myth. Contrary to popular belief, calcium is not leached from a mother's teeth while pregnant or nursing. The calcium the fetus needs is provided through the mother's diet and not by her teeth. When calcium intake is deficient, your body will provide calcium from stores in your bones, not your teeth. Calcium-rich foods are primarily found in dairy products, so drink your milk and help your little one grow strong bones and teeth.

CHAPTER 6

Late Pregnancy Nutrition (Third Trimester)

THE THIRD TRIMESTER lasts from week 26 until term, which is usually around 40 weeks of gestation. This is the time of your pregnancy when the fetus puts on most of its weight, storing fat and appearing more rounded. In the last month of your pregnancy, between week 36 and week 40, the fetus will gain about $\frac{1}{2}$ lb (250 g) each week, so you can see that each week a baby remains in utero can make a significant difference in the eventual birth weight of your newborn. Close to term, the head should be facing down and the fetus will keep its arms and legs tucked in close to his body. As you near your due date, there is less and less room in the uterus for baby to move around, but you should still continue to feel active movement every day.

During the third trimester, many women feel more energetic and generally excited about the prospect of giving birth. However, many may also experience leg cramps and swelling of the legs, ankles and feet. You need to be especially cautious about your blood pressure because gestational hypertension (pre-eclampsia) can be a problem at this stage in your pregnancy. Your nutrition needs are similar to the second trimester — an extra 300 calories a day beyond pre-pregnancy needs and adequate iron (27 mg per day), calcium (1,000 mg per day) and folic acid (600 mcg per day). During the third trimester, the fetus begins to store iron.

Leg Cramps

Pregnant women sometimes experience leg cramps or muscle contractions in their feet and calves. These cramps often occur in the middle of the night and can be extremely painful. Leg cramps may be caused by calcium deficiency. Adequate calcium intake, along with a warm bath before bed and stretching out calf muscles, may help to avoid these leg cramps. If a leg cramp does happen during the night, try stretching out calf muscles by lifting your toes toward the sky and massaging the affected calf muscle. Walking around to stretch out the muscle and improve circulation to the area may also help.

Third Trimester Growth and Development

- At week 26, the fetus weighs about 1½ to 2 lbs (700 to 900 g) and by week 36 about 5½ lbs (2,500 g). By the time the baby is due to be born at 40 weeks, the baby weighs between 6½ and 9 pounds (3,000 and 4,000 g).

- By week 28, the brain forms its characteristic bumps and grooves. The amount of brain tissue continues to develop throughout the third trimester.

- If you are expecting a boy, the testes will now descend from the abdomen into the scrotum.

- The hair on the head continues to grow, and the fingernails reach the fingertips.

- By week 36, the lungs are actively producing surfactant, a chemical needed by the lungs to prevent respiratory distress syndrome and for the baby to breathe on its own.

- By week 39, the large intestine is filled with dark green, sticky meconium that the baby will pass as its first stool. The fine, downy lanugo hair and white vernix have virtually disappeared as your baby prepares for the birth process.

Swelling of Legs, Ankles and Feet

Sometime during the second trimester, many women complain about swelling in their ankles and feet. Swelling (edema) tends to get worse over the course of the day and then dissipates by morning, only to start all over again. This swelling happens because your body retains extra fluid during pregnancy. A pregnant woman's blood volume increases by 40% over the course of her pregnancy. Progesterone also encourages fluid retention, and the growing uterus puts additional pressure on the veins that carry blood back to the heart from the lower portion of your body.

The extra fluid pools in your feet, ankles and calves. This condition can worsen in warm weather or in women who spend much of the day on their feet. There should not be any pain associated with this type of swelling.

Did You Know ...

Pre-eclampsia

A small amount of swelling in your ankles and feet is normal and common. However, swelling of the hands and face may indicate a more serious condition, known as gestational hypertension.

Tips for Reducing Leg Swelling

To help reduce the swelling in your legs, ankles and feet try these strategies:

- Get adequate exercise involving your legs.
- Try not to cross your legs.
- Sit with your feet up.
- Try lying down with your feet on some pillows. Feet should be raised above the level of your heart as much as possible to encourage blood return to the heart.
- Do not stand for long periods of time.
- Wear support hose.
- Avoiding socks with tight elastics around the top.
- Increase fluid intake because dehydration can sometimes make fluid retention worse.
- Limit, but don't eliminate, salt intake.

Did You Know ...

High Blood Pressure Risks

Gestational hypertension, or pre-eclampsia, is one of the leading causes of death in pregnant women and a major morbidity factor for the mother and the fetus. It is estimated that about 7% of expectant mothers will develop pre-eclampsia.

Gestational Hypertension

Gestational hypertension, also known as toxemia or pre-eclampsia, most commonly occurs in the third trimester but can happen at any time. Gestational hypertension is different from the high blood pressure that occurs when a woman is not pregnant. You are considered to have high blood pressure when your blood pressure is greater than 140/90 mmHg. Normal blood pressure levels should be less than 120 mmHg for the top number (systolic pressure) and less than 80 mmHg for the bottom number (diastolic pressure).

If gestational hypertension becomes severe, problems can arise in the mother's kidneys, liver and brain. Pre-eclampsia can then lead to eclampsia, where a woman may suffer seizures because of changes in the brain. Left untreated, severe gestational hypertension can lead to death.

Risk Factors for Gestational Hypertension

- First-time mothers
- Previous high blood pressure before pregnancy
- Multiple gestation (expecting twins or triplets)
- Family history of pre-eclampsia
- Having diabetes or other diseases that may affect kidney function
- Age (younger than 18 or older than 35 years)

Signs of Gestational Hypertension (Pre-eclampsia)

If you have any of these symptoms, be sure to see your doctor right away.

- Pain in upper right part of abdomen
- Constant severe or changing headaches
- Spots in front of your eyes
- Blurred vision
- Unusual swelling, especially around the face
- Weight gain that is sudden and more than 1 lb (250 g) per day
- High blood pressure, greater than 140/90
- Generalized edema or swelling of the hands, face, feet and ankles
- Protein in your urine

(**Source:** *Healthy beginnings: Your handbook for pregnancy and birth.* 2nd edition. Reproduced by permission of the Society of Obstetricians and Gynaecologists of Canada.)

During pregnancy, high blood pressure can also cause extra protein to spill into your urine. This is why your doctor has you test a sample of your urine on a stick when you visit her. She is checking to see if there is protein or sugar in your urine.

Because gestational hypertension causes the blood vessels to constrict, it can reduce the blood supply to the placenta, which, in turn, can lead to a reduction in the blood supply to the fetus. This reduction of blood supply can limit fetal growth.

Fortunately, that happens very rarely in North America because of the superb prenatal care that most pregnant women receive. However, when gestational hypertension cannot be controlled, the baby may have to be delivered prematurely. Early delivery may be the only way to decrease blood pressure when other methods, such as bed rest and medication, have failed.

 ## Is pre-eclampsia caused by being overweight?

Current literature does not suggest a link between excessive weight gain or obesity and the development of pre-eclampsia. In fact, pre-eclampsia often occurs in women who are underweight at conception or who fail to gain adequate weight early in their pregnancy.

Studies have shown that women who have routine exercise plan during pregnancy may experience less difficulty during childbirth and have a quicker recovery period than more sedentary women. This is likely explained by the increase in muscle tone and conditioning. Although the physical size of the fetus and its weight may make it more difficult to perform previously tolerated exercises, most women can modify their exercise routines and are able to continue with them during the last trimester of pregnancy.

Management of Gestational Hypertension

The goal when a pregnant woman's blood pressure is elevated is to keep the fetus inside the uterus for as long as possible. This can happen as long as there is no significant maternal or fetal risk.

When pregnancy-induced hypertension is mild, treatment is primarily activity restriction. This usually brings down blood pressure when it is only slightly elevated. Mothers used to be asked to restrict their weight gain to manage high blood pressure. This is now thought to be unwise and risky for the health of the baby.

When gestational hypertension is severe, a mother may be hospitalized and given medication in addition to bed rest to help lower her blood pressure. If medications still cannot control blood pressure, then, as a last resort, the baby may have to be delivered, sometimes earlier than desired.

Declining Energy Levels

As your pregnancy draws to an end and the birth of your baby nears, you may have extra energy or you may notice some of the fatigue you experienced in your first trimester returning. Your expanding belly and the general demands of pregnancy may cause you to feel more tired and to move slower than you did earlier in your pregnancy. You may also be sleeping less well during the night because of general discomfort and frequent trips to the bathroom.

Although there is nothing you can do nutritionally to help battle the fatigue you may be experiencing, eating a well-balanced diet will help you feel better and provide the energy you need to get through your remaining days. Rest when you can, and appreciate the sleep you are able to get now, because in the first few weeks after your baby is born, sleep is a precious commodity.

Can stretch marks be prevented?

Stretch marks are reddish-colored marks that happen when the skin is stretched beyond its natural limits. They are most common on the breasts, thighs and stomach of pregnant women. Although they usually fade over time, stretch marks rarely disappear completely. Unfortunately, stretch marks are just a reality for some women. Many women like to use vitamin E, cocoa butter or lanolin oils. Two studies recently suggested that certain creams containing vitamin E may help reduce the appearance of stretch marks. These creams are not harmful to your unborn baby, and can be used to help the itchy, dry skin that is sometimes associated with being pregnant. They will not, however, necessarily prevent the development of stretch marks.

CHAPTER 7

Post-Partum Nutrition and Breastfeeding

DECIDING TO BREASTFEED your baby is a significant nutritional decision you will need to make during your pregnancy. Ideally, you will have become well informed about the benefits of breastfeeding before pregnancy. Most health-care providers recommend breast milk rather than "formula," not only because breast milk is highly nutritious, but also because it offers immunity from many childhood diseases. Women's bodies are well prepared to provide breast milk for their babies.

Many nutrient requirements are higher during lactation than they were during pregnancy. A well-balanced diet is particularly important after the birth of your baby to support the needs of breastfeeding — and to help get your body back to its pre-pregnant size. Good nutrition will also help you to combat fatigue and promote general well-being.

In this book, we have provided over 150 recipes to help you prepare nutritious meals. Many of these can be made ahead and frozen during pregnancy to provide healthy and ready-to-go meals in minutes for the first few months after your baby is born, when healthy nutrition may be the last thing on your mind.

Breastfeeding

Lactation

Understanding the basic physiology of lactation provides a foundation for breastfeeding successfully.

Hormone Actions

Lactation (breast milk production) is under hormonal control. Once the levels of the hormone progesterone drop off after delivery, breast milk production is encouraged. After delivery, another hormone, prolactin, is secreted to stimulate the production of the milk. Prolactin ensures synthesis of milk. If breast milk release is not stimulated through feeding or through removal of breast milk by pumping, then prolactin levels will drop and reach non-pregnant levels by 7 days after birth.

Oxytocin, another hormone, plays a role in the release of the milk from the breast, which is commonly known as "letdown." Oxytocin also causes the uterus to contract. Women in the first few days post-partum may feel these contractions or cramping during breastfeeding. The contraction of the uterus means that its size is decreasing, allowing the abdomen to return to its more normal pre-pregnancy size.

Mature human milk is produced about 50 to 59 hours after birth (ranging from 38 to 98 hours after birth). As breastfeeding becomes established, the amount of minerals, vitamins and other nutrients reaches a steady amount by about 3 weeks after birth.

Colostrum Production

The breast glands produce water, amino acids (small parts of proteins), fats, vitamins, lactose (sugar), minerals and other substances that they take from the mother's blood to produce milk. In the first few days of lactation, milk is referred to as colostrum. Thick and sticky, colostrum can be clear to yellow-orange in color. It is rich in protein and minerals and lower in carbohydrate, fat and some vitamins than mature milk (which is white in color). Colostrum is also rich in immunoglobulins that protect the infant from many different types of infections. These immunoglobulins work mainly in the intestine, protecting the infant from bacterial infections. The newborn has a relatively immature immune system; this early breast milk provides added protection.

Nutrient Composition of Breast Milk

Human breast milk provides all of the energy and nutrients that a full-term infant requires for normal growth and development. Preterm infants may need extra minerals and vitamins.

Ninety percent of mature breast milk is water, which is essential for the hydration of the infant. Breast milk is composed of macronutrients — carbohydrates (lactose),

Did You Know …

Vitamin D Supplements

In the United States, the American Pediatric Society recommends that all breastfed infants receive 200 IU of vitamin D every day. The Dietitians of Canada, the Canadian Pediatric Society and Health Canada all suggest that breastfed infants receive 400 IU per day of vitamin D. Breastfed babies living in northern Canadian communities should receive 800 IU per day. Parents can purchase a vitamin D supplement appropriate for newborn infants at any local pharmacy.

Did You Know …

Breast Milk Production

Studies show that about 500 mL per day of breast milk is produced 3 to 4 days after delivery, going up to about 800 mL per day (with a wide range of 550 mL to 1.2 L per day).

proteins and fats — as well as micronutrients — vitamins, minerals, hormones and enzymes. Its caloric content is about 68 calories for every 3 oz (100 mL).

Carbohydrates

Lactose is the main carbohydrate found in human milk. Lactose is a disaccharide, a sugar made up of two sugar molecules. Lactose helps to increase calcium and iron absorption. It provides a large amount of energy to the rapidly growing brain of the infant. Infants have the ability to digest lactose into monosaccharides — galactose and glucose. It is very rare for infants to have a lactase deficiency. Lactase is the enzyme found in the small intestine that breaks down the lactose into galactose and glucose.

Proteins

The high-quality protein found in breast milk meets all of the infant's needs for growth. Casein and whey are among the many proteins in breast milk. Breast milk contains more whey than formulas do. Whey is easier to digest, while casein requires more energy for digestion. As milk matures, there is a higher proportion of whey to casein. Other components of the proteins are amino acids and nucleotides. These are important for many metabolic functions.

Fats

Fat makes up about one-half of the calories of breast milk. Breast milk provides the essential fatty acids, including docosahexaenoic acid (DHA) and arachidonic acid (AA), which were also important for brain and retina (visual) development in the fetus. The total fat of the mother's diet does not affect the amount of fat in breast milk, but the type of fat consumed in the mother's diet will affect the type of fat in breast milk. Limit dietary intake of trans fats and increase intake of omega 3 fats. The fat component of milk is higher in the hindmilk, the milk produced as the breast is emptied.

 Doesn't breast milk have higher levels of cholesterol than formula?

Yes, there is a greater proportion of cholesterol in breast milk than there is in formula. However, studies suggest this early exposure to cholesterol in breast milk may have a protective effect against coronary heart disease later in life.

Foremilk vs. Hindmilk

If a baby receives only the initial milk, or the foremilk, of a feeding and then is put on the other breast for more foremilk, the baby may not be receiving enough of the richer, fatty hindmilk. Foremilk is high in sugar, or carbohydrate, while the hindmilk, or end part of the feeding, is rich in fat. Switching breasts during breastfeeding before the first one is emptied may cause a baby to have increased gas and looser, usually green and watery stools because of the higher sugar load.

It is important to ensure that the hindmilk is received by the infant. Gently compressing or squeezing the breast during the feed will empty the breast and release more of the hindmilk, ensuring a good mix of foremilk and hindmilk. This may help decrease the gas and eliminate looser or watery stools caused by the high carbohydrate load of the foremilk. When the baby still appears hungry but is no longer swallowing on the first breast, offer the second breast.

Vitamins

Breast milk contains both fat-soluble vitamins (A, D, E and K) and water-soluble vitamins (Bs and C). While the fat-soluble vitamins are not really affected by the mother's diet, the water-soluble vitamins are.

For mothers who consume a well-balanced diet, the supplementation of vitamins for exclusively breastfed infants up to 6 months of age is not required, with the exception of vitamin D. Breast milk usually does not contain enough vitamin D to prevent deficiency, possibly due to health warnings to decrease exposure to the sun and to the increased use of sunscreens by the mother. Vitamin D is a fat-soluble vitamin, produced by the body in the presence of adequate sunlight. It is important for the development of healthy bones and teeth. Inadequate vitamin D intakes may result in rickets. In northern latitudes, most infants will not receive adequate sunlight to make sufficient vitamin D. Therefore, all exclusively breastfed infants less than 6 months of age should receive a vitamin D supplement until an adequate dietary source of vitamin D is introduced.

Vitamin K is found in small but adequate amounts in breast milk. In the newborn, vitamin K is usually given at birth, by needle, to prevent hemorrhage, or uncontrolled bleeding. Bacteria in the intestine are not yet present in the newborn, and this becomes an important source of vitamin K as the infant grows.

Did You Know ...

Calorie Requirements

Calorie requirements during lactation are about 200 to 500 calories per day higher than they were during pre-pregnancy. This means that an average woman needs between 2,200 and 2,900 calories daily. Incorporating 200 to 500 calories into your diet is easy. Listen to your body. Eat when you feel hungry and drink when you feel thirsty. Fluid needs are increased as well. While breastfeeding, include 15 cups (3.8 L) of fluid in your diet every day, including milk, water, soup and fruit juice.

Minerals

Breast milk provides all of the minerals required by the infant for normal growth and development. These include sodium, calcium, iron, zinc and magnesium, among others. Although the content of iron is low in breast milk, it is easily absorbed. The diet of the mother has little influence on the mineral content of breast milk, as maternal body stores regulate the amount of minerals in human breast milk.

General Guidelines for Breastfeeding

In the first few days and weeks after your baby is born, you may have many questions about breastfeeding. We have tried to provide some general guidelines for breastfeeding and answers to some of the more common questions you may have. If you feel you need additional breastfeeding support, contact your hospital or local public health office. They will be able to provide you with information about how to find qualified lactation support in your neighborhood.

1. **Make sure your baby is getting a good latch:** This is priority number one in the first few days after birth. Breastfeeding can be initially stressful for a mother who has never breastfed before. It is a new skill that neither you nor your baby has done before, and it can take some time to master. Learning your baby's feeding cues and making sure the baby latches properly are important to decrease some of the initial discomfort. Be patient and ask for help if you need it. Some of the breastfeeding issues that we discuss later in this chapter hinge on having a good latch.

   Make sure that your baby opens his mouth wide before putting him to the breast and that most of your areola (at least 1½ inches and not just the nipple) is in your baby's mouth while feeding. Both lips should be rolled out.

   Mothers may find it difficult to determine if the baby has a good latch on their own, so you might consider asking a breastfeeding professional to check your baby's latch before you leave the hospital.

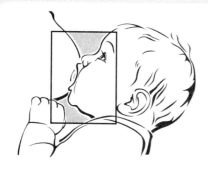

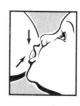

| mouth opening | pause (mouth wide) | mouth closing |

Most breastfed infants have sufficient iron stores for the first 6 months of life. After this time, introduction of an iron-containing food is recommended to supplement the breast milk because the iron stores of the infant become depleted by this time. Iron is required for this rapid period of growth. Both lactose and vitamin C help with the absorption of iron.

2. **Feed your baby often:** A newborn infant should feed on demand, at least 8 times in a 24-hour period. It is common for babies to feed 10 to 12 times a day. Look for your baby to give you cues that she is hungry, like moving her lips or putting her hands in her mouth. Crying is a late indicator that your baby is hungry. A newborn's stomach is very small and cannot handle a large volume of fluid. She will require frequent feeds. Breast milk is also more easily digested than formula, so breastfed babies will feel full for a shorter period of time and will feed more often.

3. **Offer and keep your baby on one breast until your baby has come off the breast on his own:** This will ensure that your baby receives the calorie-dense, fatty hindmilk every feed. If he indicates that he is still hungry for more milk, you can then offer your other breast.

4. **Don't watch the clock:** This is a mistake that many new mothers make, thinking there hasn't been enough time between feeds. "Little Johnny can't be hungry again, I just fed him 2 hours ago." Use your baby as the indicator for hunger and not the clock. Breastfed babies can feed often during the course of the day, especially in the early evening. Your baby may be telling you that she is hungry by crying or being fussy, munching on her hands or fingers or opening her mouth wide as you gently touch her cheek. Frequent evening feedings begin to prepare an infant to sleep through the night.

5. **Avoid the use of artificial nipples, pacifiers, infant formula, water or glucose feeds in the first 2 to 4 weeks of life:** Your baby is learning to breastfeed, which can take some time. Using pacifiers or bottle nipples can make it more difficult for your newborn to learn to breastfeed. The exception to this rule is premature infants, who may benefit from sucking on a pacifier or artificial nipple when they are not able to take feeds by mouth.

6. **Learn ways to recognize if your baby is getting enough milk:** This includes listening for swallows and counting the number of stools and wet diapers your baby makes in a day. In a 24-hour period, you can expect six to eight wet diapers and two or more yellow seedy stools during the first 6 weeks of life. After this, the stool pattern may change.

Benefits of Breastfeeding

Without a doubt, breastfeeding is the best form of nutrition for a newborn baby. Breast milk is nature's perfect food. It is designed to meet 100% of a healthy infant's nutritional requirements, with the exception of vitamin D, until a baby is 6 months old.

Nevertheless, some mothers choose not to breastfeed at all, and although we encourage breastfeeding as an optimal source of nutrition, a mother's decision not to breastfeed needs to be respected. For women who choose not to breastfeed, formula feeding is an adequate alternative. There are many different formulas available on the market, and all are subject to strict regulations, so any choice of formula will be nutritionally balanced, though not as well as balanced as breast milk. A cow's milk–based formula is usually recommended as the first choice for mothers who choose not to breastfeed their infant.

FOR BABY

1. **Enhanced immunity:** Breast milk provides immunities, including enzymes, immunoglobulins and leukocytes (white blood cells), which help infants fight infection. The longer a baby breastfeeds, the greater the protective effect against illness. Studies have shown that exclusively breastfed babies have lower rates of many illnesses, including:

   - Diarrhea (gastroenteritis): Many studies have demonstrated that breastfeeding helps prevent diarrheal disease. Breastfeeding helps to reduce the rates of diarrhea by providing protective factors, as well as decreasing the exposure to other foods or water that may have been contaminated with disease-causing pathogens.

   - Ear infections (otitis media): Many studies have demonstrated that breastfeeding helps to prevent ear infections. The exact reason for this preventive effect is not known, but it is thought that immunologic factors, feeding position and lack of irritation from cow's milk formula may all play a role.

   - Respiratory illness: There is strong evidence to suggest that breastfeeding offers protection against the development of RSV (respiratory syncytial virus) infection, which is a common and potentially life-threatening infection that infants are particularly susceptible to. The studies on breastfeeding and the prevention of other respiratory illnesses, including childhood asthma, are inconclusive.

   - Allergies and atopic disease: As with respiratory illness, studies on the preventive effect that breastfeeding has on the development of childhood food allergies and eczema are inconclusive. The strongest predictor for the development of food allergies is family history. However, the rates of allergy to cow's milk protein found in formula are significantly higher than allergy to the proteins found in breast milk.

- **Chronic disease prevention:** Studies are beginning to show that breastfeeding offers long-term protection against the development of many chronic diseases, such as diabetes, celiac disease and multiple sclerosis.

- **Childhood cancer:** A study found that children who were never breastfed or who were breastfed on a short-term basis had an increased risk of developing Hodgkin's disease versus children who were breastfed for at least 6 months.

2. **Convenience:** Breastfeeding is very convenient. It is possible to breastfeed anytime, anywhere. Breast milk is always fresh and at the perfect temperature. There is no worrying about where you will heat up a bottle in the shopping mall or at the park.

3. **Cleanliness:** Breast milk does not require preparation or sterilization techniques that are dependent on a clean water supply.

FOR MOTHERS

1. **Uterine involution:** Breastfeeding helps to stimulate the production of the hormone oxytocin, which causes the uterus to contract (uterine involution) and helps the uterus return more quickly to its pre-pregnancy size.

2. **Disease prevention:** Research suggests that breastfeeding can help a woman prevent chronic diseases later in life, including pre-menopausal breast cancer, ovarian cancer and osteoporosis.

3. **Unwanted pregnancies:** The absence of a menstrual period during breastfeeding, called lactational amenorrhea, can also prevent additional unwanted pregnancies in the first 6 months for mothers who are exclusively breastfeeding. Of course, this is not foolproof. If you really do not want to become pregnant again, be sure to discuss with your doctor other methods of contraception.

4. **Bonding between mother and child:** Breastfeeding can provide a wonderful bonding experience between a mother and her newborn child.

5. **Environmental benefits:** Breast milk is delivered without the additional packaging or processing involved in the making of infant formula. The reduction of waste from leftover cans and containers of formula, as well as the reduction of the waste involved in processing infant formula, helps to contribute to the health of our planet.

6. **Economy:** The costs of breastfeeding, including such items as nursing bras and pads, do not come close to the cost of formula. It is estimated that the average cost of infant formula is about $100 to $150 per month. This does not include the cost of bottles, caps and nipples. Specialty allergy formulas can reach as high as $300 to $400 per month.

Hormones

Human growth factors, insulin, prolactin, thyroxine cholecystokinin and cortisol are hormones found in human breast milk. They help to strengthen the intestine of the infant, promote digestion and enhance the immune system.

Enzymes

Lipase and amylase are enzymes found in breast milk. Along with an infant's pancreatic enzymes, they help an infant digest fat and polysaccharides (long-chain carbohydrates).

Protective Factors

There is also a range of other protective factors found in breast milk. Research has shown that these protective factors, along with the immunoglobulins, help to decrease the

 How do I know if my baby is getting enough milk?

Often in the first few days of your child's life, when you are initiating breastfeeding and learning your baby's feeding cues, you may be concerned that your newborn is not getting enough breast milk. It is difficult to know for sure how much an infant is drinking when there is no measurement available for the amount of fluid consumed.

There are four ways to ensure that your baby is getting enough breast milk. First, make sure your baby has a comfortable latch and you hear a rhythmic suck and swallow. Second, count the number of wet diapers each day. Third, count the number of bowel movements each day. Fourth, weight gain is the best indicator that your baby is getting enough breast milk, but this is not always practical and babies don't get weighed every day at home.

Try keeping a list of your baby's feedings and wet diapers and stools for the first week of life, when dehydration can happen quickly and your level of exhaustion can make it difficult to keep everything straight.

1. **Latch and suck:** Your baby's mouth should be wide open and the lips should be turned out while your baby is sucking at the breast. Most of your areola should be in the baby's mouth. Your baby is sucking well if, after a period of rapid sucks to send the message to the breast to release the milk, the sucks become longer and deeper, with audible swallowing. A mother's milk comes out in waves called letdowns, and the baby will alternate between faster sucking and slower rhythmic sucks as more milk becomes available. It is normal for a baby to suck properly and then nibble. Nibbling happens when pauses are short, steady and even. There is no swallowing heard when a baby is nibbling at the breast. When a baby nibbles, she is not getting enough milk from the breast. You can express some breast milk during a feed to help encourage your baby to swallow.

incidence of otitis media (ear infections), bacterial infections, gastroenteritis and respiratory illness in breastfed infants.

Maternal Nutrient Requirements

Many maternal nutrient requirements are higher during lactation than they were even during pregnancy. Increased energy is required to support a mother's nutritional needs in the post-partum period and to support breast milk production, which, in turn, promotes the optimum growth and development of your newborn baby.

This increase in caloric requirement must be tempered by the fact that most women want to return to their pre-pregnant size and are trying to lose, not gain, additional weight. Many women are also less active in the weeks and months following

2. **Wet diapers:** In the first 2 to 3 days after birth, there will only be a small amount of urine produced. Urine should be clear in color, but may appear pink. If you do see a pink tinge to the urine, make sure that baby is latching well and that you feed your baby slightly more often, for example, every 2 hours. If this does not increase the number of wet diapers produced, you need to speak with your doctor. Your newborn may require additional breast milk or fluid. By days 4 to 5 of life, a breastfeeding baby should have a minimum of six wet, soaking diapers. The diapers should feel heavy and full. Urine should be clear or pale yellow in color and should have no smell.

3. **Bowel movements:** In the first few days of life, your newborn baby will be passing meconium (baby's first stool). Meconium is dark green or black in color and is sticky like tar. By day 4 or 5 of life, exclusively breastfed babies should have stool that resembles a seedy, yellowy-green liquid or paste. If the baby is not receiving any formula, the stools should have little or no smell. By 4 or 5 days of life, there should be at least two bowel movements each day. If your baby is still passing meconium by day 5 of life, you should speak with your doctor. This may indicate that the baby is not getting enough milk at the breast.

4. **Weight gain:** This is the best way to determine whether or not baby is getting enough milk. Weight gain should be checked often in the first month of life. All babies should visit their doctor 3 days after leaving the hospital and then about once a week until the baby is 1 month old, at which time breastfeeding should be well established. Your baby should regain birth weight by 2 to 3 weeks of age. Weight should be checked on the same scale at each visit because small differences in weight on a scale can have a large significance when talking about the weight of a tiny infant.

the birth of their baby than they were before becoming pregnant and don't have the same means of burning off calories as they did before.

A mother's diet does not have to be perfect to support breastfeeding. In fact, the quality of a mother's diet has only a modest effect on the amount and quality of breast milk produced. It is, however, to a mother's advantage to eat as well as she can while breastfeeding for both her health and her child's health.

 ## Quick Guide to Breastfeeding Sufficiency

Baby's 1st Week	Number of Feeds	Number of Stools	Number of Wet Diapers
Day 1–2	Number of feeds will increase each day. Should feed 8 to 12 times a day	Dark green or black meconium; may only have 1 sticky stool	1 to 3 wet diapers, increasing in fullness each day
Day 3–4	8 to 12 times per day, every 2 to 3 hours	Day 3 stool may still be black. Day 4 stool will be lighter in color (greenish brownish yellow; may have 2 stools)	3 to 4 soaked diapers
Day 5–6	8 to 12 times per day	Minimum of 2 bowel movements per day; will be yellowish in color and seedy in texture	6 or more heavily soaked diapers; will continue to have this many diapers for many months

If my breasts feel full after feedings, does this mean my baby has not eaten enough?

The way your breasts feel is not a good indication of whether or not your baby is feeding well. The firmness of your breasts has nothing to do with the amount of milk you have produced. By day 3 or 4 of your baby's life, your breasts may be very full, tender and swollen. This is your body's response to beginning milk production. The swelling will subside over a few days. After that, your breasts will still feel full before feedings, and this, too, will subside as the weeks go on (unless you miss a feeding). Eventually, your breasts will adapt to making milk and will no longer always feel full before feeds. This does not mean you are making less milk.

Expressing and Freezing Breast Milk

Breast Pumps

Breast pumps have been devised for expressing breast milk. A simple hand-held or battery-operated pump can cost between $40 and $65, while more efficient electric pumps sell for $250 to $350. Some hospitals and pharmacies rent commercial grade electric breast pumps for home use at a nominal cost. Some pumps manufactured by food, bottle or infant formula companies are poorly designed and not recommended for more than occasional use. We suggest using a breast pump made by a company that specializes in breastfeeding equipment. Your birth hospital or public health professional can also help provide you with this information.

Pumping Procedure

1. Before pumping your breast milk, be sure to wash your hands thoroughly with soap and water. Breast milk is relatively free of bacteria, but care must be taken not to contaminate the breast milk with bacteria from your hands or dirty equipment. Breast pump kits should also be washed well with hot soapy water and air-dried between pumpings. Follow the manufacturer's instructions.

2. Pump each breast for 10 to 15 minutes or until milk stops flowing. If you are exclusively feeding your baby pumped breast milk, then pumping should be done as often as you would feed your infant — every 2 to 3 hours for newborns, with longer periods between feedings for older infants.

3. If you are pumping to store some additional breast milk for an occasional feeding, pumping can be done as often as you like. Remember, the more often you pump, the more breast milk you will produce. You can pump both breasts after you breastfeed your baby, or if you breastfeed on one side per feeding, then you can pump the other breast after a feed.

Breastfeeding Positions

There are four common positions to breastfeed your baby. Each position has its own benefits and drawbacks. Some mothers choose to feed in one position only, while other mothers like to use a combination of positions at different feedings. Experiment with positions as you gain experience. Many mothers may also find a breastfeeding pillow helpful. Keep in mind that these are just illustrations, and a lactation consultant or breastfeeding expert should help you with positioning, especially for twins.

1. **Madonna (cradle) position:**
   This position is most commonly associated with breastfeeding and the position most frequently used by experienced mothers. The cradle position can be difficult to master because mothers may feel they have poor control over their newborn's head.

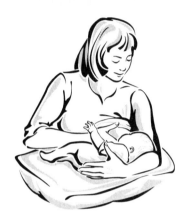

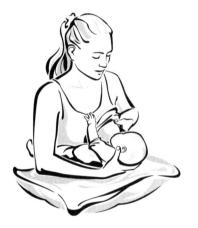

2. **Cross-cradle position:** In this position, mothers feel they have more control of their baby's head. If you are feeding on the left breast, support the breast with your left hand, while your right arm and hand support the baby's head at the breast.

3. **Football (clutch) hold position:**
   In this position, your baby's legs are tucked under your arm on the same side of the body as the feeding breast. This position gives you the best control over your baby's head. It is an excellent choice after a caesarean section (C-section) because no pressure from the weight of the baby is put on the mother's belly. It is also a common choice for mothers who are breastfeeding twins in tandem (or at the same time).

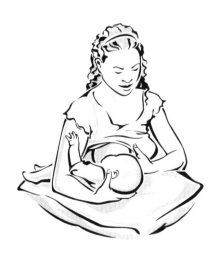

4. **Side-lying position:** This position is done in bed while you are lying down. It allows you to rest while breastfeeding. This position can also be slightly more difficult to master than the football hold.

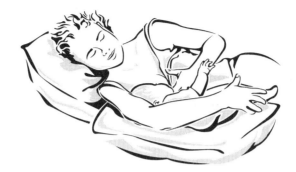

5. **Positions for feeding multiples:** You can breastfeed two babies at one time. It takes a little time and a lot of patience. Breastfeeding two babies at the same time can cut feeding time in half and give a mother a few extra spare minutes in the day. Multiples can be fed in the football position, cradle position or a combination of the two. A lactation consultant will be a helpful resource for any mother who wants to breastfeed twins, triplets or more.

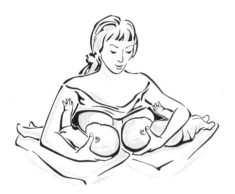

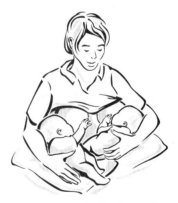

a. Football position

b. Cradle position

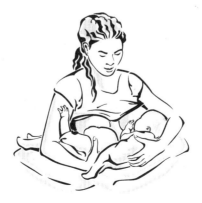

c. Combination position

Storing Expressed Milk

1. Expressed milk can be stored in the refrigerator or freezer in glass or hard plastic bottles or containers. There are also freezer bags made for the storage of breast milk. If using a plastic bottle liner or freezer bag not specifically designed for freezing breast milk, parents will want to double-bag the milk to avoid breakage.

2. Frozen breast milk should be stored in small portions, about 2 to 4 oz (60 to 120 mL) in volume. Smaller portions will defrost quickly and cause less waste if baby doesn't drink all the breast milk that was thawed.

3. Once milk is collected in clean containers, it should be labeled clearly with the date and time of expression so that the baby can consume the milk in the order it was pumped.

4. When freezing breast milk, be sure to leave some space at the top of the storage container because the milk will expand as it freezes.

Defrosting Expressed Breast Milk

1. Defrosting can be done overnight in the refrigerator. It will take approximately 8 to 12 hours for the milk to thaw completely. Frozen milk can also be defrosted by placing it under warm running water or in a dish of warm water. Boiling water should not be used as it can affect the milk's immunologic (infection-fighting) properties. Breast milk should never be heated in a microwave or put back in the freezer after the milk has thawed. Microwaving changes the composition of breast milk and can cause hot spots that can burn a baby's mouth.

2. Once thawed, breast milk should be refrigerated and consumed within 24 hours. Freshly pumped breast milk can be stored for up to 72 hours in the refrigerator and up to 6 months in a deep-freezer if frozen using the proper techniques.

3. Discard any breast milk that the baby does not consume during a feeding.

How do I know if my baby is thriving and growing normally?

Growth and weight gain are the best indicators of whether or not a baby is getting adequate nutrition. Your family physician or pediatrician will monitor the growth of the baby at regular visits in the early months of life to ensure that your baby is growing at an appropriate rate. Growth charts that reflect normal growth of the population are used to plot the height and weight of the baby. Any deviation will be recognized by the physician and assessment of diet intake may then be required.

Breastfeeding Issues

For breastfeeding to be successful, education of the mother before pregnancy, as well as support from health-care workers with breastfeeding expertise, is recommended. Some mothers have no older-generation family members or friends who have breastfed to teach them about normal baby behaviors. With the appropriate support from trained health-care workers, in most cases, issues regarding breastfeeding can be resolved. Nevertheless, complications can arise in breastfeeding that may require medical attention and perhaps supplementing breastfeeding with formula feeding.

Contraindications to Breastfeeding

Rare cases where breastfeeding is not possible or not recommended include infants with an inborn error of metabolism called galactosemia. Breastfeeding is also contraindicated for mothers who are HIV positive or who are using illegal drugs. Infants who are born extremely premature and weigh less than 4.4 lbs (2,000 g) should receive breast milk that is fortified with extra nutrients. Most prescription and over-the-counter drugs are compatible with breastfeeding. Talk to your doctor for a complete list of these medications. The Motherisk program at The Hospital for Sick Children is also an invaluable resource. See the Resources section in this book for contact information.

Poor Breast Milk Supply

A small proportion of women are not able to make enough breast milk for their infant, but the majority of these women are still able to breastfeed. You may need to alter feeding

Did You Know ...
Feeding Frenzy

One of the common reasons for women to discontinue breastfeeding is that they feel they are unable to produce enough milk for the baby to grow. Babies do have "growth spurts." During these times, feeding demand is greater. Women may describe these more frequent feedings as a "feeding frenzy", but this should not be confused with a lack of adequate milk supply. The nutritional needs of babies change as they grow.

patterns and supplement with formula. Speak with a lactation consultant, a professional trained in the art of breastfeeding, for advice.

Factors in Insufficient Milk Supply

- Congenital insufficient breast gland tissue
- Breast reduction
- Post-partum hemorrhage
- Anemia

Tips for Increasing Milk Supply

- Feed your baby often, a minimum of 8 times in a 24-hour period. The more often you empty the breast, the more you will signal your breasts to make more milk.

- Compress your breasts during feeds to help increase milk intake by your baby. Better emptying or removal of milk can help to increase supply. Pumping after feeds can also help to increase breast milk supply.

- Herbal preparations are drugs and should be used with caution. Many herbs have unknown purity, making dosage levels difficult to gauge. Speak with your doctor or lactation consultant before starting any herbal therapy while breastfeeding.

- Consult with your doctor about using prescription drugs, such as metoclopramide (used in the United States) and domperidone (used primarily in Canada), which have also been shown to increase milk supply. Drugs and herbal preparations should only be used when other factors contributing to poor milk supply have been evaluated and ruled out. Milk supply is usually established by day 7.

- If you are taking estrogen-containing birth control pills, this may also decrease your milk supply. Breastfeeding mothers should be switched to a birth control pill with a low level of estrogen or use another form of contraception. Speak to your physician about your options.

Too Much Breast Milk

Insufficient breast milk production is more common than milk oversupply. However, mothers who have an overabundant milk supply may experience a forceful letdown of milk at feeds. The baby may have frequent watery stools due to the large amount of sugary foremilk consumed and may develop a diaper rash from the frequent stooling. If you have an overactive letdown reflex, you might want to see a lactation consultant for additional strategies for breastfeeding.

My newborn baby sleeps through the night without feeding. Is this normal?

Your baby should not be sleeping through the night in the first month of life. Although you may be happy to get some much-needed rest, a newborn baby feeds about every 2½ to 3 hours and should have only one period of up to 5 hours of continuous sleep. It is important to remember that breast milk empties from the stomach faster due to its easy digestion, so your baby may get hungry more often. If your baby is sleeping through the night in the first month, he needs to be woken for feeds. If he falls asleep shortly after you put him at the breast to feed, this may indicate that baby is tired and lethargic from a lack of energy. He may not be getting enough breast milk.

Tips for Decreasing Milk Supply when Overabundant

- Feed only one breast per feed. If baby stops feeding and then wants to return to the breast within an hour of the last feed, place her on the same breast.

- Feed lying down or leaning back so gravity isn't also causing milk to flow more quickly.

- Avoid pumping or expressing additional breast milk unless this is absolutely necessary for comfort. Pumping will only cause an increase in milk production.

Breast Reduction and Augmentation (Implants)

Many women who have had a breast reduction or implants wonder whether or not they will be able to breastfeed. The answer lies in how much breast tissue was damaged during surgery.

Reduction surgery can interfere with a mother's capacity to produce milk. Most women who have had breast reduction surgery are able to breastfeed, although the baby may require additional supplementation with infant formula. This can be achieved with a lactation aid tube at the breast or by bottle. Close monitoring of the baby's growth is required until breast milk supply is determined.

Most women who have had breast implant surgery are also able to breastfeed, provided that the implants were not inserted through an incision in the areola. No evidence suggests that silicone from implants will harm the baby; the benefits of breastfeeding greatly outweigh the perceived risk.

Mastitis

Mastitis (breast infection) is a rare complication of breastfeeding caused by the bacterium *Staphylococcus aureus*. Fortunately, it is easily treatable. Mastitis may result from plugged ducts, cracked or bleeding nipples, missed breast feedings or prolonged times between breast feedings. Women with mastitis often complain that part or all of one breast is very tender, red and hot. Along with these symptoms of inflammation, women may have a fever and may feel run down and achy, much like symptoms of the flu. A mother may feel as if the symptoms are getting worse instead of better.

Mastitis should be treated early enough so that symptoms do not get so severe that the mother decides to discontinue breastfeeding. Mastitis is treated with antibiotics, and symptoms usually resolve within 24 hours of treatment. By breastfeeding and keeping milk flowing, mastitis will resolve.

Tips for Preventing Mastitis

- Ensure that breasts are emptied with each feeding.
- Try not to let prolonged periods of time go by without breastfeeding.
- Express milk if a breast becomes engorged or very full because milk that is not released may result in a thicker milk that can clog up the ducts.
- Get plenty of rest because stress and fatigue may affect the immune system, making you more likely to develop mastitis.
- Eat a balanced diet to help strengthen the immune system.
- Apply cold or warm compresses to the tender area.
- Massage the tender area in a gentle fashion to help relieve the pain.

Did You Know ...

Thrush Prevention

Both mother and baby should receive treatment together or one may continue to reinfect the other. Frequent diaper changes and frequent handwashing are recommended strategies to prevent thrush.

Thrush

Thrush (candida) is caused by a yeast infection. This candidiasis yeast grows in warm, moist environments, such as the nipple or the baby's mouth or buttocks. It results in persistently sore nipples for the mother and mouth or buttock irritation for the child. White patches in the baby's mouth may or may not be present. Babies may be exposed to the yeast during delivery (from the mother's genital tract). Thrush may occur in a mother or a baby treated with antibiotics, which disrupt the normal flora of the body. Thrush is usually treated with an oral or topical agent.

Sore or Cracked Nipples

Many breastfeeding mothers develop some soreness when they begin to breastfeed their newborn because the nipple is a sensitive area for most women. This is most common in first-time moms and should resolve after about a week. Nipple soreness that lasts longer than the first week of life is not normal, and chronic pain is an indicator that something is wrong. Sore nipples are often cited as a reason why women stop breastfeeding before they had originally intended.

If you are experiencing chronic nipple soreness and are not getting relief, speak with a lactation consultant, who will be able to provide you with more information and strategies to help correct the problem. To find a lactation consultant in your neighborhood, contact your local public health office.

Treatment should not include shortening the length of a feed to prevent nipple soreness. This will only delay the pain. It also prevents baby from receiving nutrient-rich hindmilk, which, over an extended period, can contribute to poor weight gain.

Tips for Treating Sore Nipples

If you are able to fix latch problems, you will also be able to fix nipple soreness.

- **Poor latch or suck:** Babies learn to suck properly when they have a proper latch. In many cases, however, the baby is only sucking on the nipple and not the entire areola. Sucking on the nipple only does not stimulate the breast fully, which causes the baby to suck harder, which ultimately increases the amount of nipple soreness. Make sure your baby opens her mouth wide (like a yawn) and that her tongue is down before putting her to the breast. This will allow her to get more of the areola into her mouth and should provide a better latch and less soreness. Also be sure to release your baby's suction from the breast before taking her off the breast. This can also contribute to sore, cracked nipples.

If your baby appears to have a good latch and suck and you are still experiencing nipple pain, the pain may have other causes.

- **Engorgement:** When a breast becomes engorged, it becomes physically hard and the nipple becomes flat. When the baby tries to feed, he has trouble latching and may damage nipple tissue. Expressing or pumping off some breast milk for a few minutes will soften the areola and make latching easier.

- **Nipple infection:** This can occur when nipples are cracked and can delay healing. Treatment with oral or topical antibiotics may be required.

- **Thrush:** This can cause nipples to become red and sore and is often associated with a burning sensation. Nystatin, an antifungal drug, can be used to treat candida infection of the breast.

- **Biting behaviors:** Biting can be due to excessive soother use or bottle feeding with a short, soft nipple.

Inverted Nipples

Another rare complication may be inverted nipples. Inverted nipples do not prevent a mother from breastfeeding. A baby will learn to feed on inverted nipples. By providing the mother with adequate support and effective intervention techniques, breastfeeding can be successful. Time also helps improve symptoms.

Blocked or Plugged Ducts

A hard, painful swelling of a small to significant part of the breast may indicate a blocked duct. Symptoms of blocked ducts include tenderness, warmth and possible redness in one area of the breast. If the blockage is located in a duct close to the skin, you may also feel a defined lump. Occasionally, you may also see a small, white "milk plug" at the opening of the duct on the nipple. Be aware that plugged ducts can lead to mastitis if untreated or ignored. Have your physician check any lumps in your breast that you are concerned about.

It is not known why blocked ducts happen or what causes them, but it is thought that they may be caused by skipping feedings, a constricting bra, poor maternal nutrition and stress. Blocked ducts are often found in mothers with an abundant milk supply who may not be adequately draining the breast with feeds. Plugged ducts also seem to be more common in the winter months; this is thought to be due to either the restrictive clothing worn in the winter.

Tips for Treating Blocked Ducts

- While feeding on the blocked side, massage the area of blocked duct toward the nipple with as much pressure as you can tolerate. This seems to be the best way to relieve blocked ducts and helps stimulate milk flow.

- Try massaging breasts in a warm shower or bath before a feeding.

- Apply a warm, damp compress to the area of blockage several times a day to help get milk flowing.

- Offer your baby the breast a minimum of 8 times in a 24-hour period. Feeding on the affected breast will help encourage the breast to drain.

- Point the baby's chin right below or next to the area of blockage, if possible. Keep in mind that this is sometimes not a practical position to feed your baby.

- Try changing your baby's position during a feed to ensure complete drainage of the breast.

- Avoid the use of constricting bras or clothing, including underwire bras and the straps from an infant carrier.

Breast Engorgement

Breast engorgement is not the same thing as breast fullness, which is normal between the second and fourth day of a newborn's life. From time to time, breastfeeding mothers will commonly have breast fullness, which generally lasts less than 24 hours, during which time the mother will still be able to breastfeed comfortably. Breast fullness does not prevent baby from breastfeeding, and breastfeeding helps to relieve fullness. Breasts may be tender and sensitive but should still be soft to the touch.

Engorgement, however, is often caused by not managing breast fullness well, by either restricting the length or delaying the frequency of breastfeeding. During breast engorgement, breasts will be beyond being full and the breast will be so engorged that the baby will find it very difficult, if not impossible, to latch onto the nipple. This state of engorgement usually happens when breastfeeding has not been effective up until this point and the latch was never well established. It can also happen when a baby has not been allowed to feed often enough. When a baby is unable to feed, the mother's nipple tissue can become so stretched that even the leaking of breast milk is not possible. The breasts will be painful, swollen and red.

Tips for Treating Breast Engorgement

- Soften the areola first before feeding. This will help promote the letdown of breast milk. You can do this by hand, expressing some milk before offering the breast to your baby.
- Make sure the baby is latched on well at the breast. If you need help, call your public health department to find out about lactation services in your neighborhood. In Canada, lactation consulting services are often offered free of charge.
- Offer your breast to your baby a minimum of 8 times in a 24-hour period, but don't watch the clock to know when it is time to feed. Watch your baby for cues or signs of hunger, such as increased fussiness, munching on hands and crying.
- Apply cold compresses on the breasts after feeding to help relieve engorgement.
- Compress breasts during feeds to help get your milk flowing.
- Apply cabbage leaves. No, this is not a joke. Refrigerated green cabbage (not red) leaves placed around the breasts two to three times a day for about 20 minutes or until leaves wilt will help relieve engorgement. Stop cabbage leaf treatment when engorgement subsides, because continual use of cabbage leaves can decrease milk supply.

Further Breastfeeding Issues

Many women have questions about the safety of drugs, alcohol, caffeine and environmental contaminants while breastfeeding. The Motherisk program at The Hospital for Sick Children is an excellent source of information on these issues. See the Resources section in this book for contact information.

Prescription Drug Use during Breastfeeding

Many mothers have been told in the past by their doctors or family members to stop breastfeeding when they are given a prescription medication because of fears that the medication may get into the breast milk and harm the baby. You may worry that a drug that was unsafe to take during pregnancy will have a similar toxic effect during breastfeeding. In many cases, this concern is unwarranted. Very few drugs are actually contraindicated during breastfeeding.

Of course, there are many factors that affect how much of the drug is actually absorbed into the baby's body. These include how quickly a drug is metabolized by a mother's body, the dose of the drug and how a drug is taken (for example, orally or by injection), as well as how old the infant is, how often a baby feeds and whether breast milk is the only source of food for the infant.

Discuss any concerns about medication you may be taking while breastfeeding with your doctor. If the drug you are taking is not safe to take while breastfeeding, your doctor may be able to recommend an alternative medication that is compatible with nursing.

Alcohol Intake during Breastfeeding

Many women want to know if it is okay to have the occasional glass of wine or beer after 9 months of completely avoiding alcohol. Social drinking is not generally considered a problem while breastfeeding. Most breastfeeding professionals would prefer that a woman have an occasional drink while breastfeeding rather than giving up breastfeeding altogether and thus prevent giving her baby all the benefits of breast milk. The occasional drink is the key factor here.

If you choose to have a glass of alcohol while you are breastfeeding, you may wish to keep in mind that peak levels of alcohol are found in breast milk 30 to 60 minutes after a

Did You Know ...

Breast Barrier

While the placenta allows drugs to cross freely from mother to fetus, the breast serves as a filter of sorts and acts as a barrier to many common prescription drugs. Most drugs do pass into breast milk. The presence of a drug in breast milk does not necessarily mean the baby will absorb it. Many drugs are, in fact, absorbed very poorly by a baby's digestive system. Almost all drugs appear in very small amounts in breast milk, usually less than 1% of the maternal dose.

mother drinks on an empty stomach or 60 to 90 minutes after drinking and eating. You may wish to have a drink soon after breastfeeding so that at least 2 hours have passed before putting your baby back at the breast.

Caffeine Intake during Breastfeeding

As with most other drugs, only a very small amount of caffeine consumed by a mother makes its way into breast milk. One study found that as little as 0.06% to 1.5% of a mother's intake of caffeine actually appears in breast milk and that no caffeine at all makes it into the urine up to 5 hours after the initial nursing period. Another study found that even 5 cups of coffee a day for 5 days did not affect infant heart rates or sleep time.

These studies suggest that caffeine in moderate amounts presents no significant problem for normal full-term infants. So you can go ahead and enjoy your favorite cup of latte.

Environmental Contaminant Exposure during Breastfeeding

Pollution is a problem for everyone on this planet. While there is little evidence that the environmental contaminants found in human milk are harmful for babies, some mothers are concerned about the potential risks of pollutants in their breast milk. Breast milk is undeniably nature's perfect food, and although some contaminants may get into breast milk, there may ultimately be some risk from environmental contamination in whatever you choose to feed your infant, including infant formula.

Eventually, children will eat the same foods as the rest of the family and will be exposed to the same contaminants. The risk of contaminants in breast milk is generally considered to be low, but lactating women may choose to take nutrition-related precautions to minimize the amount of contaminants passed into their breast milk.

Tips for Avoiding Contaminants

- Avoid eating freshwater fish from waters known to be contaminated.
- Wash all fruits and vegetables well before eating.
- Trim all visible fat from meats before eating.
- Avoid or eat no more than one meal per month of top-predator fish, such as fresh or frozen tuna, shark and swordfish.

Did You Know ...

Alcohol Risks

Studies have shown that breastfeeding mothers who drink alcohol on a frequent regular basis can have babies whose motor development is impaired. Alcohol is known to decrease levels of the hormone prolactin and blocks the release of oxytocin. When combined, this can mean a decrease in the amount of milk produced. Another study found that when nursing women drank alcohol, their babies' suck behavior at the breast changed. Babies were found to suck more, but they ultimately obtained less milk.

Did You Know ...

MSG

Monosodium glutamate (MSG) is a sodium salt formed with the amino acid glutamate, and used to enhance the flavor of some foods. It appears that MSG cannot cross the placenta, so is considered safe to eat while pregnant. For a mother who is breastfeeding, it poses no risk to the infant.

Food Allergies and Breastfeeding

High-Risk Infants

An infant is considered to be at high risk for allergies when at least one parent or a sibling has an allergy.

Medical professionals and research scientists continue to study the extent that breastfeeding prevents, reduces or increases the development of food allergies. Here are answers to the most frequently asked questions about breastfeeding and allergies in the mother and the child.

Can I prevent food allergies by breastfeeding my baby?

Exclusive breastfeeding for a minimum of 6 months may help to prevent the development of a food allergy. Some studies have suggested that there is a critical time in early infancy when a high-risk infant (at least one parent or a sibling has an allergy) is at even greater risk for becoming sensitized to ingested food allergens. Studies looking at the prevention of food allergies have primarily been beneficial for babies who are at high risk for developing atopic diseases (including a food allergy, eczema and asthma). Babies are considered at high risk for developing a food allergy if there is a strong family history of atopic disease, meaning that one parent or sibling also has a food allergy.

Should I eliminate certain foods from my diet while breastfeeding to prevent an allergy to these foods?

Food allergens can be detected in breast milk, which may lead to early sensitization to certain foods in babies who are exclusively breastfed. However, studies are inconclusive about whether or not avoiding specific foods during breastfeeding will help to prevent the development of a food allergy in the child. The American Academy of Pediatrics (AAP) currently suggests that mothers who are breastfeeding high-risk infants may want to avoid eating peanuts while they are nursing. The avoidance of peanuts will not necessarily prevent the development of a peanut allergy, but it is a small change that does not affect the overall nutrient composition of a mother's diet and will not lead to nutrient deficiencies.

Avoiding or eliminating certain foods while breastfeeding has not been shown to prevent the development of food allergies. Elimination diets can be nutritionally incomplete.

What should I do if I have a food allergy?

If you are breastfeeding and are allergic to a specific food, it is important that you continue to avoid whatever foods cause you to experience a reaction. Your baby may or may not develop a food allergy, and if he does develop food allergies, they may or may not be the same foods that you are allergic to. It is atopic disease in general (including diseases such as asthma, allergies and eczema) that is hereditary and not the specific food allergy. If you have multiple food allergies and need to avoid many foods, you may want to speak with a registered dietitian about ensuring that you are meeting the nutritional needs for you and your baby.

 # What should I do if my baby develops a food allergy?

If your infant has been diagnosed with a food allergy, you should avoid eating the food that causes the allergy while breastfeeding. When an infant is very young, the food causing the allergy may not yet be determined and you may be put on a trial elimination diet that may include avoiding all milk, egg, fish, peanut and nut products. This takes an intense commitment on a mother's part because milk and eggs can be found in a countless number of food products. Complete avoidance of these foods is necessary to prevent an allergic reaction in some breastfed infants. Nutrition counseling by a registered dietitian should be a part of the protocol to ensure that all of your nutritional needs (and ultimately your baby's) are being met. Supplemental calcium, among other vitamins, may be required.

If this elimination diet is not successful in preventing the symptoms of allergy in a breastfed infant, it may be suggested that you use a specialty allergy formula. These infant formulas have extensively broken down proteins to prevent an allergic reaction in infants. Soy formulas may be suggested if the allergy seems to be IgE-mediated. IgE-mediated allergy is a specific subtype of allergy. Other milks, such as goat's milk and sheep's milk, should not be given to an allergic infant because they are very similar in makeup to cow's milk and will also likely cause a similar allergic reaction. Alternative milks can be nutritionally unsatisfactory as a calorie source for infants under the age of 1 year.

Duration of Breastfeeding

Exclusive breastfeeding for 6 months, with supplemental foods being introduced at 6 months or after, and the continuation of breastfeeding until 12 months or beyond is seen as the gold standard for infant nutrition. This may not be possible for some mothers because of work demands, fatigue or other factors that may come into play. It is up to individual parents to determine how long to breastfeed their infant.

 Ten Common Breastfeeding Questions & Answers

1. **Will a glass of beer help to bring my milk in?**

   There is no evidence that drinking a glass of beer or alcohol will help bring your milk in. Your milk should come in about 2 to 3 days after birth regardless of whether or not you have something alcoholic to drink.

2. **Do I need to give my baby a vitamin supplement while I am breastfeeding?**

   Health Canada and the Canadian Pediatric Society recommend that exclusively breastfed babies in Canada receive a daily vitamin D supplement of 10 mcg (400 IU) until the infant's diet includes 10 mcg (400 IU) of vitamin D per day from other dietary sources or until the baby is 1 year old. The American Pediatric Society suggests a daily vitamin D supplement of 5 mcg (200 IU).

3. **Should I continue to take my multivitamin during lactation?**

   If your diet is balanced, you should not need to take a multivitamin while breastfeeding. However, if your diet is lacking or you are concerned that you are not eating as well as you should, a multivitamin can ensure that you are receiving sufficient amounts of vitamins and minerals, such as iron and calcium. A multivitamin should never replace healthy eating habits.

4. **How much tuna or fish is safe to eat while breastfeeding?**

   The guidelines for eating tuna and fish while breastfeeding are the same as during pregnancy. You should avoid or limit your intake of fresh or frozen tuna and other fish that may be high in mercury to about one meal per month. Continue to enjoy fish that may be low in mercury, including canned light tuna, up to two 6-oz (175 g) servings a week.

5. **Does my breastfed baby need extra water in the hot weather?**

   You do not need to give your baby additional water in the hot weather. Breast milk has a very high water content, and giving a young infant (under 6 months) water can lead to nutritional deficiencies. Breastfeeding your infant on a regular basis will provide your baby with all the fluid needed to stay hydrated and grow.

There are many factors to consider when deciding when to wean an infant off the breast. Each woman's circumstances are different. If an infant is weaned off the breast prior to the introduction of homogenized milk at around 12 months, both the Canadian and American pediatric societies recommend the use of an iron-fortified, cow's milk–based infant formula as a safe nutritional alternative to breastfeeding.

6. Do I need to eat more or drink lots of fluid to breastfeed?

Energy requirements are higher during breastfeeding than during pregnancy, but you do not necessarily need to eat more to support breastfeeding. Eat a well-balanced diet and let your hunger guide you. Eat when you are hungry and stop when you are full. The same advice goes for fluid. Some women find themselves very thirsty while nursing. Let your thirst guide how much to drink. While breastfeeding, consume 15 cups (3.8 L) of fluid every day, including milk, fruit juice and water.

7. Can I have a glass of wine with dinner while breastfeeding?

Having the occasional glass of wine or alcohol while breastfeeding should not pose a risk for your baby. Alcohol is present in very small amounts in breast milk, and there is no need for you to "pump and dump" your breast milk after having a glass of wine. However, heavy, regular drinking can affect your infant and should be avoided.

8. Can I drink coffee while breastfeeding?

It is safe to drink coffee while nursing. Caffeine passes into the breast milk in very small amounts. Studies have shown that even 5 cups of coffee a day does not appear to affect infants.

9. Should I avoid eating peanuts while breastfeeding?

For mothers whose infants are at high risk of developing a food allergy only (for example, one or both parents have an allergy, or a parent and a sibling have a food allergy), the American Academy of Pediatrics suggests that avoiding peanuts while breastfeeding may prevent an infant from becoming sensitized to peanut protein.

10. Where can I find a lactation consultant in my neighborhood?

Call your local public health office or your birth hospital. Both should be able to put you in contact with a lactation consultant in your neighborhood. Many communities have drop-in breastfeeding services provided by lactation consultants free of charge.

Maternal Weight Loss

Getting back into shape after giving birth is a high priority for many women. The benefits of returning to your usual weight and achieving a healthy BMI are not only physical, but also psychological.

However, returning to a normal weight does not occur within days after birth, but usually within a few months to 1 year. The amount of weight lost after delivery depends on several factors, principally your weight status before pregnancy and the amount of weight you gained during pregnancy. Diet most certainly plays as role as well: it is the fine balance of caloric intake and output that determines weight changes. Some women may return to their usual weight within a few weeks or months, while many take up to 1 year or longer to get back to their normal weight post-partum.

Weight Loss Rates

Research reveals that most women retain about 7 to 15 lbs (3 to 7 kg) of the weight that they gained during pregnancy at 6 weeks postpartum. The most significant cause of this weight retention is overall weight gain during pregnancy.

Women who gain more than the recommended amount of weight during their pregnancy or who have a BMI that is over 27 in pre-pregnancy are more likely to retain excess weight at 1 year postpartum. Women who do retain more weight after pregnancy and whose BMI is above the normal healthy range are at greater risk of developing coronary heart disease, Type 2 diabetes and stroke. Lifestyle factors have a large influence on weight retention post-partum. These include, but are not limited to, attitudes toward diet and exercise before pregnancy, family support and social influences.

To assist with efforts to lose weight post-partum, a diet that includes lower-fat or leaner meats, low-fat dairy products, plenty of fruits and vegetables and whole grains is recommended. Follow the USDA MyPyramid food guide or Canada's Food Guide to Healthy Eating to meet your daily nutrient and calorie needs.

Breastfeeding and Weight Loss

Breastfeeding may promote weight loss due to the higher energy demands required by lactation. Body fat stores start to decrease by day 15 after giving birth in breastfeeding women. Weight loss with lactation is especially true for younger women and those who gained the expected amount of weight during their pregnancy.

Weight loss of about ½ to 1 lb (250 to 500 g) per week will not compromise breastfeeding in women with a normal BMI pre-pregnancy.

Exercise during Post-Pregnancy

The level of exercise after giving birth will depend on individual factors, such as the type of delivery (vaginal or cesarean section), how fit the mother was before and during pregnancy and the overall health of the mother. Women who have been active throughout pregnancy and who gained the recommended amount of weight during the pregnancy usually have an easier time losing weight than those who did not exercise or who gained an excess amount of weight during the pregnancy. In one study, women with varying BMIs were able to return to their pre-pregnancy fitness level and strength by 27 weeks after delivery. Not all women return to their pre-pregnancy weight or size as readily, if ever.

Benefits of Post-partum Exercise

- Helps speed up recovery from the delivery process
- Increases energy levels
- Reduces stress levels and depression
- Increases possibility that the routine of daily exercise will be passed on to the child, encouraging increased activity as a lifelong habit

Cesarean Section

For women who had a cesarean section, any type of exercise should be avoided in the first 3 days after delivery. Most physicians will recommend that women avoid strenuous exercise and avoid carrying heavy objects for 6 weeks after a cesarean section.

Recommended Exercises

Your doctor or health-care provider will be able to guide you in the type of exercises that are recommended at different time periods during post-partum. In the first few days after delivery, plenty of rest is usually recommended while the body recovers from the strain of the delivery. Ligaments and joints are softened following birth (for up to 3 months), so high-impact exercises and excessive stretching may not be recommended. As the uterus contracts after delivery, which may take a few weeks, the abdomen will return to its more flattened shape. Breastfeeding assists with the process of uterine contraction.

Walking versus driving in the car to local destinations is one simple method to include exercise in the daily routine. Other exercises, such as swimming, yoga, cycling and low-impact aerobic workouts, are often recommended. Pelvic floor exercises, called Kegel exercises, in the immediate post-partum period are recommended for most women by the Society of Obstetricians and Gynaecologists of Canada to help reduce the incidence of urinary incontinence. These exercises may also be recommended during pregnancy.

Exercise and Breastfeeding

Breastfeeding women trying to lose weight in post-partum can be encouraged to exercise with no detrimental effects to the infant. The nutrients in breast milk remain unchanged with exercise. There may be an increase in lactic acid (an end product of exercising that is passed from the mother into the breast milk) after the mother has exercised. This has been reported in some studies to make the milk taste sour. Some women report their infants do not like to nurse after they have exercised, but other studies did not prove this to be true.

Although studies in this area are lacking, exercise during lactation may help maintain healthy bones and prevent osteoporosis. It is known that breastfeeding may decrease the bone mineral content of mothers. This loss is regained, however, after weaning.

Postpartum Depression

Postpartum depression affects about 5% to 10% of women. The degree of symptoms can be quite variable, and you should inform your doctor if you feel you may have postpartum depression. The following dietary and lifestyle changes may help to prevent or relieve symptoms:

- Increasing intake of foods rich in iron or taking an iron supplement to correct low hemoglobin levels (low hemoglobin levels may be a risk factor for depression);
- Eating a diet rich in carbohydrates (decreased insulin levels may contribute to symptoms of postpartum depression);
- Increasing intake of food rich in omega 3 fatty acids;
- Participating in a regular exercise routine to increase energy levels and to help return to a normal BMI.

Did You Know ...

Omega 3 Treatment

Some studies indicate that increasing omega 3 fatty acids in the diet helps to prevent and reduce symptoms of post-partum depression.

CHAPTER 8

Good Nutrition for Life

GOOD NUTRITION IN INFANCY lays the foundation for good nutrition throughout your child's life. If growth is normal, breastfeeding on demand or feeding your baby recommended amounts of formula provides all the nutritional support needed for growth in the first 6 months of life. The stage of development from age 6 months to 2 years is also very important as your child makes the transformation from breast milk or formula to eating solid foods. Good eating habits developed at this stage can last for a lifetime.

In our previous book, Better Baby Food, *we describe the nutritional needs of young children and make recommendations for good nutrition. For nutritional advice on feeding your child from age 2 to 6, you may want to consult our book* Better Food for Kids. *We wish you good luck in guiding your child and yourself in eating nutritiously.*

Recommendations for Feeding a Young Child

- Introduce solids at 6 months: Iron-fortified cereals are a recommended first choice because they provide a good source of iron, a nutrient needed by this age.

- Gradually introduce different solid foods one at a time: Preparing homemade foods is recommended to provide more variety. Homemade foods are also less expensive than commercial baby foods. Either form should provide a variety of foods and nutrients as solids gradually replace some of the calories and nutrients of milk in your child's diet.

- Ensure that your child receives iron-containing foods daily (fortified cereals, meat, chicken, tofu) after 1 year of age, when breast milk or formula may be replaced by whole milk, which is not a good source of iron.

- Continue to provide a large variety of foods to the toddler. Food variety encourages the intake of different foods as the child grows and may help prevent "picky eating."

- Always serve fresh fruits and cooked or fresh vegetables as snacks. Just make sure they are appropriate for his age. Some may cause choking in the early years.

- Start educating your child about the importance of good nutrition. The idea of balancing foods will help encourage variety.

- Encourage your child by example to eat nutritious food and to be physically active. Childhood obesity is on the rise. It is up to parents to help prevent this disease.

PART 2

Better Recipes for Pregnancy

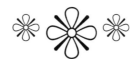

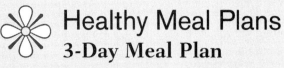

Healthy Meal Plans
3-Day Meal Plan

In the following 3-day meal plan, we provide examples of well-balanced menus that meet the guidelines for pregnant women set by the USDA MyPyramid and Canada's Food Guide to Healthy Eating.

DAY 1

Breakfast	Bran cereal (raisin bran)	1 cup (250 mL) with ½ cup (125 mL) skim milk
	Skim milk	1 cup (250 mL)
	Whole wheat toast	1 slice with 2 tsp (10 mL) peanut butter
Snack	Apple	1 whole
	Cheddar cheese	1 oz (30 g)
	Bottled water	2 cups (500 mL)
Lunch	*Ginger Chili Sweet Potato Soup* (page 168)	1 serving
	Whole wheat roll	1 small with 1 tsp (5 mL) butter
	Skim milk	1 cup (250 mL)
	Banana	1 whole
Snack	Digestive cookies	2
	Apple juice	¾ cup (175 mL)
Dinner	*Beef Fajitas* (page 232)	2 fajitas
	Tossed salad	1 cup (250 mL)
	Raspberry Basil Vinaigrette (page 193)	1 tbsp (15 mL)
	Water	1 cup (250 mL) with lemon
Snack	Low-fat strawberry yogurt	¾ cup (175 mL)

DAY 2

Breakfast	Oatmeal	¾ cup (175 mL) with ½ cup (125 mL) skim milk & 1 tsp (5 mL) brown sugar
	Whole wheat toast	1 slice with 1 tsp (5 mL) margarine
	Blueberries	¼ cup (50 mL)
	Orange juice	½ cup (125 mL)
Snack	*Banana Oat Bran Muffins* (page 153)	1 muffin
	Skim milk	1 cup (250 mL)

Lunch	Tuna fish sandwich on whole wheat bread with lettuce and tomato	
	Cucumber slices	2 tbsp (25 mL)
	Vanilla yogurt	¾ cup (175 mL)
	Chocolate milk	1 cup (250 mL)
Snack	Celery sticks with cream cheese	4 with 2 tbsp (25 mL) cream cheese
	Skim milk	1 cup (250 mL)
Dinner	Grilled chicken breast	4 oz (125 g)
	Baked potato	1 with 1 tsp (5 mL) margarine and 1 tbsp (15 mL) low-fat sour cream
	Steamed broccoli	½ cup (125 mL)
	Tossed salad	1 cup (250 mL) with 1 tbsp (15 mL) salad dressing
	Milk	1 cup (250 mL)
Snack	Popcorn	2 cups (500 mL)
	Skim milk	1 cup (250 mL)

DAY 3

Breakfast	*Fiber-Full Bran Pancakes* (page 144)	2 pancakes with 2 tbsp (25 mL) table syrup
	Sliced strawberries	½ cup (125 mL)
	Skim milk	1 cup (250 mL)
Snack	Almonds	¼ cup (50 mL)
	Chocolate milk	1 cup (250 mL)
Lunch	Chicken noodle soup	1 cup (250 mL)
	Tasty Bean Salad (page 188)	½ cup (125 mL)
	Saltine crackers	4
	Orange	1 whole
	Water	1 cup (250 mL)
Snack	*Granola* (page 163)	1 serving
	Skim milk	1 cup (250 mL)
Dinner	*Beef Souvlaki* (page 234)	1 serving
	Tzatziki Sauce (page 159)	¼ cup (50 mL)
	Steamed basmati rice	½ cup (125 mL)
	Green beans	½ cup (125 mL)
	Water	1 cup (250 mL)
	Fruit cocktail (in its own juice)	1 cup (250 mL)
Snack	Whole wheat raisin toast	1 slice with 1 tsp (5 mL) margarine
	Cheddar cheese	1 oz (30 g)

❀ Nutritional Analysis of Meal Plans

Day	Energy (kcal)	Protein (g)	Fat (g)	Carbohydrate (g)	Fiber (g)	Calcium (mg)	Iron (mg)	Folate (mcg)
Day 1	2,300	99	62	352	26	1,593	20	250
Day 2	2,000	109	58	262	26	2,055	11	328
Day 3	2,600	124	81	384	37	1,859	20	353

❀ Daily Recommended Intakes (DRIs)*

Energy (cal)	Protein (g) (RDA)	Fat (g)	Carbohydrate (g) (RDA)	Fiber (g) (AI)	Calcium (mg) (AI)	Iron (mg) (RDA)	Folate (mcg) (RDA)
DURING PREGNANCY							
1st Trimester: approximately 2,100–2,500;** *2nd and 3rd Trimesters:* approximately 2,300–2,700**	71	20–35% of total energy intake	175	28	1,000	27	600
DURING LACTATION							
2,500–2,900**	71	20–35% of total energy intake	210	29	1,000	9	500

*Water needs (AI) are 12 cups (3 L) a day during pregnancy and 15 cups (3.8 L) a day during lactation (this is water from all sources, including food and drinks).

**Needs vary depending on pre-pregnancy BMI and activity level. Consult your doctor to discuss your energy requirements.

Best Recipes for Vital Nutrients

Power Recipes

The following recipes are excellent sources of all four of the key nutrients highlighted in this book:

White Bean Soup with Swiss Chard (page 171)
Chicken Tacos (page 211)
Chickpea Tofu Stew (page 251)
Spinach Frittata (page 264)

The following recipes are excellent sources of three of the four key nutrients highlighted in this book:

Fassolada (page 170)
Savory Red Lentil Soup (page 172)
Lemony Lentil Soup with Spinach (page 173)
Rice and Bean Salad (page 187)
Turkey Chili (page 214)
Salmon with Roasted Vegetables (page 219)
20-Minute Chili (page 235)
Mixed Winter Beans (page 248)
Vegetarian Chili (page 252)
Spaghetti with Zucchini Balls and Tomato Sauce (page 254)
Lentil Spaghetti Sauce (page 255)
Falafel in Pita (page 260)
Swiss Chard Frittata in a Pita (page 263)
Mushroom-Spinach Lasagna with Goat Cheese (page 278)

Calcium

EXCELLENT SOURCE

Sunny Orange Shake (page 142)
Banana Berry Wake-Up Shake (page 142)
Breakfast Muesli to Go (page 143)
Healthy Cheese 'n' Herb Bread (page 146)
White Bean Soup with Swiss Chard (page 171)
Hot and Sour Chicken Soup (page 175)
Chicken Tacos (page 211)
Salmon with Roasted Vegetables (page 219)
Salmon Burgers (page 223)
Grilled Tofu (page 250)
Sweet and Tasty Tofu (page 250)
Chickpea Tofu Stew (page 251)

Spinach Frittata (page 264)
Mushroom-Spinach Lasagna with Goat Cheese (page 278)

GOOD SOURCE

Creamy Microwave Oatmeal (page 144)
Sonoma Chicken Salad (page 183)
Chicken Nuggets (page 212)
Sole and Spinach Casserole (page 224)
Parmesan-Crusted Snapper with Tomato Olive Sauce (page 226)
Mixed Winter Beans (page 248)
Vegetarian Shepherd's Pie with Peppered Potato Topping (page 256)
Swiss Chard Frittata in a Pita (page 263)
Rapini with Balsamic Vinegar (page 267)
Cauliflower Casserole (page 270)
Pasta with Goat Cheese, Snow Peas and Tomato Coulis (page 272)
Hoisin Stir-fried Vegetables and Tofu over Rice Noodles (page 274)

SOURCE

Fiber-Full Bran Pancakes (page 144)
Big-Batch Bran Muffins (page 150)
Banana Oatmeal Muffins (page 154)
Cottage Cheese Herb Dip (page 156)
Eggplant Dip (page 157)
Tofu and Chickpea Garlic Dip (page 158)
Tzatziki Sauce (page 159)
Portobello Mushrooms with Goat Cheese (page 161)
Granola (page 163)
Carrot Orange Soup (page 166)
Ginger Chili Sweet Potato Soup (page 167)
Fassolada (page 170)
Savory Red Lentil Soup (page 172)
Lemony Lentil Soup with Spinach (page 173)
Borscht (page 174)
Mandarin Orange Salad with Almonds (page 181)
Crunchy Broccoli Salad (page 182)
Greek Summer Salad (page 184)
Beet and Feta Salad (page 186)
Rice and Bean Salad (page 187)
Tasty Bean Salad (page 188)

Tuscan Bean Salad (page 190)
Lentil Salad (page 191)
Warm Chickpea Salad (page 193)
Bulgur Salad (page 194)
Mediterranean Potato Salad (page 195)
Chicken Salad Amandine (page 196)
Thai-Style Beef Salad (page 198)
Best-Ever Baked Chicken (page 200)
Baked Chicken and Potato Dinner (page 201)
Yogurt-Marinated Chicken (page 202)
Pesto Chicken Thighs (page 204)
Sticky Sesame Chicken (page 209)
Curried Chicken (page 210)
Turkiaki Fiesta (page 213)
Turkey Chili (page 214)
Baked Fish with Tomatoes and Roasted
   Red Pepper (page 217)
Honey Dill Salmon with Dijon (page 220)
Baked Lemon Salmon with Mango Salsa
   (page 221)
Soy-Glazed Salmon (page 222)
Parmesan Herb-Baked Fish Fillets
   (page 226)
The Narrows Crab Cakes (page 227)
Sweet and Spicy Shrimp with Broccoli
   (page 228)
Garlic Chili Shrimp (page 229)
Coconut Shrimp Curry (page 230)
Beef Fajitas (page 232)
Beef Stroganoff (page 233)
20-Minute Chili (page 235)
Meatball Pasta Sauce (page 237)
Meatloaf "Muffins" with Barbecue Sauce
   (page 239)
Quick and Easy Cabbage Rolls (page 241)
Orange Ginger Pork and Vegetables
   (page 244)
Stir-fried Vegetables with Tofu (page 249)
Vegetarian Chili (page 252)
Spaghetti with Zucchini Balls and Tomato
   Sauce (page 254)
Chickpea-Herb Burgers (page 253)
Zucchini, Mushroom and Bean Loaf with
   Tomato Sauce (page 257)
Roasted Yam Fajitas (page 258)
Falafel in Pita (page 260)
Spinach Risotto (page 261)
Egg and Mushroom Fried Rice (page 262)
Green Beans with Cashews (page 268)

Pasta Fagioli Capra (page 273)
Spaghetti with Broccoli (page 275)
Tuna Garden Pasta (page 277)
Cinnamon Baked Pears (page 282)
Autumn Crumble (page 283)
Vanilla Custard (page 293)
Orange Crème Caramel (page 294)

Folate

EXCELLENT SOURCE

Sunny Orange Shake (page 142)
Black Bean Salsa (page 159)
Cauliflower Popcorn Snack (page 162)
Fassolada (page 170)
White Bean Soup with Swiss Chard
   (page 171)
Savory Red Lentil Soup (page 172)
Lemony Lentil Soup with Spinach (page 173)
Borscht (page 174)
Mandarin Orange Salad with Almonds
   (page 181)
Rice and Bean Salad (page 187)
Tasty Bean Salad (page 188)
White Bean Salad with Lemon-Dill Vinaigrette
   (page 189)
Tuscan Bean Salad (page 190)
Lentil Salad (page 191)
Warm Chickpea Salad (page 193)
Thai-Style Beef Salad (page 198)
Chicken Tacos (page 211)
Turkey Chili (page 214)
Salmon with Roasted Vegetables (page 219)
20-Minute Chili (page 235)
Mixed Winter Beans (page 248)
Chickpea Tofu Stew (page 251)
Vegetarian Chili (page 252)
Spaghetti with Zucchini Balls and Tomato
   Sauce (page 254)
Lentil Spaghetti Sauce (page 255)
Zucchini, Mushroom and Bean Loaf with
   Tomato Sauce (page 257)
Falafel in Pita (page 260)
Spinach Risotto (page 261)
Swiss Chard Frittata in a Pita (page 263)
Spinach Frittata (page 264)
Rapini with Balsamic Vinegar (page 267)
Pasta Fagioli Capra (page 273)

Hoisin Stir-fried Vegetables and Tofu over Rice Noodles (page 274)
Spaghetti with Broccoli (page 275)
Linguine with Tuna, White Beans and Dill (page 276)
Mushroom-Spinach Lasagna with Goat Cheese (page 278)
Penne with Tuna and Peppers (page 280)

GOOD SOURCE

Breakfast Muesli to Go (page 143)
Carrot Bran Muffins (page 151)
Tofu and Chickpea Garlic Dip (page 158)
Black and White Bean Salsa (page 160)
Ginger Chili Sweet Potato Soup (page 168)
Sweet Green Pea Soup (page 169)
Mango, Strawberry and Cucumber Salad (page 179)
Greens with Strawberries (page 180)
Crunchy Broccoli Salad (page 182)
Sonoma Chicken Salad (page 183)
Spinach and Rice Salad (page 185)
Beet and Feta Salad (page 186)
Tabbouleh (page 192)
Mediterranean Potato Salad (page 195)
Curried Chicken (page 210)
Chicken Nuggets (page 212)
Baked Lemon Salmon with Mango Salsa (page 221)
Soy-Glazed Salmon (page 222)
Salmon Burgers (page 223)
Sole and Spinach Casserole (page 224)
Sweet and Spicy Shrimp with Broccoli (page 228)
Meatballs with Teriyaki Sauce (page 236)
Quick and Easy Cabbage Rolls (page 241)
Orange Ginger Pork and Vegetables (page 244)
Stir-fried Vegetables with Tofu (page 249)
Vegetarian Shepherd's Pie with Peppered Potato Topping (page 256)
Roasted Yam Fajitas (page 258)
Egg and Mushroom Fried Rice (page 262)
Green Beans with Cashews (page 268)
Green Beans and Tomato (page 269)
Cauliflower Casserole (page 270)
Pasta with Goat Cheese, Snow Peas and Tomato Coulis (page 272)
Tuna Garden Pasta (page 277)

SOURCE

Banana Berry Wake-Up Shake (page 142)
Muesli Mix (page 143)
Creamy Microwave Oatmeal (page 144)
Fiber-Full Bran Pancakes (page 144)
Banana Bread (page 145)
Healthy Cheese 'n' Herb Bread (page 146)
Apricot Bran Bread (page 147)
Zucchini Nut Loaf (page 148)
Coffee Cake (page 149)
Big-Batch Bran Muffins (page 150)
Banana Oatmeal Muffins (page 154)
Lentil Dip (page 156)
Eggplant Dip (page 157)
Hummus (page 158)
Portobello Mushrooms with Goat Cheese (page 161)
Granola (page 163)
No-Bake Trail Mix (page 164)
Carrot Orange Soup (page 166)
Southwestern Sweet Potato Soup (page 167)
Hot and Sour Chicken Soup (page 175)
Asian Turkey and Noodle Soup (page 176)
Mango-Cucumber Salad (page 178)
Asian Cucumber Salad (page 179)
Greek Summer Salad (page 184)
Bulgur Salad (page 194)
Chicken Salad Amandine (page 196)
Vietnamese Chicken and Rice Noodle Salad (page 197)
Best-Ever Baked Chicken (page 200)
Baked Chicken and Potato Dinner (page 201)
Pesto Chicken Thighs (page 204)
Crispy Chicken (page 205)
Greek Lemon Chicken (page 208)
Turkiaki Fiesta (page 213)
Parmesan Herb-Baked Fish Fillets (page 216)
Baked Fish with Tomatoes and Roasted Red Pepper (page 217)
South Side Halibut (page 218)
Honey Dill Salmon with Dijon (page 220)
Parmesan-Crusted Snapper with Tomato Olive Sauce (page 226)
The Narrows Crab Cakes (page 227)
Garlic Chili Shrimp (page 229)
Coconut Shrimp Curry (page 230)
Beef Fajitas (page 232)
Beef Stroganoff (page 233)
Beef Souvlaki (page 234)

Meatball Pasta Sauce (page 237)
Homestyle Meatloaf (page 238)
Meatloaf "Muffins" with Barbecue Sauce (page 239)
Beef Lettuce Wraps (page 240)
Spiced Veal Stir-fry (page 242)
Just Peachy Pork (page 243)
Teriyaki Pork Chops (page 245)
Grilled Tofu (page 250)
Sweet and Tasty Tofu (page 250)
Couscous (page 266)
Cinnamon Baked Pears (page 282)
Autumn Crumble (page 283)
Buttermilk Oat-Banana Cake (page 284)
Chocolate Cupcakes (page 285)
Sunflower Cookies (page 287)
Lemony Biscotti (page 290)
Almond Crescents (page 291)
Berry Oatmeal Squares (page 292)
Vanilla Custard (page 293)
Orange Crème Caramel (page 294)

Iron

EXCELLENT SOURCE

Big-Batch Bran Muffins (page 150)
Carrot Bran Muffins (page 151)
Granola (page 163)
Fassolada (page 170)
White Bean Soup with Swiss Chard (page 171)
Savory Red Lentil Soup (page 172)
Lemony Lentil Soup with Spinach (page 173)
Hot and Sour Chicken Soup (page 175)
Rice and Bean Salad (page 187)
Curried Chicken (page 210)
Chicken Tacos (page 211)
Chicken Nuggets (page 212)
Turkey Chili (page 214)
Salmon with Roasted Vegetables (page 219)
Beef Fajitas (page 232)
Beef Stroganoff (page 233)
Beef Souvlaki (page 234)
20-Minute Chili (page 235)
Meatballs with Teriyaki Sauce (page 236)
Meatloaf "Muffins" with Barbecue Sauce (page 239)
Mixed Winter Beans (page 248)
Stir-fried Vegetables with Tofu (page 249)
Grilled Tofu (page 250)
Sweet and Tasty Tofu (page 250)

Chickpea Tofu Stew (page 251)
Vegetarian Chili (page 252)
Spaghetti with Zucchini Balls and Tomato Sauce (page 254)
Lentil Spaghetti Sauce (page 255)
Roasted Yam Fajitas (page 258)
Falafel in Pita (page 260)
Swiss Chard Frittata in a Pita (page 263)
Spinach Frittata (page 264)
Pasta with Goat Cheese, Snow Peas and Tomato Coulis (page 272)
Pasta Fagioli Capra (page 273)
Hoisin Stir-fried Vegetables and Tofu over Rice Noodles (page 274)
Mushroom-Spinach Lasagna with Goat Cheese (page 278)
Penne with Tuna and Peppers (page 280)

GOOD SOURCE

Banana Berry Wake-Up Shake (page 142)
Breakfast Muesli to Go (page 143)
Creamy Microwave Oatmeal (page 144)
Fiber-Full Bran Pancakes (page 144)
Apricot Bran Bread (page 147)
Tofu and Chickpea Garlic Dip (page 158)
Black Bean Salsa (page 159)
Portobello Mushrooms with Goat Cheese (page 161)
No-Bake Trail Mix (page 164)
Ginger Chili Sweet Potato Soup (page 168)
Asian Turkey and Noodle Soup (page 176)
Crunchy Broccoli Salad (page 182)
Sonoma Chicken Salad (page 183)
Tasty Bean Salad (page 188)
White Bean Salad with Lemon-Dill Vinaigrette (page 189)
Tuscan Bean Salad (page 190)
Lentil Salad (page 191)
Warm Chickpea Salad (page 193)
Mediterranean Potato Salad (page 195)
Chicken Salad Amandine (page 196)
Thai-Style Beef Salad (page 198)
Baked Chicken and Potato Dinner (page 201)
Pesto Chicken Thighs (page 204)
Turkiaki Fiesta (page 213)
Baked Fish with Tomatoes and Roasted Red Pepper (page 217)
Salmon Burgers (page 223)
Sole and Spinach Casserole (page 224)

Sweet and Spicy Shrimp with Broccoli (page 228)
Garlic Chili Shrimp (page 229)
Coconut Shrimp Curry (page 230)
Meatball Pasta Sauce (page 237)
Homestyle Meatloaf (page 238)
Beef Lettuce Wraps (page 240)
Quick and Easy Cabbage Rolls (page 241)
Just Peachy Pork (page 243)
Orange Ginger Pork and Vegetables (page 244)
Teriyaki Pork Chops (page 245)
Savory Lamb Chops (page 246)
Chickpea-Herb Burgers (page 253)
Vegetarian Shepherd's Pie with Peppered Potato Topping (page 256)
Zucchini, Mushroom and Bean Loaf with Tomato Sauce (page 257)
Spinach Risotto (page 261)
Egg and Mushroom Fried Rice (page 262)
Green Beans with Cashews (page 268)
Spaghetti with Broccoli (page 275)
Linguine with Tuna, White Beans and Dill (page 276)
Tuna Garden Pasta (page 277)
Autumn Crumble (page 283)

SOURCE

Muesli Mix (page 143)
Banana Bread (page 145)
Healthy Cheese 'n' Herb Bread (page 146)
Zucchini Nut Loaf (page 148)
Coffee Cake (page 149)
Cranberry Oat Muffins (page 152)
Banana Oat Bran Muffins (page 153)
Banana Oatmeal Muffins (page 154)
Eggplant Dip (page 157)
Cauliflower Popcorn Snack (page 162)
Carrot Orange Soup (page 166)
Southwestern Sweet Potato Soup (page 167)
Sweet Green Pea Soup (page 169)
Borscht (page 174)
Mango, Strawberry and Cucumber Salad (page 179)
Asian Cucumber Salad (page 179)
Mandarin Orange Salad with Almonds (page 181)
Greek Summer Salad (page 184)
Spinach and Rice Salad (page 185)
Beet and Feta Salad (page 186)
Tabbouleh (page 192)
Bulgur Salad (page 194)
Vietnamese Chicken and Rice Noodle Salad (page 197)
Best-Ever Baked Chicken (page 200)
Yogurt-Marinated Chicken (page 202)
Ginger, Soy and Lime Chicken (page 203)
Crispy Chicken (page 205)
Grilled Honey-Ginger Chicken Breasts (page 206)
Honey Dijon Chicken (page 207)
Greek Lemon Chicken (page 208)
Sticky Sesame Chicken (page 209)
Parmesan Herb-Baked Fish Fillets (page 216)
South Side Halibut (page 218)
Honey Dill Salmon with Dijon (page 220)
Baked Lemon Salmon with Mango Salsa (page 221)
Soy-Glazed Salmon (page 222)
Parmesan-Crusted Snapper with Tomato Olive Sauce (page 226)
The Narrows Crab Cakes (page 227)
Spiced Veal Stir-fry (page 242)
Couscous (page 266)
Rapini with Balsamic Vinegar (page 267)
Green Beans and Tomato (page 269)
Cauliflower Casserole (page 270)
Cinnamon Baked Pears (page 282)
Buttermilk Oat-Banana Cake (page 284)
Chocolate Cupcakes (page 285)
Date Oatmeal Cake with Mocha Frosting (page 286)
Sunflower Cookies (page 287)
Reverse Chocolate Chip Cookies (page 288)
Grandma's Rolled Oat Cookies (page 289)
Lemony Biscotti (page 290)
Almond Crescents (page 291)
Berry Oatmeal Squares (page 292)
Vanilla Custard (page 293)
Orange Crème Caramel (page 294)

Fiber

EXCELLENT SOURCE

Breakfast Muesli to Go (page 143)
Muesli Mix (page 143)
Big-Batch Bran Muffins (page 150)
Black Bean Salsa (page 159)
Fassolada (page 170)
White Bean Soup with Swiss Chard (page 171)
Savory Red Lentil Soup (page 172)

Lemony Lentil Soup with Spinach (page 173)
Rice and Bean Salad (page 187)
Tasty Bean Salad (page 188)
White Bean Salad with Lemon-Dill Vinaigrette (page 189)
Tuscan Bean Salad (page 190)
Lentil Salad (page 191)
Warm Chickpea Salad (page 193)
Chicken Tacos (page 211)
Turkey Chili (page 214)
20-Minute Chili (page 235)
Mixed Winter Beans (page 248)
Chickpea Tofu Stew (page 251)
Vegetarian Chili (page 252)
Chickpea-Herb Burgers (page 253)
Spaghetti with Zucchini Balls and Tomato Sauce (page 254)
Lentil Spaghetti Sauce (page 255)
Vegetarian Shepherd's Pie with Peppered Potato Topping (page 256)
Zucchini, Mushroom and Bean Loaf with Tomato Sauce (page 257)
Falafel in Pita (page 260)
Roasted Yam Fajitas (page 258)
Swiss Chard Frittata in a Pita (page 263)
Spinach Frittata (page 264)
Pasta Fagioli Capra (page 273)

GOOD SOURCE

Creamy Microwave Oatmeal (page 144)
Carrot Bran Muffins (page 151)
Ginger Chili Sweet Potato Soup (page 168)
Crunchy Broccoli Salad (page 182)
Bulgur Salad (page 194)
Curried Chicken (page 210)
Turkiaki Fiesta (page 213)
Salmon with Roasted Vegetables (page 219)
Green Beans with Cashews (page 268)
Pasta with Goat Cheese, Snow Peas and Tomato Coulis (page 272)
Hoisin Stir-fried Vegetables and Tofu over Rice Noodles (page 274)
Spaghetti with Broccoli (page 275)
Linguine with Tuna, White Beans and Dill (page 276)
Mushroom-Spinach Lasagna with Goat Cheese (page 278)
Penne with Tuna and Peppers (page 280)
Cinnamon Baked Pears (page 282)

SOURCE

Fiber-Full Bran Pancakes (page 144)
Healthy Cheese 'n' Herb Bread (page 146)
Apricot Bran Bread (page 147)
Banana Oat Bran Muffins (page 153)
Banana Oatmeal Muffins (page 154)
Lentil Dip (page 156)
Eggplant Dip (page 157)
Tofu and Chickpea Garlic Dip (page 158)
Black and White Bean Salsa (page 160)
Portobello Mushrooms with Goat Cheese (page 161)
Granola (page 163)
Carrot Orange Soup (page 166)
Southwestern Sweet Potato Soup (page 167)
Sweet Green Pea Soup (page 169)
Asian Turkey and Noodle Soup (page 176)
Mango, Strawberry and Cucumber Salad (page 179)
Mandarin Orange Salad with Almonds (page 181)
Sonoma Chicken Salad (page 183)
Greek Summer Salad (page 184)
Beet and Feta Salad (page 186)
Tabbouleh (page 192)
Mediterranean Potato Salad (page 195)
Thai-Style Beef Salad (page 198)
Baked Chicken and Potato Dinner (page 201)
Salmon Burgers (page 223)
Sole and Spinach Casserole (page 224)
Beef Souvlaki (page 234)
Meatloaf "Muffins" with Barbecue Sauce (page 239)
Quick and Easy Cabbage Rolls (page 241)
Spiced Veal Stir-fry (page 242)
Just Peachy Pork (page 243)
Orange Ginger Pork and Vegetables (page 244)
Stir-fried Vegetables with Tofu (page 249)
Spinach Risotto (page 261)
Egg and Mushroom Fried Rice (page 262)
Couscous (page 266)
Rapini with Balsamic Vinegar (page 267)
Green Beans and Tomato (page 269)
Cauliflower Casserole (page 270)
Tuna Garden Pasta (page 277)
Autumn Crumble (page 283)
Buttermilk Oat-Banana Cake (page 284)
Date Oatmeal Cake with Mocha Frosting (page 286)
Grandma's Rolled Oat Cookies (page 289)
Berry Oatmeal Squares (page 292)

Breakfasts

Sunny Orange Shake. 142

Banana Berry Wake-Up Shake 142

Breakfast Muesli to Go 143

Muesli Mix 143

Creamy Microwave Oatmeal 144

Fiber-Full Bran Pancakes. 144

Banana Bread 145

Healthy Cheese 'n' Herb Bread 146

Apricot Bran Bread 147

Zucchini Nut Loaf. 148

Coffee Cake 149

Big-Batch Bran Muffins 150

Carrot Bran Muffins 151

Cranberry Oat Muffins 152

Banana Oat Bran Muffins. 153

Banana Oatmeal Muffins 154

Sunny Orange Shake

MAKES 1 SERVING

This shake, like the Banana Berry Wake-Up Shake (see recipe, below), is packed with bone-building calcium.

¾ cup	low-fat vanilla yogurt	175 mL
½ cup	orange juice	125 mL
2 tbsp	skim-milk powder	25 mL

1. In a blender, combine yogurt, orange juice and skim-milk powder; blend until smooth.

NUTRITIONAL ANALYSIS PER SERVING

| Energy: 206 kcal | Fat: 1 g | Fiber: 0.1 g | Iron: 0.3 mg |
| Protein: 16 g | Carbohydrate: 35 g | Calcium: 532 mg | Folate: 86 mcg |

Banana Berry Wake-Up Shake

MAKES 2 SERVINGS

This creamy shake, which can be made the night before, is a great way to use up ripe bananas that have been frozen. When bananas start to get brown, pop them in the freezer and take out as needed.

1	banana	1
1 cup	fresh or frozen berries (any combination)	250 mL
1 cup	milk or vanilla-flavored soy milk	250 mL
¾ cup	low-fat vanilla yogurt (or other flavor that complements berries)	175 mL

1. In a blender, liquefy banana and berries with a small amount of the milk. Add remaining milk and yogurt; blend until smooth. If shake is too thick, add extra milk or soy milk to achieve desired consistency.

NUTRITIONAL ANALYSIS PER SERVING

| Energy: 200 kcal | Fat: 3 g | Fiber: 2.8 g | Iron: 0.5 mg |
| Protein: 10 g | Carbohydrate: 35 g | Calcium: 348 mg | Folate: 38 mcg |

Breakfast Muesli to Go

1 cup	large-flake or 3-minute oats (not instant)	250 mL
1 cup	low-fat plain yogurt	250 mL
½ cup	2% milk	125 mL
2 tbsp	liquid honey or pure maple syrup	25 mL
1 cup	assorted berries (fresh or frozen)	250 mL
1	large banana, sliced	1

1. In a plastic container, combine oats, yogurt, milk and honey; gently fold in berries. Add banana before serving or add to sealable container before taking muesli on the go.

NUTRITIONAL ANALYSIS PER SERVING

Energy: 409 kcal	Fat: 5 g	Fiber: 7.6 g	Iron: 2.4 mg
Protein: 18 g	Carbohydrate: 78 g	Calcium: 370 mg	Folate: 53 mcg

Health Tip

Oats are a great source of soluble fiber, which can help prevent constipation and decrease the risk of developing hemorrhoids. The fiber in oats can also help to keep blood sugar levels lower.

Excellent source of:
- Calcium and fiber

Good source of:
- Folate and iron

MAKES 2 SERVINGS

This complete breakfast works well for people on the go as it is best if made the night before. Divide into 2 sealable containers and leave room to add some banana.

TIP

For variety, try serving this muesli with different types of yogurt and fresh fruit in season. If using vanilla or fruit-flavored yogurt, you can omit the honey or reduce the amount you use.

Muesli Mix

4 cups	quick-cooking rolled oats	1 L
1 cup	dried cranberries	250 mL
½ cup	flax seeds	125 mL
½ cup	wheat germ	125 mL
½ cup	oat bran	125 mL
½ cup	wheat bran	125 mL

1. In a large bowl, mix together oats, cranberries, flax seeds, wheat germ, oat bran and wheat bran. Pour into an airtight container. Store in a cool, dry place.

NUTRITIONAL ANALYSIS PER SERVING

Energy: 180 kcal	Fat: 5 g	Fiber: 6.8 g	Iron: 2.0 mg
Protein: 7 g	Carbohydrate: 31 g	Calcium: 34 mg	Folate: 28 mcg

Excellent source of:
- Fiber

Source of:
- Folate and iron

MAKES 14 SERVINGS

TIPS

Store flax seeds and wheat germ in the refrigerator because of their high fat content.

To add even more fiber and nutrients to this high-fiber cereal, try serving it with peaches and blueberries, topped with yogurt.

Good source of:
- Calcium, iron and fiber

Source of:
- Folate

MAKES 1 SERVING

This breakfast provides both soluble fiber from oatmeal and insoluble fiber from wheat bran. Including both types of fiber in your diet is beneficial to long-term health.

TIP

Here's an easy way to boost your calcium intake: When preparing hot cereal, substitute milk for half of the water called for in the package directions.

Creamy Microwave Oatmeal

½ cup	milk or soy milk	125 mL
2 tbsp	raisins	25 mL
1 tsp	wheat bran	5 mL
Pinch	salt	Pinch
½ cup	quick-cooking rolled oats	125 mL
¼ tsp	ground cinnamon	1 mL

1. In a 4-cup (1 L) microwave-safe bowl, combine ½ cup (125 mL) water, milk, raisins, bran and salt. Microwave on High for 2 minutes. Stir in oats and cinnamon; microwave on High for 3 to 4 minutes, stirring at 1-minute intervals, or until oatmeal has thickened. Cover and let stand for 1 minute. Serve with brown sugar or maple syrup and milk.

NUTRITIONAL ANALYSIS PER SERVING			
Energy: 278 kcal	Fat: 5 g	Fiber: 5.5 g	Iron: 2.5 mg
Protein: 12 g	Carbohydrate: 48 g	Calcium: 199 mg	Folate: 22 mcg

Good source of:
- Iron

Source of:
- Calcium, folate and fiber

MAKES 8 PANCAKES

These flavorful pancakes can help boost your fiber intake. They are especially delicious with maple syrup or fruit preserves.

Fiber-Full Bran Pancakes

¾ cup	whole wheat flour	175 mL
½ cup	bran cereal flakes, crushed	125 mL
¼ cup	wheat germ	50 mL
1½ tsp	baking powder	7 mL
Pinch	salt	Pinch
1	egg	1
1	egg white	1
1 cup	milk	250 mL
1 tbsp	vegetable oil	15 mL

1. In a medium bowl, combine flour, bran flakes, wheat germ, baking powder and salt. Set aside.

2. In a small bowl, blend together egg, egg white, milk and oil; stir into bran mixture until combined. Heat nonstick griddle or skillet over medium heat. For each pancake, pour about ¼ cup (50 mL) batter onto griddle. Cook, turning once, for about 1 to 2 minutes per side or until golden.

NUTRITIONAL ANALYSIS PER SERVING (2 PANCAKES)			
Energy: 222 kcal	Fat: 7 g	Fiber: 5.2 g	Iron: 4.2 mg
Protein: 10 g	Carbohydrate: 31 g	Calcium: 116 mg	Folate: 44 mcg

Banana Bread

- Preheat oven to 350°F (180°C)
- 9- by 5-inch (2 L) loaf pan, greased

1¼ cups	all-purpose flour	300 mL
1 tsp	baking soda	5 mL
½ tsp	baking powder	2 mL
1	egg	1
1	egg white	1
¾ cup	granulated sugar	175 mL
¼ cup	low-fat plain yogurt	50 mL
¼ cup	vegetable oil	50 mL
1 tsp	vanilla	5 mL
1 cup	mashed ripe bananas (about 2 to 3 medium)	250 mL

1. In a bowl, sift together flour, baking soda and baking powder. Set aside.

2. In a large mixing bowl, blend egg, egg white, sugar, yogurt, oil and vanilla. Blend in bananas. Add dry ingredients; mix until just combined. Pour batter into prepared pan. Bake in preheated oven for 1 hour or until a tester inserted in center of loaf comes out clean.

Variation

Banana Muffins: To make a muffin version of this recipe, spoon batter into 12 greased or paper-lined muffin cups. Bake at 350°F (180°C) for 18 to 22 minutes or until firm to the touch.

NUTRITIONAL ANALYSIS PER SERVING (1 OF 12 SLICES)			
Energy: 163 kcal	Fat: 5 g	Fiber: 0.8 g	Iron: 0.7 mg
Protein: 3 g	Carbohydrate: 27 g	Calcium: 15 mg	Folate: 12 mcg

Source of:
- Folate and iron

MAKES 1 LOAF

For variety, try adding a handful of fresh blueberries, frozen cranberries or chocolate chips to the batter when baking this family favorite.

TIPS

As this loaf freezes well, why not make an extra one and freeze it for later use? You can also slice and freeze individual servings and have them ready to include in lunch bags.

To increase the fiber content of this recipe, substitute up to ½ cup (125 mL) whole wheat flour for the same quantity of all-purpose flour. If your bananas are extremely ripe, you can reduce the sugar to ½ cup (125 mL).

MAKES 1 LOAF

Containing cheese, milk and sesame seeds, this delicious bread is a great way to add calcium to your diet. Serve with a hearty soup for an easy lunch or light supper.

TIP

If you're out of sesame seeds, sprinkle this loaf with chopped walnuts before baking.

Healthy Cheese 'n' Herb Bread

- Preheat oven to 400°F (200°C)
- 8-inch (20 cm) round pan, nonstick or lightly greased

2 cups	all-purpose flour	500 mL
1 cup	whole wheat flour	250 mL
½ cup	rolled oats	125 mL
1 tbsp	granulated sugar	15 mL
2 tsp	baking powder	10 mL
1 tsp	dried basil	5 mL
½ tsp	baking soda	2 mL
½ tsp	dried oregano	2 mL
½ tsp	salt	2 mL
¼ cup	cold butter or margarine	50 mL
1 cup	shredded Swiss cheese	250 mL
1	egg	1
1 cup	buttermilk	250 mL
2 tbsp	sesame seeds	25 mL

1. In a medium bowl, combine all-purpose flour, whole wheat flour, oats, sugar, baking powder, basil, baking soda, oregano and salt. Using a pastry blender, cut in butter until mixture resembles fine crumbs. Stir in cheese.

2. Beat together egg and buttermilk; add to butter mixture, stirring with fork to make a soft moist dough. Place dough in prepared pan. Sprinkle with sesame seeds. Bake in preheated oven for 25 to 30 minutes or until tester inserted in center comes out clean. Cut into 10 wedges to serve.

NUTRITIONAL ANALYSIS PER SERVING (1 OF 10 SLICES)			
Energy: 306 kcal	Fat: 13 g	Fiber: 3.1 g	Iron: 2.0 mg
Protein: 13 g	Carbohydrate: 35 g	Calcium: 277 mg	Folate: 20 mcg

Apricot Bran Bread

- Preheat oven to 350°F (180°C)
- 8- by 4-inch (1.5 L) loaf pan, nonstick or lightly greased

2 cups	bran cereal flakes	500 mL
¾ cup	chopped dried apricots	175 mL
½ cup	all-purpose flour	125 mL
½ cup	whole wheat flour	125 mL
½ cup	packed brown sugar	125 mL
2 tsp	baking powder	10 mL
1 tsp	grated orange zest	5 mL
½ tsp	salt	2 mL
½ tsp	ground nutmeg	2 mL
1	egg, lightly beaten	1
½ cup	skim milk	125 mL
½ cup	freshly squeezed orange juice	125 mL
¼ cup	vegetable oil	50 mL

1. Crush cereal flakes to make ¾ cup (175 mL) crumbs. In a large bowl, combine cereal, apricots, all-purpose flour, whole wheat flour, brown sugar, baking powder, orange zest salt and nutmeg.

2. In a second bowl, beat together egg, milk, orange juice and oil; stir into dry ingredients until well combined. Pour into prepared pan. Bake in preheated oven for about 55 minutes or until tester inserted in center comes out clean. Cool for 10 minutes before removing from pan. Cool completely on wire rack.

NUTRITIONAL ANALYSIS PER SERVING (1 OF 14 SLICES)

Energy: 140 kcal	Fat: 4 g	Fiber: 2.4 g	Iron: 2.5 mg
Protein: 3 g	Carbohydrate: 25 g	Calcium: 35 mg	Folate: 29 mcg

Health Tip

Apricots are an excellent source of vitamins A and C. Vitamin A is important for healthy sight and for healing wounds, while vitamin C is an antioxidant, keeping cells healthy and strong.

Good source of:
- Iron

Source of:
- Folate and fiber

MAKES 1 LOAF

This tasty and nutritious quick bread freezes well. Keep some in the freezer for unexpected guests.

TIPS

Freeze this and other quick breads in individually wrapped single slices. Pop them into lunch bags. They will be defrosted by the time lunch comes around.

Although we tend to think of bran as a cereal and breakfast food, it can be used to add flavor as well as nutrition to many different dishes. Try using bran in meat loaf, instead of bread crumbs, or as a coating for baked chicken or fish, as well as in its more traditional roles in muffins and breads.

Apricots are a great snack — carry some in your purse for an energy boost. Try them mixed with nuts and seeds.

Zucchini Nut Loaf

MAKES 1 LOAF

This classic quick bread freezes well. Wrap individual slices in plastic wrap and freeze. Pop into the toaster to defrost.

TIP

To reduce the fat in this recipe, substitute ½ cup (125 mL) chopped fruit or raisins for the nuts.

• Preheat oven to 350°F (180°C)
• 8- by 4-inch (1.5 L) loaf pan, greased

1½ cups	all-purpose flour	375 mL
1 tsp	ground cinnamon	5 mL
½ tsp	baking soda	2 mL
½ tsp	salt	2 mL
½ tsp	ground nutmeg	2 mL
¼ tsp	baking powder	1 mL
1	egg	1
¾ cup	granulated sugar	175 mL
⅓ cup	vegetable oil	75 mL
2 tbsp	2% milk	25 mL
1 cup	shredded zucchini (unpeeled)	250 mL
½ cup	chopped walnuts or pecans	125 mL
½ tsp	grated lemon zest (optional)	2 mL

1. In a large bowl, combine flour, cinnamon, baking soda, salt, nutmeg and baking powder.

2. In a medium bowl, beat egg; whisk in sugar, oil and milk. Stir in zucchini, nuts and lemon zest (if using); stir zucchini mixture into dry ingredients.

3. Pour batter into prepared pan. Bake in preheated oven for 50 minutes or until tester inserted in center comes out clean. Cool for 10 minutes in pan. Turn out onto rack to cool completely.

NUTRITIONAL ANALYSIS PER SERVING (1 OF 10 SLICES)			
Energy: 307 kcal	Fat: 12 g	Fiber: 1.8 g	Iron: 1.9 mg
Protein: 6 g	Carbohydrate: 45 g	Calcium: 22 mg	Folate: 19 mcg

Health Tip

Zucchini is a good source of vitamin C. Vitamin C is a powerful antioxidant, which means that it protects cells and tissue from damage caused by oxidation (a natural process that occurs as the body ages). Vitamin C also helps the body absorb iron.

Coffee Cake

- Preheat oven to 350°F (180°C)
- 8-inch (2 L) glass baking dish, greased

¾ cup	all-purpose flour	175 mL
¼ cup	whole wheat flour	50 mL
2 tsp	baking powder	10 mL
1 tsp	baking soda	5 mL
1 cup	granulated sugar	250 mL
½ cup	butter, softened	125 mL
2	eggs	2
1 tsp	vanilla	5 mL
1 cup	plain yogurt	250 mL
½ cup	packed brown sugar	125 mL
½ cup	chopped pecans	125 mL
2 tsp	ground cinnamon	10 mL

1. In a small bowl, combine all-purpose flour, whole wheat flour, baking powder and baking soda.

2. In a large bowl, cream sugar and butter until light and fluffy. Beat in eggs and vanilla. Beat in flour mixture and yogurt. Pour about half the batter into baking dish.

3. In the same small bowl, combine brown sugar, pecans and cinnamon. Sprinkle half of the nut mixture evenly on top of the batter. Pour in the remaining batter and sprinkle with the remaining nut mixture.

4. Bake in preheated oven for about 40 minutes, or until a tester inserted in the center comes our clean. Let cool on a wire rack.

NUTRITIONAL ANALYSIS PER SERVING (1 OF 12 SLICES)			
Energy: 269 kcal	Fat: 13 g	Fiber: 1.0 g	Iron: 1.1 mg
Protein: 3 g	Carbohydrate: 35 g	Calcium: 54 mg	Folate: 12 mcg

Source of:
- Folate and iron

MAKES 12 SERVINGS

Try this delicious light cake at any time of the day.

TIP

For added fiber, use ½ cup (125 mL) all-purpose flour and ½ cup (125 mL) whole wheat flour. The cake will be slightly heavier in texture.

Make ahead

Wrap in plastic wrap, then foil, and store at room temperature for up to 2 days or in the freezer for up to 2 months.

MAKES 24 MUFFINS

Eating bran muffins for breakfast, or as a snack anytime during the day, is a great way to add fiber to your diet. Bran promotes regularity and a healthy digestive system. Pack these muffins with a shake for a quick meal to go.

TIP

Sour milk can be used instead of buttermilk. To prepare, combine 3 tbsp (45 mL) freshly squeezed lemon juice or vinegar with 4 cups (1 L) milk and let stand for 5 minutes.

Make ahead

This batter can be prepared and stored for up to 2 weeks in the refrigerator. Pour batter into prepared muffin tins and bake as needed. Or you can bake the whole batch and keep extras in the freezer.

Big-Batch Bran Muffins

• Preheat oven to 375°F (190°C)
• Two 12-cup muffin tins, greased or paper-lined

5½ cups	100% bran cereal	1.375 L
5 cups	all-purpose flour	1.25 L
2 cups	packed brown sugar	500 mL
1 cup	chopped dates or raisins	250 mL
1 tbsp	baking soda	15 mL
1 tbsp	ground cinnamon	15 mL
4	eggs	4
4 cups	buttermilk or sour milk (see tip, at left)	1 L
1 cup	vegetable oil	250 mL

1. In a large bowl, combine cereal, flour, brown sugar, dates, baking soda and cinnamon.

2. In another large bowl, mix together eggs, buttermilk and oil. Stir into dry ingredients and mix until moistened.

3. Spoon batter into muffin cups, filling to the top. Bake in preheated oven for 25 to 30 minutes or until golden brown. Cool in pans for 5 minutes; remove muffins. Cool on a wire rack. Store in airtight containers; freeze, if desired.

NUTRITIONAL ANALYSIS PER SERVING (1 MUFFIN)			
Energy: 366 kcal	Fat: 12 g	Fiber: 8.1 g	Iron: 7.7 mg
Protein: 8 g	Carbohydrate: 63 g	Calcium: 97 mg	Folate: 18 mcg

Health Tip

Bran cereal is an excellent source of fiber and is also loaded with B vitamins, iron and zinc.

Carrot Bran Muffins

- Preheat oven to 400°F (200°C)
- One 12-cup muffin tin, greased or paper-lined

1¼ cups	whole wheat flour	300 mL
1¼ cups	high-fiber bran cereal	300 mL
1 tsp	baking powder	5 mL
1 tsp	baking soda	5 mL
1 tsp	ground cinnamon	5 mL
½ tsp	ground nutmeg	2 mL
½ tsp	salt	2 mL
2	eggs	2
1 cup	grated carrots	250 mL
¾ cup	buttermilk	175 mL
⅓ cup	packed brown sugar	75 mL
¼ cup	vegetable oil	50 mL
½ cup	raisins	125 mL

1. In a large bowl, combine flour, cereal, baking powder, baking soda, cinnamon, nutmeg and salt.

2. In a separate bowl, beat eggs thoroughly; blend in carrots, buttermilk, brown sugar and vegetable oil. Add to dry ingredients, stirring just until moistened. Stir in raisins.

3. Spoon batter into prepared muffin cups, filling about three-quarters full. Bake in preheated oven for about 20 minutes or until tops of muffins spring back when lightly touched.

MAKES 12 MUFFINS

Two favorites, carrot and bran, are combined in this tasty muffin. A great start to any day!

TIPS

When making these muffins, keep wet and dry ingredients separate until you're ready to mix, then mix just enough to blend the two components. This produces a coarse crumb that is just fine for these muffins.

Start your day right by eating one of these muffins for fiber accompanied by a Banana Berry Wake-Up Shake (see recipe, page 142) for calcium and vitamins. The bran in these muffins provides insoluble fiber, which aids in regularity. As you increase your fiber intake, remember to drink more fluids to help the fiber work more effectively.

NUTRITIONAL ANALYSIS PER SERVING (1 MUFFIN)			
Energy: 168 kcal	Fat: 5 g	Fiber: 4.5 g	Iron: 3.6 mg
Protein: 5 g	Carbohydrate: 29 g	Calcium: 50 mg	Folate: 43 mcg

Cranberry Oat Muffins

**MAKES
12 MUFFINS**

These tart, tasty muffins can be enjoyed year-round if you freeze fresh cranberries when they are available in the fall. It is unnecessary to thaw cranberries before using in this recipe.

TIPS

If fresh or frozen cranberries are not available, try soaking ¾ cup (175 mL) dried cranberries in ½ cup (125 mL) orange juice or water for about 15 minutes, or replace cranberries with blueberries.

These tangy muffins, along with fresh fruit, cottage cheese and a glass of milk, make a great get-up-and-go start to the day; you get fiber, calcium and many other valuable vitamins and minerals.

• Preheat oven to 400°F (200°C)
• One 12-cup muffin tin, greased or paper-lined

¾ cup	old-fashioned rolled oats	175 mL
1½ cups	all-purpose flour, divided	375 mL
1 cup	granulated sugar	250 mL
2 tsp	baking powder	10 mL
½ tsp	salt	2 mL
½ cup	butter or margarine	125 mL
1½ cups	fresh or frozen cranberries, chopped	375 mL
1	egg, beaten	1
⅔ cup	2% milk	150 mL
2 tsp	grated lemon zest	10 mL

Topping

2 tsp	ground cinnamon	10 mL
2 tsp	granulated sugar	10 mL

1. In a food processor or blender, process oats until very fine. Combine oats, flour (except for 2 tbsp/25 mL), sugar, baking powder and salt. Cut in butter with a pastry blender or food processor until mixture resembles coarse crumbs.

2. Toss cranberries with reserved flour; stir into flour mixture.

3. Combine egg, milk and lemon zest; mix thoroughly. Add to dry ingredients, stirring just until moistened; do not overmix. Spoon into lightly greased or paper-lined muffin cups, filling three-quarters full.

4. *Prepare the topping:* Combine cinnamon and sugar; sprinkle over muffins.

5. Bake in preheated oven for 20 to 24 minutes or until tops of muffins spring back when lightly touched.

NUTRITIONAL ANALYSIS PER SERVING (1 MUFFIN)			
Energy: 240 kcal	Fat: 9 g	Fiber: 1.2 g	Iron: 1.5 mg
Protein: 3 g	Carbohydrate: 36 g	Calcium: 38 mg	Folate: 9 mcg

Health Tip

Cranberries provide vitamin C, an important antioxidant, and are a good source of vitamin K, which plays an important role in blood clotting and bone metabolism.

Banana Oat Bran Muffins

Source of:
• Folate, iron and fiber

MAKES 12 MUFFINS

- Preheat oven to 400°F (200°C)
- 12-cup muffin tin, lightly greased

¾ cup	oat bran	175 mL
½ cup	quick-cooking rolled oats	125 mL
½ cup	natural wheat bran	125 mL
½ cup	whole wheat flour	125 mL
½ cup	all-purpose flour	125 mL
½ cup	lightly packed brown sugar	125 mL
1 tbsp	baking powder	15 mL
½ tsp	baking soda	2 mL
½ tsp	ground cinnamon	2 mL
Pinch	salt	Pinch
2	eggs, lightly beaten	2
1 cup	mashed ripe bananas (about 3)	250 mL
½ cup	skim milk	125 mL
½ cup	butter, melted	125 mL

This is a terrific recipe for expectant moms who need a little fiber boost. These muffins aren't too sweet and are really quick to prepare, so they're an excellent on-the-go breakfast or snack choice. They also freeze very well, which means they're always fresh when you eat them!

1. In a large bowl, combine oat bran, oats, wheat bran, whole wheat flour, all-purpose flour, brown sugar, baking powder, baking soda, cinnamon and salt.

2. In a medium bowl, whisk together eggs, bananas, milk and butter. Add to flour mixture and mix with a wooden spoon until just combined. Pour evenly into prepared muffin cups.

3. Bake in preheated oven for 20 minutes or until a toothpick inserted in the center of a muffin comes out clean. Let cool on a wire rack.

TIP

Natural wheat bran and oat bran can both be found in most large grocery stores. They are usually kept in the hot cereal aisle.

Make ahead

Wrap in plastic wrap, then place in a freezer bag and store in the freezer for up to 2 months.

NUTRITIONAL ANALYSIS PER SERVING (1 MUFFIN)			
Energy: 216 kcal	Fat: 10 g	Fiber: 3.7 g	Iron: 1.7 mg
Protein: 5 g	Carbohydrate: 31 g	Calcium: 48 mg	Folate: 21 mcg

MAKES 6 MUFFINS

Although muffins can be frozen, they are always best when freshly baked. The toaster oven is perfect for making small batches.

Banana Oatmeal Muffins

• Preheat toaster oven to 400°F (200°C)
• 6-cup muffin tin, lightly greased

1 cup	all-purpose flour	250 mL
½ cup	old-fashioned rolled oats	125 mL
⅓ cup	packed brown sugar	75 mL
¾ tsp	baking powder	4 mL
½ tsp	baking soda	2 mL
½ tsp	ground cinnamon	2 mL
¼ tsp	salt	1 mL
1	egg	1
½ cup	mashed ripe banana (about 1)	125 mL
½ cup	buttermilk	125 mL
¼ cup	vegetable oil	50 mL
½ tsp	vanilla	2 mL

Topping

2 tbsp	packed brown sugar	25 mL
1 tbsp	old-fashioned rolled oats	15 mL

1. In a large bowl, combine flour, oats, brown sugar, baking powder, baking soda, cinnamon and salt.

2. In a separate bowl, beat egg. Stir in mashed banana, buttermilk, oil and vanilla.

3. Add wet ingredients to dry ingredients. Stir just to combine. Spoon batter into muffin cups.

4. *Prepare the topping:* In a small bowl, combine brown sugar and rolled oats. Sprinkle topping over muffins.

5. Bake in preheated toaster oven for 18 to 20 minutes, or until tops of muffins spring back when lightly touched in center. Turn pan halfway through cooking time. Cool muffins in pan for 5 minutes before turning out onto a rack.

Variation

Banana Chocolate Chip Muffins: Add ½ cup (125 mL) chocolate chips to dry ingredients.

NUTRITIONAL ANALYSIS PER SERVING (1 MUFFIN)			
Energy: 277 kcal	Fat: 10 g	Fiber: 2.1 g	Iron: 2 mg
Protein: 5 g	Carbohydrate: 43 g	Calcium: 69 mg	Folate: 17 mcg

Appetizers and Snacks

Cottage Cheese Herb Dip 156

Lentil Dip 156

Eggplant Dip 157

Tofu and Chickpea Garlic Dip 158

Hummus. 158

Tzatziki Sauce 159

Black Bean Salsa 159

Black and White Bean Salsa. 160

Portobello Mushrooms with Goat Cheese 161

Cauliflower Popcorn Snack 162

Granola 163

No-Bake Trail Mix 164

MAKES 1½ CUPS (375 ML)

This dip will enhance any lazy summer afternoon. For best results, prepare ahead of time and refrigerate.

Cottage Cheese Herb Dip

1 cup	low-fat cottage cheese	250 mL
½ cup	low-fat plain yogurt	125 mL
1	green onion, chopped	1
½ tsp	garlic powder	2 mL
½ tsp	celery seed	2 mL
¼ tsp	dry mustard	1 mL
¼ tsp	Worcestershire sauce	1 mL
Pinch	freshly ground black pepper	Pinch
Dash	hot pepper sauce	Dash

1. In a food processor or blender, cream cottage cheese and yogurt until very smooth. Stir in onion, garlic powder, celery seed, mustard, Worcestershire sauce, pepper and hot pepper sauce. Chill overnight.

NUTRITIONAL ANALYSIS PER SERVING (¼ CUP/50 ML)			
Energy: 44 kcal	Fat: Trace	Fiber: 0.1 g	Iron: 0.2 mg
Protein: 6 g	Carbohydrate: 3 g	Calcium: 70 mg	Folate: 8 mcg

MAKES 1½ CUPS (375 ML)

This high-fiber dip can be enjoyed with tortilla chips, vegetables or fresh bread.

Make ahead

Place in an airtight container and store in the refrigerator for up to 2 days.

Lentil Dip

1 cup	red lentils, rinsed	250 mL
1	clove garlic, minced	1
⅓ cup	olive oil	75 mL
¼ cup	freshly squeezed lemon juice	50 mL
2 tbsp	minced onion	25 mL
1 tsp	ground cumin	5 mL
½ tsp	salt	2 mL

1. In a small saucepan, bring 1½ cups (375 mL) water and lentils to a boil over high heat and boil for 4 minutes. Remove from heat. Cover and let stand until lentils are tender and water is absorbed, about 15 minutes.

2. In a food processor, process lentils, garlic, olive oil, lemon juice, onion, cumin and salt until smooth and creamy.

NUTRITIONAL ANALYSIS PER SERVING (1 TBSP/15 ML)			
Energy: 53 kcal	Fat: 3 g	Fiber: 2.3 g	Iron: 0.6 mg
Protein: 2 g	Carbohydrate: 5 g	Calcium: 6 mg	Folate: 37 mcg

Eggplant Dip

- Preheat oven to 450°F (230°C)

1	eggplant (about 1 lb/500 g)	1
1 tsp	vegetable oil	5 mL
2	cloves garlic, roughly chopped	2
½ cup	chopped onion	125 mL
¼ cup	packed chopped fresh parsley	50 mL
1 tbsp	freshly squeezed lemon juice	15 mL
1 tsp	red wine vinegar	5 mL
1 tsp	Dijon mustard	5 mL
½ tsp	dried basil	2 mL
½ tsp	dried oregano	2 mL
¼ cup	olive oil	50 mL
	Salt and freshly ground black pepper	
¼ cup	whole black olives (about 8)	50 mL

1. Brush eggplant lightly with vegetable oil. Using a fork, pierce the skin lightly at 1-inch (2.5 cm) intervals. Place on a baking sheet and bake for 1 hour, or until eggplant is very soft and the skin is dark brown and caved in.

2. Transfer eggplant to a working surface. Cut off 1 inch (2.5 cm) at the stem end and discard (this part never quite cooks through). Peel the eggplant by picking at an edge from the cut end, then pulling upward. The skin should come off easily in strips.

3. Cut the eggplant lengthwise and place each half with the interior facing you. With a spoon scoop out the tongues of seed-pods, leaving as much of the flesh as possible. To remove the additional seed-pods hiding inside, cut each piece of eggplant in half and repeat the deseeding procedure. Once deseeded, let cleaned eggplant sit to shed some of its excess water.

4. Put garlic, onions, parsley, lemon juice, vinegar, mustard, basil and oregano into the bowl of a food processor; process at medium and then at high speed, until ingredients are homogenized. With motor still running, add olive oil through feed tube in a very thin stream until emulsified.

5. Add deseeded eggplant flesh to the food processor; pulse on and off, just until incorporated. Transfer to a serving bowl, season to taste with salt and pepper and garnish with black olives.

NUTRITIONAL ANALYSIS PER SERVING

Energy: 167 kcal	Fat: 14 g	Fiber: 3.9 g	Iron: 1.3 mg
Protein: 2 g	Carbohydrate: 11 g	Calcium: 72 mg	Folate: 32 mcg

Source of:
- Calcium, folate, iron and fiber

MAKES 4 SERVINGS

Creamy and vibrantly flavored, this version of baked eggplant purée — and there are many, from Indian to Greek — is refreshing and memorable.

Make ahead

Cover and keep at room temperature for up to 2 hours. If refrigerated, let it come back to room temperature and give it a couple of stirs before serving.

**MAKES
6 TO 8 SERVINGS**

Tofu combined with beans, such as the chickpeas used here, gives the dip a butter-like texture. Serve with vegetables, crackers or bread.

TIP

Make sure to buy tofu that has been coagulated with calcium sulfate or calcium chloride. Read the ingredient list on the label for the coagulant. Otherwise, you won't get nearly as much calcium out of this recipe.

Tofu and Chickpea Garlic Dip

8 oz	soft (silken) tofu, drained	250 g
1 cup	rinsed and drained canned chickpeas	250 mL
2 tbsp	tahini (see tip, below left)	25 mL
2 tbsp	freshly squeezed lemon juice	25 mL
1 tsp	minced garlic	5 mL
1/4 cup	chopped fresh dill (or 1 tsp/5 mL dried)	50 mL
1/4 cup	chopped green onions	50 mL
1/4 cup	chopped green olives	50 mL
1/4 cup	chopped red bell peppers	50 mL
1/4 tsp	freshly ground black pepper	1 mL

1. In a food processor, combine tofu, chickpeas, tahini, lemon juice and garlic; purée. Stir in dill, green onions, olives, red peppers and pepper. Cover and refrigerate for up to 1 day. Stir before serving.

NUTRITIONAL ANALYSIS PER SERVING (1 OF 8)			
Energy: 87 kcal	Fat: 5 g	Fiber: 2.2 g	Iron: 2.7 mg
Protein: 5 g	Carbohydrate: 8 g	Calcium: 121 mg	Folate: 41 mcg

**MAKES 1 CUP
(250 ML)**

TIPS

Tahini is a Middle Eastern condiment found in the specialty section of some supermarkets. If you can't find it, use smooth peanut butter instead.

Surround the dip with crackers, fresh vegetable sticks or pita bread pieces.

Hummus

1 cup	drained canned chickpeas	250 mL
1/4 cup	tahini	50 mL
2 tbsp	freshly squeezed lemon juice	25 mL
4 tsp	olive oil	20 mL
3/4 tsp	crushed garlic	4 mL
1 tbsp	chopped fresh parsley	15 mL

1. In a food processor, combine chickpeas, 1/4 cup (50 mL) water, tahini, lemon juice, oil and garlic; process until creamy and smooth.
2. Transfer to a serving dish and sprinkle with parsley.

NUTRITIONAL ANALYSIS PER SERVING (1 TBSP/15 ML)			
Energy: 48 kcal	Fat: 3 g	Fiber: 1.1 g	Iron: 0.6 mg
Protein: 2 g	Carbohydrate: 4 g	Calcium: 21 mg	Folate: 21 mcg

Tzatziki Sauce

½ cup	peeled, coarsely shredded English cucumber	125 mL
1 cup	yogurt	250 mL
2	cloves garlic	2
	Salt	
1 tsp	extra-virgin olive oil	5 mL
Pinch	cayenne pepper or paprika	Pinch

1. Drain cucumber through a strainer, pressing by hand to extract as much juice as possible (you can save this juice and use it as an astringent for the face).

2. In a bowl, stir together cucumber shreds and yogurt. Press garlic through a garlic press directly into bowl; mix in. Season to taste with salt.

3. Transfer sauce to a serving bowl and let rest for 30 minutes. Drizzle with olive oil and sprinkle with cayenne (for spicy) or paprika (for mild) just before serving.

NUTRITIONAL ANALYSIS PER SERVING (¼ CUP/50 ML)

| Energy: 40 kcal | Fat: 2 g | Fiber: 0.1 g | Iron: 0.1 mg |
| Protein: 2 g | Carbohydrate: 3 g | Calcium: 62 mg | Folate: 5 mcg |

Source of:
• Calcium

MAKES 1⅓ CUPS (325 ML)

A relative (and a descendant) of Afghani/Indian raitas, this soothing yogurt-based sauce is a lovely complement to Greek-style fried zucchini and a wonderful dip for raw vegetables.

TIP

Tzatziki sauce is best when made ahead, but after 3 days it gets too garlicky.

Make ahead

Cover and store in the refrigerator for up to 3 days. Bring to room temperature before serving.

Black Bean Salsa

1	can (19 oz/540 mL) black beans, drained and rinsed	1
1 cup	drained canned corn kernels	250 mL
1 cup	diced tomatoes	250 mL
2 tbsp	freshly squeezed lime juice or cider vinegar	25 mL
2 tbsp	finely chopped fresh cilantro or parsley	25 mL
1 tbsp	extra-virgin olive oil	15 mL
½ tsp	minced garlic	2 mL
Pinch	freshly ground black pepper	Pinch

1. In a medium bowl, gently toss together beans, corn, tomatoes, lime juice, cilantro, oil, garlic and pepper.

NUTRITIONAL ANALYSIS PER SERVING (½ CUP/125 ML)

| Energy: 133 kcal | Fat: 3 g | Fiber: 6.8 g | Iron: 2.3 mg |
| Protein: 7 g | Carbohydrate: 22 g | Calcium: 24 mg | Folate: 102 mcg |

Excellent source of:
• Folate and fiber

Good source of:
• Iron

MAKES ABOUT 3 CUPS (750 ML)

Eating more meals with beans and corn is one way to increase your intake of fiber and folic acid. Serve this zesty salsa with baked tortilla chips or as a condiment for any plain grilled or baked meat, fish or chicken.

**MAKES 3 CUPS
(750 ML)**

*Serve over salad,
over grains such as
couscous or rice, or
with fish or chicken.*

TIP

Keep beans in your
cupboard for a quick and
easy addition to salads,
pastas and soups.

Make ahead

Spoon into an airtight
container and store in the
refrigerator for up to 1 day.
Stir well before serving.

Black and White Bean Salsa

1 cup	rinsed and drained canned black beans	250 mL
1 cup	rinsed and drained canned navy beans	250 mL
1 cup	chopped plum tomatoes	250 mL
½ cup	drained canned corn	125 mL
⅓ cup	chopped fresh cilantro	75 mL
⅓ cup	chopped green onions	75 mL
⅓ cup	chopped red bell peppers	75 mL
2 tbsp	freshly squeezed lime juice	25 mL
1½ tbsp	olive oil	22 mL
1½ tsp	chili powder	7 mL
1 tsp	minced garlic	5 mL
	Freshly ground black pepper	

1. In a bowl, combine black beans, navy beans, tomatoes, corn, cilantro, green onions, red peppers, lime juice, olive oil, chili powder and garlic; mix well. Season to taste with pepper.

NUTRITIONAL ANALYSIS PER SERVING (¼ CUP/50 ML)			
Energy: 64 kcal	Fat: 2 g	Fiber: 3.2 g	Iron: 0.8
Protein: 3 g	Carbohydrate: 10 g	Calcium: 18 mg	Folate: 44 mcg

Health Tip

Black beans and navy beans are good sources of fiber, protein and folate. A healthy intake of fiber (more than 25 g a day) can help reduce the risk of developing diabetes and help keep blood cholesterol levels lower.

Portobello Mushrooms with Goat Cheese

- Preheat broiler
- Baking sheet

2 tbsp	olive oil	25 mL
6 oz	portobello mushrooms, trimmed and sliced ½ inch (1 cm) thick	175 g
1 tbsp	finely chopped garlic	15 mL
2 tsp	balsamic vinegar, divided	10 mL
¼ tsp	salt	1 mL
Pinch	freshly ground black pepper	Pinch
¼ tsp	drained green peppercorns (optional)	1 mL
2 oz	goat cheese	60 g
2 tsp	pine nuts	10 mL
	Several lettuce leaves	
2 tsp	olive oil	10 mL

1. In a nonstick skillet, heat oil over high heat for 1 minute. Add mushroom slices in one layer; cook 2 to 3 minutes or until nicely browned (they will absorb all the oil). Turn and cook second side for under a minute. Add garlic, 1 tsp (5 mL) of the vinegar, salt and pepper; continue cooking for 1 minute to brown the garlic somewhat.

2. Remove from heat. Arrange on baking sheet in 2 flat piles about 3 inches (7.5 cm) wide. Sprinkle evenly with peppercorns (if using). Divide goat cheese in two; make each half into a thick disk, about 1 inch (2.5 cm) wide. Place a disk of cheese on each pile of mushrooms. Sprinkle pine nuts evenly over the piles, some on the cheese and some on the surrounding mushrooms.

3. Broil the mushrooms for just under 4 minutes or until the cheese is soft and a little brown, and the pine nuts are dark brown.

4. Line 2 plates with lettuce. Carefully lift each pile off the baking sheet and transfer as intact as possible onto the lettuce. Sprinkle about 1 tsp (5 mL) olive oil and ½ tsp (2 mL) vinegar over each portion and serve immediately.

NUTRITIONAL ANALYSIS PER SERVING			
Energy: 308 kcal	Fat: 27 g	Fiber: 3.0 g	Iron: 2.3 mg
Protein: 10 g	Carbohydrate: 9 g	Calcium: 119 mg	Folate: 31 mcg

Good source of:
- Iron

Source of:
- Calcium, folate and fiber

MAKES 2 SERVINGS

Exotic-sounding name notwithstanding, portobello mushrooms are nothing more than overgrown regular mushrooms. But for some alchemical reason their taste is very different (more meaty) from those lowly buttons. As a result they are usually associated with "wild" (or "fancy") mushrooms and are very much in demand. Luckily, they are available everywhere and often, quite conveniently, already trimmed and sliced into attractive ½-inch (1 cm) slices.

TIP

Green peppercorns are sold packed in brine; leftovers will keep if refrigerated in their original brine. While optional, they are delicious in this recipe.

Make ahead

Prepare through Step 2, cover and keep at room temperature for up to 1 hour.

MAKES 10 CUPS (2.5 L)

You must try this one — it's a great healthy snack, but there won't be any left!

TIP

Use leftover cauliflower the next day, steamed with broccoli for a colorful side dish.

Make ahead

Place in an airtight container and store in the refrigerator for up to 3 days.

Cauliflower Popcorn Snack

• Preheat oven to 450°F (230°C)
• Baking sheet, lined with foil

6 tbsp	olive oil	90 mL
2 tsp	granulated sugar	10 mL
1 tsp	salt	5 mL
½ tsp	paprika	2 mL
½ tsp	ground turmeric	2 mL
¼ tsp	onion powder	1 mL
¼ tsp	garlic powder	1 mL
2	heads cauliflower, cut into florets (about 10 cups/2.5 L)	2

1. In a large resealable plastic bag, combine olive oil, sugar, salt, paprika, turmeric, onion powder and garlic powder. Add cauliflower florets and shake well to coat cauliflower. Spread in a single layer on prepared baking sheet.

2. Bake in preheated oven for 30 to 35 minutes, or until the larger pieces are easy to pierce with a knife or fork.

NUTRITIONAL ANALYSIS PER SERVING (1 CUP/250 ML)			
Energy: 118 kcal	Fat: 9 g	Fiber: 1.5 g	Iron: 1.0 mg
Protein: 3 g	Carbohydrate: 9 g	Calcium: 52 mg	Folate: 114 mcg

Health Tip

Cauliflower is loaded with nutrients, including protein, fiber, folate, B vitamins, vitamin C and vitamin K. This is one snack that should be made often!

Granola

- Preheat oven to 325°F (160°C)
- Large roasting pan

5 cups	large-flake rolled oats	1.25 L
2 cups	barley flakes	500 mL
1½ cups	raw unsalted nuts (almonds, filberts, pecans), chopped	375 mL
1 cup	sesame seeds	250 mL
1 cup	raw unsalted shelled sunflower seeds	250 mL
1 cup	raw unsalted pumpkin seeds	250 mL
1 cup	skim-milk powder	250 mL
1 cup	wheat germ	250 mL
1 cup	unsweetened coconut	250 mL
¾ cup	olive oil or canola oil	175 mL
½ cup	molasses	125 mL
½ cup	liquid honey	125 mL
1 tbsp	ground cinnamon	15 mL
2 cups	dried fruit (raisins, apricots, mango, pineapple, banana), chopped	500 mL

1. In a large roasting pan, combine oats, barley flakes, raw nuts, sesame, sunflower and pumpkin seeds, skim-milk powder, wheat germ and coconut.
2. Combine oil, molasses, honey and cinnamon. Stir thoroughly into oat mixture. Bake in preheated oven for about 30 minutes or until golden brown; stir frequently. Cool; stir in fruit. Store, covered, in a cool, dry location.

NUTRITIONAL ANALYSIS PER SERVING

Energy: 253 kcal	Fat: 15 g	Fiber: 2.8 g	Iron: 3.6 mg
Protein: 8 g	Carbohydrate: 26 g	Calcium: 109 mg	Folate: 36 mcg

Excellent source of:
- Iron

Source of:
- Calcium, folate and fiber

MAKES 40 SERVINGS

This is probably one of the best granola recipes you will ever make! Enjoy as a cereal, with yogurt, over fruit or as a snack.

TIPS

You can vary the taste and texture of this granola by trying different grains and adding dried fruits such as apples, pears and dates.

Although sunflower and pumpkin seeds provide fiber, they are also high in fat. This means they become rancid quickly. Be sure to buy them from a store with high turnover, use them quickly and store in the refrigerator.

**MAKES 6 CUPS
(1.5 L)**

Here's a quick and easy snack to make up and take along for a high-carbohydrate energy boost.

Make ahead

Store at room temperature in an airtight container. Mixture will be less crisp after 1 or 2 days.

No-Bake Trail Mix

4 cups	Shreddies-type cereal	1 L
1 tsp	ground cinnamon	5 mL
1½ cups	chopped mixed dried fruit	375 mL
1 cup	shredded coconut (optional)	250 mL
½ cup	whole almonds, toasted	125 mL

1. In a large bowl, combine cereal and cinnamon; mix in dried fruit, coconut (if using) and almonds.

NUTRITIONAL ANALYSIS PER SERVING (½ CUP/125 ML)			
Energy: 162 kcal	Fat: 5 g	Fiber: 0.9 g	Iron: 3.3 mg
Protein: 4 g	Carbohydrate: 27 g	Calcium: 41 mg	Folate: 17 mcg

Health Tip

Almonds are a great source of iron, calcium and vitamin E, an important antioxidant. Keep some in your cupboard for when you get the munchies.

Soups

Carrot Orange Soup 166

Southwestern Sweet Potato Soup 167

Ginger Chili Sweet Potato Soup 168

Sweet Green Pea Soup 169

Fassolada 170

White Bean Soup with Swiss Chard 171

Savory Red Lentil Soup 172

Lemony Lentil Soup with Spinach 173

Borscht 174

Hot and Sour Chicken Soup 175

Asian Turkey and Noodle Soup 176

Carrot Orange Soup

**MAKES
6 SERVINGS**

The delicious combination of orange juice and carrots makes this soup a powerhouse of beta-carotene, which is converted into vitamin A in the body. Enjoy the soup at home or heat it up and pour it into your Thermos for a healthy hot treat.

TIPS

To make a creamier soup, use evaporated milk instead of regular milk.

A hand-held blender is a convenient tool that allows you to purée the soup right in the saucepan. It also makes cleanup a snap.

2 tbsp	butter or margarine	25 mL
½ cup	chopped onion	125 mL
4 cups	sliced carrots	1 L
4 cups	chicken stock or vegetable stock	1 L
½ cup	orange juice	125 mL
½ tsp	ground nutmeg	2 mL
¼ tsp	freshly ground white pepper	1 mL
1 cup	milk	250 mL

1. In a large saucepan, heat butter over medium-high heat; add onions and cook for 4 to 5 minutes or until softened. Add carrots and chicken stock; bring to a boil. Reduce heat and simmer for 15 to 20 minutes or until carrots are very soft. Stir in orange juice, nutmeg and pepper.

2. In a food processor or blender, purée carrot mixture in batches until smooth.

3. Return soup to pan; stir in milk. Simmer over very low heat for 2 to 3 minutes or until heated through.

NUTRITIONAL ANALYSIS PER SERVING			
Energy: 126 kcal	Fat: 5 g	Fiber: 2.1 g	Iron: 0.9 mg
Protein: 6 g	Carbohydrate: 14 g	Calcium: 87 mg	Folate: 29 mcg

Health Tip

Carrots are loaded with nutrients, including fiber, potassium and vitamins A, C and K.

Southwestern Sweet Potato Soup

1 tbsp	olive oil	15 mL
½ cup	chopped onion	125 mL
2 cups	diced peeled sweet potatoes	500 mL
1 cup	diced peeled baking potatoes	250 mL
4 cups	chicken stock, vegetable stock or water	1 L
1	red bell pepper, roasted (see tip, at left), peeled, seeded and diced	1
1	jalapeño pepper, seeded and chopped	1
1 cup	fresh or frozen corn kernels	250 mL
	Salt and freshly ground black pepper	
¼ cup	chopped fresh cilantro, green onions or parsley	50 mL

1. In a large saucepan, heat oil over medium heat. Add onion and cook for 3 to 4 minutes or until softened but not browned. Add sweet potatoes and baking potatoes; cook for 2 to 3 minutes.

2. Add chicken stock; bring to a boil. Reduce heat and simmer, uncovered, for 12 to 15 minutes or until potatoes are tender.

3. In a blender or food processor, purée potato mixture in batches; return to pan. Add red pepper, jalapeño pepper and corn; cook for 3 to 4 minutes. Season to taste with salt and pepper. Serve garnished with cilantro.

NUTRITIONAL ANALYSIS PER SERVING

Energy: 155 kcal	Fat: 4 g	Fiber: 2.6 g	Iron: 1.4 mg
Protein: 6 g	Carbohydrate: 26 g	Calcium: 27 mg	Folate: 35 mcg

Good source of:
- Folate

Source of:
- Folate, iron and fiber

MAKES 6 SERVINGS

Here's a tasty and nutritious soup that capitalizes on the popularity of Southwestern cuisine. Eating dark orange and red vegetables, such as sweet potatoes and red peppers, helps to increase your intake of vitamins A and C and antioxidants.

TIP

Make your own roasted red peppers or substitute ½ cup (125 mL) bottled roasted red peppers.
To roast peppers, heat barbecue or broiler; place peppers on grill or broiling pan and cook until skins turn black. Keep turning peppers until skins are blistered and black. Place roasted peppers in large pot with lid. Steam will make them sweat and skin will be easier to peel off. Let peppers cool. Remove stems, seeds and skin.

Ginger Chili Sweet Potato Soup

MAKES 4 SERVINGS

This delicious soup features an intriguing combination of flavors. Hearty yet elegant, it makes a great prelude to a meal or a light dinner, accompanied by salad. Made with vegetable stock, it is suitable for vegetarians.

TIPS

One chopped roasted red pepper makes about 1 cup (250 mL).

Purée soup in the saucepan using a hand-held blender.

1 tbsp	vegetable oil	15 mL
1 cup	diced onion	250 mL
1 tbsp	minced garlic	15 mL
1 tbsp	minced gingerroot	15 mL
1 tbsp	chili powder	15 mL
½ tsp	salt	2 mL
	Freshly ground black pepper	
1	can (19 oz/540 mL) sweet potatoes, drained	1
1 cup	corn kernels, drained if canned or thawed if frozen	250 mL
3 cups	vegetable or chicken stock	750 mL
1	roasted red bell pepper, chopped	1
1 tbsp	freshly squeezed lemon juice	15 mL

1. In a large saucepan, heat oil over medium heat. Add onion and cook, stirring, until softened, about 3 minutes. Add garlic, ginger, chili powder, salt and pepper to taste; cook, stirring, for 1 minute. Add sweet potatoes, corn and vegetable stock. Bring to a boil. Reduce heat to low and simmer for 10 minutes. Stir in red pepper.

2. Using a slotted spoon, transfer solids to a food processor or blender. Add ½ cup (125 mL) of the cooking liquid and process until smooth. Return mixture to saucepan and stir in lemon juice. Ladle into bowls and serve immediately.

NUTRITIONAL ANALYSIS PER SERVING			
Energy: 229 kcal	Fat: 5 g	Fiber: 5.0 g	Iron: 2.2 mg
Protein: 8 g	Carbohydrate: 40 g	Calcium: 56 mg	Folate: 44 mcg

Sweet Green Pea Soup

2 tbsp	butter	25 mL
1 cup	diced onion	250 mL
½ tsp	dried tarragon or thyme	2 mL
½ tsp	salt	2 mL
	Freshly ground black pepper	
10	Boston or romaine lettuce leaves, shredded (optional)	10
1	package (12 oz/375 g) frozen sweet green peas	1
4 cups	vegetable or chicken stock	1 L
Pinch	granulated sugar	Pinch
	Finely chopped parsley or chives	

1. In a large saucepan, melt butter over medium heat. Add onion and cook, stirring, until softened, about 3 minutes. Add tarragon, salt and pepper to taste and cook, stirring, for 1 minute. Add lettuce (if using) and stir until wilted.

2. Add peas, chicken stock and sugar. Bring to a boil. Reduce heat to low and simmer until peas are tender, about 7 minutes.

3. Using a slotted spoon, remove about ¼ cup (50 mL) of the whole peas from the saucepan and set aside. Using a slotted spoon, transfer remaining solids to a food processor or blender. Add ½ cup (125 mL) of the cooking liquid and process until smooth. (You can also do this in the saucepan, using a hand-held blender.) Ladle into bowls and garnish with reserved peas and parsley.

Variations

For a richer result, stir in ½ cup (125 mL) whipping (35%) cream after the soup has been puréed. Return mixture to saucepan over low heat until heated through.

Sweet Green Pea Soup with Mint: Omit tarragon or thyme. Garnish soup with ¼ cup (50 mL) finely chopped mint, along with the whole peas.

NUTRITIONAL ANALYSIS PER SERVING

Energy: 117 kcal	Fat: 5 g	Fiber: 3.4 g	Iron: 1.7 mg
Protein: 7 g	Carbohydrate: 12 g	Calcium: 37 mg	Folate: 65 mcg

Good source of:
• Folate

Source of:
• Iron and fiber

**MAKES
6 SERVINGS**

This elegant light soup is perfect as a prelude to dinner. It is good hot or cold.

TIPS

Cooking lettuce with peas is a French technique. It adds flavor and balance to the peas and is a good way to use up lettuce that is about to pass its peak. However, this soup is quite tasty without that addition.

The flavor can easily be varied by using different herbal accents. Mint is the most common, but tarragon, parsley and chives work well, too.

**MAKES
8 SERVINGS**

The national dish of Greece, this economical, calorie-friendly, fuss-free, instantly likable soup is chock full of flavor and nutrition.

TIPS

This recipe can be easily halved; but leftovers freeze well and can be reheated with minimal loss of flavor.

This soup is meant to be fairly thick; if too thick, add 1 to 2 cups (250 to 500 mL) water, stir and bring back to boil.

Fassolada

2½ cups	dried white kidney beans	625 mL
1 tbsp	baking soda	15 mL
1	onion, diced	1
1	large carrot, diced	1
1	tomato, blanched, skinned and chopped	1
½ cup	packed chopped fresh celery leaves (or 2 stalks celery, finely chopped)	125 mL
2 tbsp	tomato paste	25 mL
1 tsp	freshly squeezed lemon juice	5 mL
¼ cup	packed chopped fresh parsley	50 mL
¼ cup	olive oil	50 mL
1 tsp	dried rosemary, basil or oregano	5 mL
1 tsp	salt	5 mL
½ tsp	freshly ground black pepper	2 mL
	Extra-virgin olive oil, olive bits, diced red onion and crumbled feta cheese as accompaniments	

1. In a large bowl, cover beans with plenty of warm water. Add baking soda and mix well. (The water will foam and remove some of the gas from the beans.) Let soak for at least 3 hours, preferably overnight, at room temperature.

2. Drain beans and transfer to a soup pot. Add plenty of water and bring to a boil. Reduce heat to medium-low and simmer for 30 minutes, occasionally skimming any foam that rises to the top.

3. Drain beans; rinse and drain again. Scrub pot, cleaning off foam stuck to the sides. Return the beans to the pot; add 12 cups (3 L) water and place over high heat. Add onion, carrot, tomato, celery leaves, tomato paste and lemon juice. Bring to a boil, stirring; reduce heat to medium-low. Cook for 1½ hours at a rolling boil, stirring very occasionally until the beans and vegetables are very tender. Add parsley, oil, rosemary, salt and pepper. Cook for another 5 minutes, stirring occasionally, and remove from heat. Cover soup and let rest for 5 to 10 minutes. If desired, season to taste with additional salt and pepper. Serve with any or all of suggested garnishes.

NUTRITIONAL ANALYSIS PER SERVING			
Energy: 262 kcal	Fat: 6 g	Fiber: 15.3 g	Iron: 5.3 mg
Protein: 14 g	Carbohydrate: 39 g	Calcium: 113 mg	Folate: 238 mcg

White Bean Soup with Swiss Chard

Excellent source of:
- Calcium, folate, iron and fiber

MAKES 4 TO 6 SERVINGS

This may be the best bean soup ever. The cooking time will depend on the freshness of the soaked beans.

2 cups	dried cannellini beans (white kidney beans) or navy beans, soaked overnight in water to cover	500 mL
1 tbsp	olive oil	15 mL
8 oz	mushrooms, finely chopped	250 g
3	cloves garlic, minced	3
1	onion, chopped	1
½ tsp	ground nutmeg	2 mL
6 cups	chicken stock	1.5 L
1 lb	Swiss chard, washed, stemmed and chopped (about 6 cups/1.5 L)	500 g
	Salt and freshly ground black pepper	
3 cups	ricotta cheese	750 mL
8	slices rustic country-style bread	8
¾ cup	grated Pecorino Romano cheese	175 mL
¼ cup	chopped flat-leaf parsley	50 mL

TIP

Don't add salt to the beans' cooking water; this toughens them and encourages them to split open.

1. Drain beans and place in a large saucepan. Add water to cover by 2 inches (5 cm); bring to a boil. Reduce heat to simmer and cook for 1½ hours or until beans are tender, skimming any foam that rises to the surface. Drain beans, discarding cooking liquid.

2. Wipe saucepan clean. Heat olive oil in saucepan over medium heat. Add mushrooms, garlic, onion and nutmeg; cook, stirring often, for 5 minutes or until vegetables are softened. Stir in cooked beans and chicken stock; bring to a boil. Reduce heat to medium-low and cook for 20 minutes. Stir in Swiss chard; cook for 2 minutes or until wilted. Season to taste with salt and pepper.

3. Preheat broiler. Spread ricotta cheese on bread slices. Top with Pecorino Romano. Broil for 2 minutes or until cheese is golden.

4. Ladle soup into soup plates. Place a piece of cheese toast in the center of each serving. Sprinkle with parsley. Serve with extra toasts on the side.

NUTRITIONAL ANALYSIS PER SERVING (1 OF 6)			
Energy: 640 kcal	Fat: 21 g	Fiber: 19.2 g	Iron: 9.3 mg
Protein: 46 g	Carbohydrate: 70 g	Calcium: 731 mg	Folate: 307 mcg

**MAKES
8 SERVINGS**

Lentils were once considered "poor man's food," but that poor person could have done worse. This prehistoric legume is extremely high in protein and is also rich in minerals.

Savory Red Lentil Soup

¼ cup	olive oil	50 mL
2	cloves garlic, chopped	2
1	large onion, chopped	1
1	large carrot, sliced	1
1 tbsp	dried marjoram	15 mL
1 tsp	dried thyme	5 mL
¼ tsp	curry powder (optional)	1 mL
5 cups	vegetable stock	1.25 L
1½ cups	red lentils	375 mL
¼ cup	chopped parsley	50 mL
3	tomatoes, chopped	3
	Salt and freshly ground black pepper	
¼ cup	red wine	50 mL
1 cup	shredded sharp Cheddar cheese (optional)	250 mL

1. In a large heavy-bottomed pot with a lid, heat oil over medium heat. Add garlic, onion, carrot, marjoram, thyme and curry powder (if using); sauté for 6 minutes or until onion is transparent.

2. Add vegetable stock, red lentils, parsley and tomatoes. Season to taste with salt and pepper. Cover and simmer for 1 hour. (Add more stock, if necessary, to achieve desired consistency.)

3. Add red wine just before serving. Garnish with cheese (if using).

NUTRITIONAL ANALYSIS PER SERVING			
Energy: 249 kcal	Fat: 7 g	Fiber: 12.4 g	Iron: 4.2 mg
Protein: 11 g	Carbohydrate: 34 g	Calcium: 56 mg	Folate: 191 mcg

Health Tip

Lentils are a great source of folate and fiber and should be part of a healthy diet. One cup (250 mL) of lentils provides more than half of the daily requirement of fiber. Fiber may help reduce the risk of heart disease.

Lemony Lentil Soup with Spinach

1 tbsp	vegetable oil	15 mL
1 cup	diced onion	250 mL
1 tbsp	minced garlic	15 mL
Pinch	cayenne pepper	Pinch
	Freshly ground black pepper	
1	package (10 oz/300 g) fresh or frozen chopped spinach, stems removed	1
1	can (19 oz/540 mL) lentils, drained and rinsed	1
5 cups	vegetable or chicken stock	1.25 L
¼ cup	freshly squeezed lemon juice	50 mL
	Salt	

1. In a large saucepan, heat oil over medium heat. Add onion and cook, stirring, until softened, about 3 minutes. Add garlic, cayenne and black pepper to taste. Cook, stirring, for 1 minute.

2. Add spinach and cook, stirring and breaking up with spoon, until thawed (if frozen) or wilted (if fresh). Add lentils and stock. Bring to a boil. Reduce heat to low and simmer for 15 minutes to cook spinach and combine flavors. Stir in lemon juice and salt to taste. Serve immediately.

Variation

Curried Lentil and Spinach Soup: Add 1 tsp (5 mL) to 1 tbsp (15 mL) curry powder, depending upon the degree of spice you prefer, along with the garlic.

NUTRITIONAL ANALYSIS PER SERVING			
Energy: 241 kcal	Fat: 6 g	Fiber: 10.7 g	Iron: 5.7 mg
Protein: 18 g	Carbohydrate: 30 g	Calcium: 130 mg	Folate: 286 mcg

Excellent source of:
- Folate, iron and fiber

Source of:
- Calcium

MAKES 4 SERVINGS

This soup is so light and refreshing it's hard to believe it's also packed with nutrition.

TIP

If you prefer, use 1 cup (250 mL) dried brown lentils, cooked, instead of the canned. Thoroughly rinse lentils under cold running water, then place in a large saucepan. Cover with 3 cups (750 mL) cold water. Bring to a boil over medium heat. Reduce heat to low and simmer until tender, about 25 minutes. Drain.

**MAKES
4 SERVINGS**

Borscht is one of those hearty peasant soups that has transcended its origins. Here's an easy-to-make version that eliminates the unpleasant job of peeling beets. The baby spinach adds a pleasant note of freshness, which is sometimes provided by the addition of beet leaves in traditional recipes. Serve hot or cold with plenty of dark rye bread.

TIPS

You can also use prepared beef, chicken or vegetable stock in this recipe. If it is not concentrated, use 2 cups (500 mL) stock and omit the water.

Top individual servings with a dollop of sour cream and/or finely chopped dill.

Borscht

1 tbsp	vegetable oil	15 mL
1 cup	diced onion	250 mL
1 tbsp	minced garlic	15 mL
1	can (14 oz/398 mL) beets, including juice	1
1	can (10 oz/284 mL) condensed beef or chicken stock (see tip, at left)	1
½	bag (10 oz/300 g) washed baby spinach	½
2 tbsp	freshly squeezed lemon juice	25 mL
	Salt and freshly ground black pepper	

1. In a large saucepan, heat oil over medium heat. Add onion and cook, stirring, until softened, about 3 minutes. Add garlic and cook, stirring, for 1 minute.

2. Add beets with juice, stock and ½ cup (125 mL) water. Bring to a boil. Reduce heat to low and simmer for 10 minutes to combine flavors. Add spinach and cook, stirring, just until wilted. Stir in lemon juice. Season with salt and pepper to taste.

3. Using a slotted spoon, transfer solids plus ½ cup (125 mL) of the liquid to a food processor or blender. Process until smooth. (You can also do this in the saucepan, using a hand-held blender.)

4. Return mixture to saucepan and stir to blend. Serve hot or chill thoroughly.

NUTRITIONAL ANALYSIS PER SERVING

Energy: 104 kcal	Fat: 4 g	Fiber: 1.8 g	Iron: 2.0 mg
Protein: 5 g	Carbohydrate: 13 g	Calcium: 64 mg	Folate: 98 mcg

Health Tip

Beets are a good source of many nutrients, including vitamin C, iron, folate and fiber. In addition to its antioxidant powers, vitamin C helps the body absorb iron, while folate helps with the production of important red blood cells.

Hot and Sour Chicken Soup

6	dried Chinese mushrooms	6
5 cups	chicken stock	1.25 L
2 cups	shredded cooked chicken (7 oz/200 g)	500 mL
1 tbsp	finely chopped gingerroot	15 mL
1	chili pepper, chopped (or ½ tsp/2 mL crushed chili flakes)	1
1 cup	diced firm tofu (see tip, at right)	250 mL
2 tbsp	white wine vinegar	25 mL
1 tbsp	sodium-reduced soy sauce	15 mL
1 tbsp	dry sherry	15 mL
1 tbsp	cornstarch	15 mL
1 tbsp	cold water	15 mL
3	egg whites, lightly beaten	3
2	shallots, thinly sliced (optional)	2

1. Cover mushrooms with hot water and soak for 10 minutes. Drain, discard stems and slice caps.

2. In a large saucepan, bring chicken stock to a boil; add mushrooms, chicken, ginger and chili pepper. Reduce heat and simmer, covered, for 5 minutes. Add tofu, vinegar, soy sauce and sherry; simmer for 2 minutes.

3. Stir cornstarch with water until smooth; gradually stir into soup and simmer for 2 to 3 minutes or until thickened slightly. Remove from heat; immediately swirl egg whites through soup. Garnish with shallots (if using).

NUTRITIONAL ANALYSIS PER SERVING

Energy: 189 kcal	Fat: 6 g	Fiber: 0.6 g	Iron: 5.7 mg
Protein: 24 g	Carbohydrate: 8 g	Calcium: 320 mg	Folate: 27 mcg

Excellent source of:
• Calcium and iron

Source of:
• Folate

MAKES 6 SERVINGS

Impress friends and family with your own version of this Chinese classic. The tofu, chicken and egg whites in this soup combine to make a good source of protein.

TIPS

Use thin green or red chilies or Thai finger chilies in this recipe rather than jalapeño chilies. If using a fresh chili pepper, wash your hands thoroughly after chopping.

Make sure to buy tofu that has been coagulated with calcium sulfate or calcium chloride. Read the ingredient list on the label for the coagulant. Otherwise, you won't get nearly as much calcium out of this recipe.

**MAKES
6 SERVINGS**

This soup tastes great made with fresh turkey breast, but you can also use leftover cooked turkey (about 1 cup/250 mL). If using cooked turkey, don't stir-fry. Add with the chicken stock in Step 1.

TIPS

Sesame oil is made from roasted sesame seeds and is used for flavoring many Asian dishes. The darker the oil, the more intense the flavor. A little goes a long way, so add it sparingly. Keep refrigerated after opening.

Grated gingerroot and chopped garlic are sold preserved in jars at most supermarkets. They are great time-savers. You can also preserve your own gingerroot. Peel and chop finely; place in a jar and cover with dry sherry or sake. Store, tightly covered, in the refrigerator.

Asian Turkey and Noodle Soup

2 tsp	vegetable oil	10 mL
8 oz	boneless skinless turkey breast, cut into strips	250 g
1 cup	sliced mushrooms	250 mL
2	cans (each 10 oz/284 mL) chicken stock	2
1 tsp	minced garlic	5 mL
1 tsp	grated gingerroot	5 mL
1 tbsp	rice wine vinegar or freshly squeezed lemon juice	15 mL
1 tbsp	soy sauce	15 mL
1 tsp	sesame oil	5 mL
¼ tsp	hot pepper sauce	1 mL
4 oz	fresh chow mein or rice noodles	125 g
1½ cups	snow peas, trimmed and cut into 1-inch (2.5 cm) pieces	375 mL
½ cup	chopped green onions	125 mL

1. In a large saucepan, heat oil over medium-high heat. Add turkey and stir-fry for 2 to 3 minutes. Add mushrooms; cook for 2 to 3 minutes. Add chicken stock, 3 cups (750 mL) water, garlic and ginger; bring to a boil. Add vinegar, soy sauce, sesame oil, hot pepper sauce and noodles; reduce heat and simmer for 3 to 4 minutes.

2. Add snow peas and green onions; simmer for 1 to 2 minutes. Serve immediately.

NUTRITIONAL ANALYSIS PER SERVING			
Energy: 156 kcal	Fat: 4 g	Fiber: 2.6 g	Iron: 2.2 mg
Protein: 19 g	Carbohydrate: 10 g	Calcium: 37 mg	Folate: 27 mcg

Health Tip

Food *and* beverages contribute to daily fluid intake. Soups are a nutritious way to increase your daily intake of fluids.

Salads

Mango-Cucumber Salad. 178

Mango, Strawberry and Cucumber Salad 179

Asian Cucumber Salad 179

Greens with Strawberries. 180

Mandarin Orange Salad with Almonds. 181

Crunchy Broccoli Salad. 182

Sonoma Chicken Salad 183

Greek Summer Salad 184

Spinach and Rice Salad. 185

Beet and Feta Salad 186

Rice and Bean Salad 187

Tasty Bean Salad 188

White Bean Salad with
    Lemon-Dill Vinaigrette 189

Tuscan Bean Salad. 190

Lentil Salad. 191

Tabbouleh 192

Warm Chickpea Salad 193

Raspberry Basil Vinaigrette 193

Bulgur Salad. 194

Mediterranean Potato Salad. 195

Chicken Salad Amandine. 196

Vietnamese Chicken and Rice Noodle Salad. . . 197

Thai-Style Beef Salad 198

Mango-Cucumber Salad

MAKES 4 TO
6 SERVINGS

This sweet-and-sour salad is extremely versatile. It combines the fundamental elements of two of Thailand's most delicious side dishes into a brand new concoction that can accompany a wide array of main courses. It also keeps well in the fridge and leftovers can be served the next day.

TIP

Here's the Thai way to create the julienne strips of mango: Hold the mango firmly in your hand and, with a sharp knife, make a number of closely spaced parallel cuts into the surface facing you, then slice thinly to get shreds. Turn over and repeat procedure with the other half. Be warned, though — this technique can lead to bloodshed if there is a slip-up.

Make ahead

Cover and keep at room temperature for up to 2 hours.

1	8-inch (20 cm) section of unpeeled English cucumber, cut lengthwise into quarters, then thinly sliced	1
1	green mango, peeled and cut into julienne strips (see tip, at left)	1
3	green onions, finely chopped	3
1	jalapeño pepper, finely chopped (with or without seeds, depending on desired hotness)	1
½	red bell pepper, cut into thin strips	½
¼ cup	slivered red onion	50 mL
2 tbsp	finely chopped fresh cilantro, divided	25 mL
2 tbsp	freshly squeezed lime juice	25 mL
2 tbsp	white vinegar	25 mL
2 tbsp	vegetable oil	25 mL
1 tbsp	granulated sugar	15 mL
	Salt	

1. Put cucumber and mango into a large bowl. Add green onions, jalapeño pepper, red pepper, red onion and half of the cilantro. Toss until well mixed.

2. In a small bowl, whisk together lime juice, vinegar, oil and sugar until emulsified. Season to taste with salt. Pour dressing over salad and toss well. Transfer to a serving bowl and garnish with the remaining cilantro.

NUTRITIONAL ANALYSIS PER SERVING (1 OF 6)			
Energy: 79 kcal	Fat: 4 g	Fiber: 1.6 g	Iron: 0.4 mg
Protein: 1 g	Carbohydrate: 11 g	Calcium: 20 mg	Folate: 11 mcg

Mango, Strawberry and Cucumber Salad

⅓ cup	rice wine vinegar	75 mL
3 tbsp	walnut or olive oil	45 mL
1 tbsp	granulated sugar	15 mL
1½ tsp	coarsely chopped fresh mint	7 mL
¼ tsp	salt	1 mL
¼ tsp	freshly ground black pepper	1 mL
2 cups	strawberries, sliced	500 mL
1	English cucumber, cut into ¼-inch (5 mm) cubes	1
1	large mango, peeled and cut into ¼-inch (5 mm) cubes	1
8 cups	mixed torn greens	2 L

1. In a large bowl, whisk together vinegar, oil, sugar, mint, salt and pepper. Add strawberries, cucumber and mango; toss gently.

2. Divide greens among 8 plates. Top with strawberry mixture.

NUTRITIONAL ANALYSIS PER SERVING			
Energy: 96 kcal	Fat: 6 g	Fiber: 2.5 g	Iron: 1.1 mg
Protein: 1 g	Carbohydrate: 12 g	Calcium: 54 mg	Folate: 42 mcg

Good source of:
• Folate

Source of:
• Iron and fiber

MAKES 8 SERVINGS

This recipe combines strawberries with mango and cucumber on top of crisp salad greens. For an added flourish, garnish each plate with a mint leaf and sliced strawberries.

TIP

When chopping fresh herbs, make sure they are well dried and use a sharp knife to ensure clean edges.

Asian Cucumber Salad

2 tbsp	rice vinegar (see tip, at right)	25 mL
1 tbsp	soy sauce	15 mL
1 tbsp	vegetable oil	15 mL
1	cucumber, peeled and sliced	1
	Salt and freshly ground black pepper	

1. In a serving bowl, combine vinegar, soy sauce and oil. Add cucumber and toss to combine. Season with salt and pepper to taste. Serve.

NUTRITIONAL ANALYSIS PER SERVING			
Energy: 86 kcal	Fat: 7 g	Fiber: 1.0 g	Iron: 0.7 mg
Protein: 2 g	Carbohydrate: 5 g	Calcium: 23 mg	Folate: 22 mcg

Source of:
• Folate and iron

MAKES 2 SERVINGS

This simple salad makes a delicious addition to any meal.

TIP

Rice vinegar, which is milder than traditional North American vinegars, is now widely available in supermarkets.

**MAKES
6 SERVINGS**

*The strawberries in
this recipe are put
to an unusual use
— in the dressing.
Combined with the
greens, they are a
great source of folate
and vitamin C.*

TIPS

Be creative when purchasing
greens for this tasty salad.
Try different combinations
of red leaf lettuce, pungent
arugula, peppery watercress
and sharp radicchio, as well
as Bibb and iceberg lettuce.
Or add a handful or two of
mesclun mix to torn romaine.

If desired, replace the
strawberries with drained
canned mandarin oranges.

Greens
with Strawberries

4 cups	assorted lettuce, torn into bite-size pieces	1 L
½ cup	sliced red onion	125 mL

Dressing

½ tsp	grated orange zest	2 mL
¼ cup	freshly squeezed orange juice	50 mL
¼ tsp	grated lemon zest	1 mL
1 tbsp	freshly squeezed lemon juice	15 mL
1 tbsp	chopped fresh mint	15 mL
1 tsp	granulated sugar	5 mL
1 cup	sliced fresh strawberries	250 mL

1. In a salad bowl, combine lettuce and onion; cover and refrigerate.

2. *Prepare the dressing:* Combine orange zest and juice, lemon zest and juice, mint and sugar. Pour over sliced strawberries; cover and refrigerate.

3. Just before serving, pour strawberry mixture over salad greens; toss gently.

NUTRITIONAL ANALYSIS PER SERVING			
Energy: 28 kcal	Fat: Trace	Fiber: 1.0 g	Iron: 0.6 mg
Protein: 1 g	Carbohydrate: 6 g	Calcium: 29 mg	Folate: 47 mcg

Mandarin Orange Salad with Almonds

8 cups	torn romaine lettuce leaves	2 L
½ cup	sliced celery	125 mL
2	green onions, chopped	2
1	can (10 oz/284 mL) mandarin orange segments, drained	1

Dressing

2 tbsp	vinegar	25 mL
4 tsp	olive oil	20 mL
1 tbsp	chopped fresh parsley (or 1 tsp/5 mL dried)	15 mL
2 tsp	granulated sugar	10 mL
¼ tsp	hot pepper sauce	1 mL
¼ tsp	salt	1 mL
	Freshly ground black pepper	
	Candied almonds (see tip, at right)	

1. In a large bowl, combine lettuce, celery, onions and mandarin oranges. Set aside.
2. *Prepare the dressing:* In a small bowl, whisk together vinegar, oil, parsley, sugar, hot pepper sauce and salt. Season with pepper to taste. Pour over salad; toss to coat.
3. Serve sprinkled with candied almonds.

NUTRITIONAL ANALYSIS PER SERVING

Energy: 157 kcal	Fat: 9 g	Fiber: 2.9 g	Iron: 1.9 mg
Protein: 4 g	Carbohydrate: 18 g	Calcium: 80 mg	Folate: 170 mcg

MAKES 4 SERVINGS

This salad is a great source of vitamin A, vitamin C and folate.

TIPS

Don't have time to wash salad greens? Plan ahead: Instead of washing only the greens you need, wash a whole head of lettuce or a bag of spinach. Toss in a salad spinner to remove extra moisture. Store lettuce in the salad spinner or wrapped in paper towels in a plastic bag until needed.

If desired, replace the canned mandarin orange segments with 2 medium oranges, peeled and sectioned, or 1 cup (250 mL) sliced strawberries in season.

To make candied almonds: In a small nonstick skillet, melt 1 tbsp (15 mL) granulated sugar over low heat. Add ¼ cup (50 mL) slivered almonds and cook, stirring constantly, for 5 to 6 minutes or until almonds are well coated with syrup and lightly browned. Cool; break apart into small pieces.

MAKES 7 CUPS (1.75 L)

A very refreshing salad, and high in fiber! You can use the delicious dressing for other salads and crudités.

Crunchy Broccoli Salad

3 cups	chopped broccoli (about 1 bunch)	750 mL
2	green onions, chopped	2
2 cups	sliced mushrooms	500 mL
½ cup	toasted sliced almonds (see tip, at left)	125 mL
¼ cup	unsalted roasted sunflower seeds	50 mL
3 tbsp	toasted sesame seeds (see tip, at left)	45 mL
2 cups	chow mein noodles	500 mL

Dressing

1	clove garlic, chopped	1
½ cup	vegetable oil	125 mL
3 tbsp	rice vinegar	45 mL
2 tbsp	sodium-reduced soy sauce	25 mL
1 tbsp	granulated sugar	15 mL
1 tsp	sesame oil	5 mL
½ tsp	freshly ground black pepper	2 mL
Pinch	salt	Pinch

1. In a medium saucepan, cover broccoli with ½ inch (1 cm) water. Cover and cook over high heat for 2 to 3 minutes, or until tender-crisp. Drain and rinse under cold water until chilled. Drain and place in a large bowl.

2. Add mushrooms, green onions, sunflower seeds, almonds, and sesame seeds to broccoli and mix well. Add chow mein noodles on top.

3. *Prepare the dressing:* In a small bowl, combine garlic, vegetable oil, vinegar, soy sauce, sugar, sesame oil, pepper and salt.

4. Pour dressing over broccoli salad and mix well.

NUTRITIONAL ANALYSIS PER SERVING (1 CUP/250 ML)			
Energy: 329 kcal	Fat: 28 g	Fiber: 4.3 g	Iron: 2.2 mg
Protein: 6 g	Carbohydrate: 18 g	Calcium: 66 mg	Folate: 60 mcg

Sonoma Chicken Salad

- Preheat barbecue to medium-high

2	boneless skinless chicken breasts	2
½	head red leaf lettuce, torn into pieces	½
¼	red bell pepper, thinly sliced	¼
½ cup	crumbled pasteurized feta cheese (2 oz/60 g)	125 mL
¼ cup	chopped peeled cucumber	50 mL
2 tbsp	diced red onion	25 mL
2 tbsp	chopped toasted almonds	25 mL
2 tbsp	chopped toasted pecans	25 mL
2 tbsp	raisins	25 mL
1 tbsp	roasted unsalted sunflower seeds	15 mL

Dressing

2 tbsp	vegetable oil	25 mL
1 tbsp	cider vinegar	15 mL
1½ tsp	granulated sugar	7 mL
Dash	hot pepper sauce (optional)	Dash
	Salt and freshly ground black pepper	

1. Place chicken breasts on preheated barbecue and grill, turning once, for 8 to 10 minutes per side, or until chicken is no longer pink inside and reaches and internal temperature of 170°F (75°C). Set aside.

2. In a large bowl, combine lettuce, red pepper, feta, cucumber and red onion.

3. *Prepare the dressing:* In a small bowl, combine oil, vinegar, sugar, hot pepper sauce (if using) and salt and pepper to taste.

4. Thinly slice chicken breasts and add to salad. Drizzle with dressing and toss to coat. Sprinkle with almonds, pecans, raisins and sunflower seeds.

NUTRITIONAL ANALYSIS PER SERVING			
Energy: 493 kcal	Fat: 32 g	Fiber: 3.6 g	Iron: 3.1 mg
Protein: 37 g	Carbohydrate: 17 g	Calcium: 233 mg	Folate: 62 mcg

Good source of:
- Calcium, folate and iron

Source of:
- Fiber

MAKES 2 SERVINGS

For a light one-dish meal, try this California-inspired chicken salad.

TIPS

Be sure to purchase pasteurized feta cheese to avoid contamination with the bacterium *Listeria monocytogenes*. Read the label carefully to determine whether the feta you wish to purchase is made from pasteurized milk.

To toast almonds, bake in preheated 350°F (180°C) oven for about 15 minutes, or until golden brown and fragrant.

Greek Summer Salad

Here's the salad everyone talks about. All the ingredients are widely available and can certainly be found in Greek or Middle Eastern establishments. The ripeness and flavor of the tomatoes is essential here.

1½ lbs	ripe tomatoes, cut into wedges (about 6 tomatoes)	750 g
1	English cucumber, sliced	1
½ cup	slivered red onion	125 mL
½ cup	whole black olives (about 16)	125 mL
¼ cup	extra-virgin olive oil	50 mL
2 tbsp	freshly squeezed lemon juice	25 mL
	Salt and freshly ground black pepper	
4 oz	feta cheese, sliced	125 g
1 tbsp	chopped fresh oregano or 1 tsp (5 mL) dried	15 mL

1. On a large serving plate, arrange tomato wedges and cucumber slices so that they just overlap. Scatter onion slivers over everything and decorate edges of the plate with olives.

2. In a small bowl, whisk together oil, lemon juice and salt and pepper to taste until emulsified. Pour dressing evenly over the salad.

3. Top the salad with the feta slices (and any feta crumbles left on your cutting board). Sprinkle oregano over everything and serve within 30 minutes.

NUTRITIONAL ANALYSIS PER SERVING (1 OF 6)			
Energy: 176 kcal	Fat: 14 g	Fiber: 2.7 g	Iron: 1.2 mg
Protein: 5 g	Carbohydrate: 10 g	Calcium: 140 mg	Folate: 29 mcg

Health Tip

Feta cheese can be made from sheep's, goat's or cow's milk, each of which has its own unique flavor. Feta is an excellent source of calcium, an important mineral for bone growth and maintenance.

Spinach and Rice Salad

Good source of:
- Folate

Source of:
- Iron

¾ cup	long-grain white rice	175 mL
2 cups	boiling water	500 mL
¼ cup	olive oil	50 mL
2 tbsp	soy sauce	25 mL
1 cup	torn spinach leaves	250 mL
½ cup	chopped green bell pepper	125 mL
¼ cup	raisins	50 mL
2 tbsp	chopped fresh parsley	25 mL
2 tbsp	chopped green onion	25 mL

Dressing

½ cup	granulated sugar	125 mL
½ cup	vinegar	125 mL
2 tsp	freshly squeezed lemon juice	10 mL
1 tsp	chopped fresh parsley	5 mL
1 tsp	dry mustard	5 mL
Pinch	paprika	Pinch
Pinch	cayenne pepper	Pinch
Pinch	garlic powder	Pinch
Pinch	salt	Pinch
Pinch	freshly ground black pepper	Pinch
1 cup	olive oil	250 mL

**MAKES
6 SERVINGS**

**MAKES 1½ CUPS
(375 ML) DRESSING**

You'll want to keep the dressing on hand for other salads, so make the entire recipe and refrigerate the extra quantity.

TIPS

Adding the oil and soy sauce while the rice is still warm keeps the grains of rice separate and ensures that they don't clump together as the rice cools.

Olive oil, like canola and peanut oil, is a monounsaturated fat choice that may help to lower cholesterol levels when included as part of healthy eating. The key is to control the total amount of fat you eat, so balance this higher-fat salad with lighter choices.

1. In a saucepan, add rice to boiling water. Cover and cook over very low heat for 20 minutes or until tender and water is absorbed. Add oil and soy sauce; cool.

2. In a large bowl, combine rice mixture, spinach, green pepper, raisins, parsley and onion.

3. *Prepare the dressing:* Whisk together sugar, vinegar, lemon juice, parsley, mustard, paprika, cayenne, garlic powder, salt and pepper. Gradually whisk in oil. Pour ¼ cup (50 mL) dressing over salad. Refrigerate remaining dressing for other salads.

NUTRITIONAL ANALYSIS PER SERVING

Energy: 228 kcal	Fat: 13 g	Fiber: 1.2 g	Iron: 0.9 mg
Protein: 2 g	Carbohydrate: 26 g	Calcium: 23 mg	Folate: 50 mcg

MAKES 4 SERVINGS

Although beets are traditionally served hot as a vegetable side dish, cold sliced or diced beets are a delicious and colorful addition to plain green salads. They combine well with a variety of salad dressings, from mayonnaise to simple vinaigrette.

TIPS

If you don't have time to chill the beet mixture, keep the canned beets refrigerated so they will be cold when you're ready to use them.

If using whole baby beets, halve before using.

Beet and Feta Salad

1	can (14 oz/398 mL) sliced beets or whole baby beets, drained	1
½ cup	finely chopped celery	125 mL
¼ cup	bottled oil and vinegar dressing	50 mL
½	bag (10 oz/300 g) washed salad greens or 2 cups (500 mL) torn lettuce, washed and dried	½
2 oz	crumbled feta cheese	60 g

1. In a salad bowl, combine beets, celery and dressing. Cover and refrigerate for at least 1 hour or overnight.

2. Add salad greens and toss well. Sprinkle feta over top and serve immediately.

Variations

Beet and Avocado Salad: Substitute ¼ cup (50 mL) finely chopped green onion for the celery and 1 avocado, cut into ½-inch (1 cm) cubes, for the feta. Cut avocado and add to greens just before tossing.

Beet and Celery Salad: Omit the feta and salad greens and increase the celery to 2 cups (500 mL), sliced. Combine beets and celery in a rectangular dish or on a platter. Mix 1 tsp (5 mL) lemon juice into the dressing and pour the mixture over the vegetables. Or, for a change, try this dressing: Mix 2 tbsp (25 mL) oil and vinegar dressing with 2 tbsp (25 mL) mayonnaise. If desired, add 1 tsp (5 mL) horseradish.

NUTRITIONAL ANALYSIS PER SERVING			
Energy: 130 kcal	Fat: 10 g	Fiber: 2.3 g	Iron: 1.8 mg
Protein: 3 g	Carbohydrate: 8 g	Calcium: 113 mg	Folate: 43 mcg

Rice and Bean Salad

1 cup	wild rice (or a mixture of wild and white rice)	250 mL
1	clove garlic, minced	1
½ cup	olive oil	125 mL
¼ cup	red wine vinegar	50 mL
1 tsp	salt	5 mL
1 tsp	freshly ground black pepper	5 mL
1 cup	drained, rinsed canned black beans	250 mL
1	red bell pepper, diced	1
1 cup	chopped fresh cilantro	250 mL

1. Cook rice according to package directions. Spread out onto a rimmed baking sheet and refrigerate until cooled. Transfer to a bowl.

2. In a small bowl, combine garlic, oil, vinegar, salt and black pepper. Pour over rice. Stir in black beans, red pepper and cilantro.

NUTRITIONAL ANALYSIS PER SERVING (1 CUP/250 ML)			
Energy: 461 kcal	Fat: 24 g	Fiber: 6.4 g	Iron: 4.5 mg
Protein: 9 g	Carbohydrate: 52 g	Calcium: 59 mg	Folate: 110 mcg

Excellent source of:
- Folate, iron and fiber

Source of:
- Calcium

MAKES 5 CUPS (1.25 L)

This colorful salad is both tasty and nutritious. It's a great high-fiber choice.

TIP

If you're not a fan of cilantro, substitute an equal amount of parsley.

Make ahead

Cover and store in the refrigerator for up to 1 day.

Tasty Bean Salad

MAKES 8 CUPS (2 L)

A very tasty salad, and high in fiber!

TIP

Keep canned chickpeas in your cupboard for an easy addition to salads, pastas and soups.

Make ahead

Cover and store in the refrigerator for up to 3 days.

4	cloves garlic, minced	4
1	can (19 oz/540 mL) chickpeas, drained	1
1	can (19 oz/540 mL) red kidney beans, drained and rinsed	1
1	can (14 oz/398 mL) cut green beans, drained	1
1	can (12 oz/341 mL) whole kernel corn, undrained	1
¼	red onion, diced	¼

Dressing

6 tbsp	olive oil	90 mL
3 tbsp	dried basil	45 mL
3 tbsp	granulated sugar	45 mL
3 tbsp	balsamic vinegar	45 mL
1 tsp	salt	5 mL
1 tsp	freshly ground black pepper	5 mL

1. In a large bowl, combine garlic, chickpeas, kidney beans, green beans, corn and onion.

2. *Prepare the dressing:* In a small bowl, combine oil, basil, sugar, vinegar, salt and pepper.

3. Pour dressing over bean mixture and stir to coat.

NUTRITIONAL ANALYSIS PER SERVING (1 CUP/250 ML)			
Energy: 242 kcal	Fat: 12 g	Fiber: 7.1 g	Iron: 2.6 mg
Protein: 6.5 g	Carbohydrate: 30 g	Calcium: 84 mg	Folate: 142 mcg

Health Tip

Chickpeas are a delicious legume, rich in protein, calcium, iron and folate.

White Bean Salad with Lemon-Dill Vinaigrette

2	cans (each 19 oz/540 mL) white kidney beans, rinsed and drained	2
2	small tomatoes, chopped	2
½ cup	finely chopped red onion	125 mL
¼ cup	chopped fresh dill, divided	50 mL
¼ cup	olive oil	50 mL
2 tbsp	freshly squeezed lemon juice	25 mL
1 tbsp	liquid honey	15 mL
¼ tsp	salt	1 mL
¼ tsp	freshly ground black pepper	1 mL

1. In a large serving bowl, combine beans, tomatoes, onion and 3 tbsp (45 mL) of the dill.

2. In a small bowl, whisk together olive oil, lemon juice, honey, salt and pepper. Add to beans; toss well. If desired, season to taste with additional salt and pepper. Serve garnished with remaining dill.

NUTRITIONAL ANALYSIS PER SERVING (1 OF 8)			
Energy: 188 kcal	Fat: 6 g	Fiber: 7.4 g	Iron: 2.9 mg
Protein: 8 g	Carbohydrate: 26 g	Calcium: 32 mg	Folate: 128 mcg

MAKES 6 TO 8 SERVINGS

Bean salads can be so disappointing. But this one is fresh-tasting and holds up well for several hours without refrigeration — perfect for a buffet table.

TIP

Dill is one of the few fresh herbs that freeze well. Simply place in a plastic bag and freeze for up to 6 months. To use, just break off what you need from the frozen bunch. For best results, add to cooked dishes rather than salads.

Make ahead

Cover and store in the refrigerator for up to 8 hours. Let stand at room temperature for 30 minutes before serving.

Excellent source of:
• Folate and fiber

Good source of:
• Iron

Source of:
• Calcium

**MAKES
4 SERVINGS**

Succulent white beans, prepared in a variety of ways, are a staple in Tuscany. Combined with tuna and a robust vinaigrette, they make a delectable salad. Served with hot crusty bread, this salad is a meal in itself.

TIPS

If you don't have sun-dried tomato pesto in your refrigerator, use 1 tbsp (15 mL) Dijon mustard or prepared basil pesto instead.

For best results, use Italian tuna packed in olive oil; it is more moist and flavorful than the paler versions packed in water.

Tuscan Bean Salad

1	can (6 oz/170 g) tuna, preferably Italian, packed in olive oil, drained	1
1	can (19 oz/540 mL) white kidney beans, drained and rinsed	1
4	finely chopped green onions (white parts only)	4
1 tbsp	prepared sun-dried tomato pesto (see tip, at left)	15 mL
½ cup	bottled oil and vinegar dressing	125 mL
	Salt and freshly ground black pepper	

1. In a bowl, combine tuna, beans, green onions and pesto. Pour in dressing and toss well. Season with salt and pepper to taste. Serve immediately or refrigerate for at least 2 hours.

Variations

Salami and White Bean Salad: Substitute 4 oz (125 g) diced salami for the tuna.

Bruschetta with Beans: Lightly brush 6 to 8 slices of country-style bread with olive oil on both sides and toast under the broiler, turning once. Spoon the bean salad evenly over the bread and serve.

NUTRITIONAL ANALYSIS PER SERVING

Energy: 361 kcal	Fat: 21 g	Fiber: 9.7 g	Iron: 2.9 mg
Protein: 20 g	Carbohydrate: 24 g	Calcium: 59 mg	Folate: 80 mcg

Health Tip

Tuna is a great source of protein and omega 3 fatty acids. It is an excellent low-fat addition to the diet. Omega 3 fatty acids have an anti-inflammatory effect, help to lower blood triglyceride levels and can lower blood pressure.

Lentil Salad

20	small cherry tomatoes, halved	20
6	radishes, chopped	6
2	cans (each 19 oz/540 mL) lentils, drained and rinsed	2
½	red onion, chopped	½
½	red bell pepper, chopped	½
½	green bell pepper, chopped	½
1½ cups	crumbled pasteurized feta cheese (6 oz/175 g)	375 mL

Dressing

¼ cup	vegetable oil	50 mL
¼ cup	white wine vinegar	50 mL
1 tsp	salt	5 mL
½ tsp	freshly ground black pepper	2 mL

1. In a large bowl, combine tomatoes, radishes, lentils, red onion, red pepper, green pepper and feta.

2. *Prepare the dressing:* In a small bowl, combine oil, vinegar, salt and pepper.

3. Drizzle dressing over salad and toss to coat. Cover and refrigerate for about 2 hours to let flavors develop.

NUTRITIONAL ANALYSIS PER SERVING			
Energy: 169 kcal	Fat: 8 g	Fiber: 6.1 g	Iron: 2.7 mg
Protein: 9 g	Carbohydrate: 17 g	Calcium: 98 mg	Folate: 139 mcg

Excellent source of:
• Folate and fiber

Good source of:
• Iron

Source of:
• Calcium

MAKES 12 SERVINGS

This crowd-pleaser is also good for you. The lentils give this salad a fiber boost, and it makes for an easy addition to an on-the-go lunch or dinner.

TIP

Although unpasteurized feta cheese is not recommended during pregnancy, many grocery stores carry pasteurized feta cheese, which is safe to consume while pregnant. Read labels carefully to ensure that feta has been made from pasteurized milk.

Make ahead

Place in an airtight container and store in the refrigerator for up to 3 days.

**MAKES
6 SERVINGS**

This may be the healthiest salad ever invented — it is certainly one of the most intriguing. Composed chiefly of parsley (normally a garnish), it is great fun to eat (random little spikes of parsley stalk and all).

TIP

If you prefer a sweeter taste, add 2 tbsp (25 mL) more oil.

Make ahead

The salad can be served immediately, but it will be better if covered and kept at room temperature for up to 2 hours. Leftover tabbouleh can be covered and kept in the refrigerator for up to 3 days. Bring back to room temperature before serving.

Tabbouleh

1	onion, finely diced	1
1	tomato, finely chopped	1
2 cups	packed chopped fresh parsley	500 mL
½ cup	bulgur wheat (about 4 oz/125 g)	125 mL
6 tbsp	freshly squeezed lemon juice	90 mL
¼ cup	olive oil	50 mL
	Salt and freshly ground black pepper	

1. In a bowl, combine onion, tomato and parsley. Mix well. Set aside.

2. In a saucepan, boil bulgur wheat in plenty of water for 6 to 8 minutes, until tender. Drain and refresh with cold water. Drain again completely and add cooked bulgur to the vegetables in the bowl. Mix well.

3. Sprinkle lemon juice and olive oil over the salad. Add salt and pepper to taste. Toss to mix thoroughly. Transfer to a serving plate.

NUTRITIONAL ANALYSIS PER SERVING			
Energy: 127 kcal	Fat: 8 g	Fiber: 3.3 g	Iron: 1.7 mg
Protein: 2 g	Carbohydrate: 14 g	Calcium: 38 mg	Folate: 48 mcg

Warm Chickpea Salad

1	can (19 oz/540 mL) chickpeas, including liquid	1
½ cup	bottled oil and vinegar dressing	125 mL
½ cup	finely chopped parsley	125 mL
¼ cup	chopped pitted black olives	50 mL
2 tbsp	prepared basil pesto sauce	25 mL

1. In a saucepan, over medium heat, bring chickpeas with liquid to a boil. Simmer for 2 minutes. Drain in a colander and rinse well in warm water.
2. Transfer chickpeas to a serving bowl. Add dressing, parsley, olives and pesto sauce. Toss well.

NUTRITIONAL ANALYSIS PER SERVING			
Energy: 360 kcal	Fat: 26 g	Fiber: 7.0 g	Iron: 3.5 mg
Protein: 9 g	Carbohydrate: 26 g	Calcium: 63 mg	Folate: 167 mcg

Excellent source of:
• Folate and fiber

Good source of:
• Iron

Source of:
• Calcium

**MAKES
4 SERVINGS**

This simple salad is delicious and very versatile. It works well as a side salad or on a buffet table. Served with warm crusty bread, it also makes a nice light meal.

Raspberry Basil Vinaigrette

1	small clove garlic, crushed	1
2 tbsp	raspberry vinegar	25 mL
1 tsp	cornstarch	5 mL
1 tsp	chopped fresh basil (or ½ tsp/2 mL dried)	5 mL
1 tsp	olive oil	5 mL
½ tsp	poppy seeds	2 mL
¼ tsp	grated lemon or orange zest	1 mL
Pinch	salt	Pinch

1. In a small saucepan, cook ½ cup (125 mL) water, garlic, vinegar and cornstarch for about 2 minutes or until thickened. Cool. In a small bowl, combine basil, oil, poppy seeds, lemon zest and salt. Stir in vinegar mixture; cover and refrigerate for at least 1 hour.

NUTRITIONAL ANALYSIS PER SERVING (1 TBSP/15 ML)			
Energy: 8 kcal	Fat: 1 g	Fiber: Trace g	Iron: 0.1 mg
Protein: Trace	Carbohydrate: 1 g	Calcium: 5 mg	Folate: Trace mcg

**MAKES ½ CUP
(125 ML)**

Most salads perk up with a special dressing that uses interesting vinegars. Raspberry, balsamic and tarragon vinegars all add extra zest to dressings.

TIP

While this vinaigrette is not in itself a source of any of the key nutrients highlighted in this book, it is delicious — and flavorful lower-fat dressing options encourage both kids and adults to consume more salads.

**MAKES
6 SERVINGS**

This salad has it all: low calories, low fat, lots of vegetables — and color and flavor to spare.

TIPS

In this recipe, using prepared fat-free Italian salad dressing adds flavor without fat.

Bulgur, or cracked wheat, is made by steaming wheat kernels, which are then dried and crushed.
It is readily available in larger supermarkets and specialty food stores.

Bulgur Salad

1 cup	bulgur	250 mL
2 cups	boiling water	500 mL
1	clove garlic, minced	1
1	tomato, seeded and diced	1
½	small zucchini, thinly sliced	½
2 tbsp	finely chopped red or Spanish onion	25 mL
½ cup	cooked corn kernels, cooled	125 mL
¼ cup	crumbled feta cheese	50 mL
¼ cup	bottled fat-free Italian dressing	50 mL
Pinch	crushed dried basil	Pinch
	Salt and freshly ground black pepper	

1. Cover bulgur with boiling water; let stand for 30 minutes. Drain.
2. In a bowl, combine bulgur, garlic, tomato, zucchini, onion and corn; stir in cheese, dressing and basil. Season with salt and pepper to taste. Cover and refrigerate for at least 1 hour.

NUTRITIONAL ANALYSIS PER SERVING

Energy: 159 kcal	Fat: 2 g	Fiber: 5.0 g	Iron: 0.9 mg
Protein: 5 g	Carbohydrate: 24 g	Calcium: 60 mg	Folate: 20 mcg

Health Tip

Bulgur is high in fiber and rich in B vitamins, as well as iron.

Mediterranean Potato Salad

1	can (6 oz/170 g) tuna, preferably Italian, packed in olive oil, drained	1
1	can (19 oz/540 mL) sliced new potatoes, drained, or 2 cups (500 mL) sliced cooked potatoes	1
¼ cup	chopped green onion	50 mL
1 tbsp	drained capers	15 mL
¾ cup	bottled oil and vinegar dressing	175 mL
1	bag (10 oz/300 g) washed salad greens or 4 cups (1 L) torn lettuce, washed and dried	1
2	hard-cooked eggs, quartered or thinly sliced (optional)	2

MAKES 4 SERVINGS

Here's a variation of salade Niçoise, a famous Provençal dish.

1. In a bowl, combine tuna, potatoes, onion and capers. Add dressing and toss to combine.
2. Arrange salad greens in a shallow serving dish or deep platter. Spoon tuna mixture over top. Garnish with sliced egg (if using).

Variation

Herb-Flavored Vinaigrette: In a bowl, combine 1 finely chopped shallot, 2 tbsp (25 mL) minced parsley or chives, 2 tbsp (25 mL) white wine vinegar and 1 tbsp (15 mL) Dijon mustard. Mix well. Whisk in ½ cup (125 mL) extra-virgin olive oil until blended.

NUTRITIONAL ANALYSIS PER SERVING

Energy: 414 kcal	Fat: 30 g	Fiber: 2.6 g	Iron: 2.4 mg
Protein: 18 g	Carbohydrate: 20 g	Calcium: 65 mg	Folate: 57 mcg

**MAKES
4 SERVINGS**

This old-fashioned recipe is a great way to use up leftover chicken. It makes a delicious luncheon dish or a light one-course dinner. The quantity of dressing may seem substantial for the amount of chicken, but it also dresses the salad greens.

TIP

To toast almonds: In a dry nonstick skillet, over medium heat, stir almonds constantly until golden brown, 3 to 4 minutes. Immediately transfer to a small bowl to prevent burning.

Chicken Salad Amandine

¼ cup	mayonnaise	50 mL
2 tbsp	olive oil	25 mL
2 tbsp	freshly squeezed lemon juice	25 mL
½ tsp	salt	2 mL
	Freshly ground black pepper	
4 cups	cubed (½ inch/1 cm) cooked chicken	1 L
½ cup	finely chopped celery	125 mL
2 tbsp	finely chopped red or green onion	25 mL
1	bag (10 oz/300 g) washed salad greens, such as hearts of romaine, or 4 cups (1 L) torn lettuce, washed and dried	1
2 tbsp	toasted slivered or sliced almonds (see tip, at left)	25 mL

1. In a bowl, combine mayonnaise, olive oil, lemon juice, salt and pepper to taste.

2. In a separate bowl, combine chicken, celery and onion. Add mayonnaise mixture. Toss to combine.

3. Spread salad greens over a deep platter. Spoon chicken mixture on top. Garnish with almonds and serve immediately.

Variation

Chicken Salad Sandwich: Omit the salad greens and almonds and use the chicken mixture as a filling for sandwiches. Add sliced tomato, lettuce and/or cucumber slices, as desired.

NUTRITIONAL ANALYSIS PER SERVING			
Energy: 403 kcal	Fat: 22 g	Fiber: 1.4 g	Iron: 2.5 mg
Protein: 45 g	Carbohydrate: 4 g	Calcium: 79 mg	Folate: 38 mcg

Vietnamese Chicken and Rice Noodle Salad

**MAKES
6 SERVINGS**

Rice noodles are an excellent alternative to pasta for people who do not include gluten in their diets. Serve this tasty salad with fruit-flavored yogurt to increase your intake of calcium.

3½ oz	wide rice noodles	99 g
12 oz	shredded cooked chicken	375 g
2 cups	diced cucumbers	500 mL
2 cups	grated carrots	500 mL
1 cup	julienned green bell peppers	250 mL
¼ cup	finely chopped fresh cilantro	50 mL

Dressing

⅓ cup	fish sauce or sodium-reduced soy sauce	75 mL
¼ cup	rice wine vinegar	50 mL
2 tbsp	freshly squeezed lime juice	25 mL
1 to 2 tbsp	curry paste	15 to 25 mL
2 tsp	granulated sugar	10 mL
1 tsp	minced garlic	5 mL
1 tsp	sesame oil	5 mL
½ cup	chopped peanuts (optional)	125 mL

1. In a large pot of boiling water, cook noodles for 5 to 8 minutes or until barely tender; drain. Rinse under cold water; drain. Transfer to a large bowl. Add chicken, cucumbers, carrots, peppers and cilantro.

2. *Prepare the dressing:* In a small bowl, blend together fish sauce, vinegar, lime juice, curry paste, sugar, garlic and sesame oil.

3. Add dressing to noodle mixture; toss to combine. Sprinkle with peanuts (if using).

TIP

Vietnamese fish sauce (nuoc nam) is an integral part of Vietnamese cooking. It is a clear, pungent liquid made by fermenting fish with salt. It takes a little getting used to, but it is a great flavor enhancer in many dishes. Fish sauce is high in sodium, so use it sparingly. Find it and curry paste in the Asian sections of some supermarkets.

NUTRITIONAL ANALYSIS PER SERVING			
Energy: 218 kcal	Fat: 3 g	Fiber: 1.8 g	Iron: 1.7 mg
Protein: 22 g	Carbohydrate: 24 g	Calcium: 35 mg	Folate: 22 mcg

Excellent source of:
• Folate

Good source of:
• Iron

Source of:
• Calcium and fiber

**MAKES
4 SERVINGS**

TIPS

In Southeast Asian countries, fish sauce, which is made from brine-covered and fermented fish, is used as widely as soy sauce in China and Japan. It is very pungent but lends an appealing note to many dishes. It is now available in the Asian food section of many supermarkets.

Use bottled preserved lemongrass for convenience. It is available in the Asian sections of many supermarkets and can be stored in the refrigerator after opening.

Thai-Style Beef Salad

¼ cup	freshly squeezed lime or lemon juice	50 mL
3 tbsp	fish sauce (see tip, at left)	45 mL
2 tsp	minced gingerroot	10 mL
2 tsp	Asian chili sauce	10 mL
4 oz	thinly sliced rare roast beef, chopped, or grilled steak, thinly sliced	125 g
2 cups	diced peeled cucumber	500 mL
1 cup	thinly sliced red or green onions (white parts only)	250 mL
¼ cup	finely chopped cilantro, divided	50 mL
1 tbsp	thinly sliced lemongrass, bottled preserved lemongrass (see tip, at left) or 1 tsp (5 mL) grated lemon zest	15 mL
1	bag (10 oz/300 g) mixed salad greens or 4 cups (1 L) arugula, washed and dried	1
12	cherry tomatoes, halved	12

1. In a bowl, combine lime juice, fish sauce, ginger and chili sauce. Mix well. Add beef, cucumber, onions, 2 tbsp (25 mL) of the cilantro and lemongrass. Toss to combine.

2. Spread salad greens over a deep platter or serving plate. Arrange meat mixture on top. Surround with cherry tomatoes and garnish with remaining cilantro. Serve immediately.

NUTRITIONAL ANALYSIS PER SERVING			
Energy: 116 kcal	Fat: 4 g	Fiber: 2.6 g	Iron: 2.6 mg
Protein: 12 g	Carbohydrate: 10 g	Calcium: 57 mg	Folate: 103 mcg

Health Tip

Beef is an excellent source of protein and iron and a great source of zinc. Zinc is needed for growth and development, for a healthy immune system and for healing wounds.

Poultry

Best-Ever Baked Chicken. 200

Baked Chicken and Potato Dinner 201

Yogurt-Marinated Chicken 202

Ginger, Soy and Lime Chicken 203

Pesto Chicken Thighs. 204

Crispy Chicken. 205

Grilled Honey-Ginger Chicken Breasts. 206

Honey Dijon Chicken. 207

Greek Lemon Chicken 208

Sticky Sesame Chicken 209

Curried Chicken 210

Chicken Tacos 211

Chicken Nuggets 212

Turkiaki Fiesta. 213

Turkey Chili. 214

MAKES 4 SERVINGS

Requiring only about 5 minutes of preparation time, this crispy baked chicken is so easy and delicious you'll never use a packaged mix again.

TIPS

Try Japanese panko, coarse packaged bread crumbs that create a particularly crunchy crust.

Add 2 tbsp (25 mL) finely chopped parsley to the bread crumb mixture in Step 2.

Best-Ever Baked Chicken

• Preheat oven to 375°F (190°C)
• Shallow baking dish

¼ cup	mayonnaise	50 mL
2 tbsp	prepared sun-dried tomato pesto	25 mL
4	skinless boneless chicken breasts (about 1 lb/500 g)	4
½ cup	bread or cracker crumbs	125 mL
¼ cup	freshly grated Parmesan cheese	50 mL

1. In a small bowl, combine mayonnaise and pesto.

2. On a plate, combine bread crumbs and cheese. Brush chicken with mayonnaise mixture on all sides, then dip into crumbs to coat thoroughly.

3. Arrange chicken in a single layer in baking dish. Bake in preheated oven until no longer pink inside, about 30 minutes.

NUTRITIONAL ANALYSIS PER SERVING			
Energy: 294 kcal	Fat: 13 g	Fiber: 0.3 g	Iron: 1.5 mg
Protein: 32 g	Carbohydrate: 11 g	Calcium: 90 mg	Folate: 11 mcg

Health Tip

The protein in chicken, like the protein from all animal sources, contains all of the essential amino acids required for growth. Chicken is also rich in B vitamins, which are important for energy metabolism.

Baked Chicken and Potato Dinner

- Preheat oven to 400°F (200°C)
- 13- by 9-inch (3 L) baking dish

4	bone-in skinless chicken breasts	4
2	unpeeled russet potatoes, cut into 1-inch (2.5 cm) cubes	2
1	onion, cut into 8 pieces	1
1 cup	chopped green and/or red bell peppers (1-inch/2.5 cm pieces)	250 mL
2 tbsp	olive oil	25 mL
¼ cup	freshly grated Parmesan cheese	50 mL
1 tsp	garlic powder	5 mL
1 tsp	Hungarian paprika	5 mL

1. Pat chicken breasts dry with paper towel; place 1 breast in each corner of baking dish. Put potatoes, onion and peppers in center of dish. Drizzle olive oil over chicken and vegetables; sprinkle with cheese, garlic powder and paprika.

2. Bake in preheated oven, stirring vegetables once halfway through cooking time, for 40 to 50 minutes or until juices run clear when chicken is pierced with a fork and vegetables are tender.

NUTRITIONAL ANALYSIS PER SERVING			
Energy: 301 kcal	Fat: 9 g	Fiber: 3.3 g	Iron: 2.3 mg
Protein: 32 g	Carbohydrate: 23 g	Calcium: 94 mg	Folate: 32 mcg

MAKES 4 SERVINGS

This recipe uses Hungarian paprika from the city of Szeged, which is available from Hungarian and fine food delicatessens. If you can't find it, regular paprika will do.

TIPS

Paprika is the mildest member of the pepper family. There are 2 main varieties, Hungarian and Spanish paprika, and both are available in sweet or hot versions.

If you need to feed a crowd, just double this recipe and use 2 baking dishes. For color contrast, use a mixture of red and green bell peppers.

**MAKES
8 SERVINGS**

Here's an interesting variation on chicken tandoori, an Indian specialty.

TIP

Instead of using chicken breasts only, you can substitute one 3-lb (1.5 kg) chicken, cut into 8 pieces; bake for 45 to 60 minutes.

Yogurt-Marinated Chicken

- Preheat oven to 350°F (180°C)
- Baking pan

1¼ cups	low-fat plain yogurt	300 mL
3	cloves garlic, minced	3
1 tbsp	minced gingerroot (or 2 tsp/10 mL ground ginger)	15 mL
1 tbsp	freshly squeezed lemon juice	15 mL
1 tbsp	vegetable oil	15 mL
2 tsp	paprika	10 mL
1 tsp	chili powder	5 mL
1 tsp	crumbled dried rosemary	5 mL
1 tsp	freshly ground black pepper	5 mL
½ tsp	turmeric	2 mL
8	boneless skinless chicken breasts (about 1½ lb/750 g)	8

1. In a large bowl, combine yogurt, garlic, ginger, lemon juice, oil, paprika, chili powder, rosemary, pepper and turmeric; whisk until smooth. Add chicken, turning to coat all over. Cover and refrigerate for 24 hours.

2. Place chicken in single layer in baking pan, reserving marinade. Bake in preheated oven for 20 to 25 minutes or until no longer pink inside, spooning additional marinade over chicken halfway through baking.

NUTRITIONAL ANALYSIS PER SERVING			
Energy: 147 kcal	Fat: 3 g	Fiber: 0.3 g	Iron: 1.0 mg
Protein: 24 g	Carbohydrate: 4 g	Calcium: 95 mg	Folate: 9 mcg

Ginger, Soy and Lime Chicken

Source of:
• Iron

**MAKES
4 SERVINGS**

The aroma from this recipe is mouthwatering — just like the grilled chicken.

• Contact grill

1	clove garlic, minced	1
2 tbsp	freshly squeezed lime juice	25 mL
2 tbsp	soy sauce	25 mL
1½ tsp	minced gingerroot	7 mL
1 tsp	packed dark brown sugar	5 mL
4	boneless skinless chicken breasts	4

1. In a small bowl, whisk together garlic, lime juice, soy sauce, gingerroot and brown sugar.

2. Place chicken breasts between two pieces of wax paper. Pound until flattened to about ½ inch (1 cm) thick and place in a shallow dish. Brush marinade on chicken, coating evenly. Cover and refrigerate for a minimum of 20 minutes or for up to 1 hour. Meanwhile, preheat contact grill.

3. Spray both sides of contact grill with vegetable cooking spray or oil. Place chicken on grill, close lid and grill for 5 to 6 minutes, or until chicken is no longer pink inside and reaches an internal temperature of 170°F (75°C).

TIPS

If your contact grill has more than one temperature setting, set it to high for this recipe.

Dark brown sugar is richer and more intensely flavored than golden brown sugar. It's a great addition to this recipe.

Make ahead

Prepare marinade, cover and store in the refrigerator for up to 1 day.

Variation

Use 8 boneless skinless chicken thighs in place of chicken breasts. Grill for same amount of time.

NUTRITIONAL ANALYSIS PER SERVING			
Energy: 142 kcal	Fat: 1 g	Fiber: 0.1 g	Iron: 1.1 mg
Protein: 28 g	Carbohydrate: 3 g	Calcium: 17 mg	Folate: 6 mcg

**MAKES
4 SERVINGS**

Your family will love this fabulous gourmet grill, but it's also an impressive meal for guests.

TIPS

If your contact grill has more than one temperature setting, set it to high for this recipe.

This recipe requires a longer grilling time to ensure the coating is crispy.

Pesto Chicken Thighs

• Contact grill

⅓ cup	pesto, homemade (see recipe, opposite) or prepared	75 mL
½ cup	dry bread crumbs	125 mL
2 tbsp	freshly grated Parmesan cheese	25 mL
¼ tsp	salt	1 mL
¼ tsp	freshly ground black pepper	1 mL
8	boneless skinless chicken thighs	8

1. Place pesto in a small bowl.
2. In a shallow bowl, mix together bread crumbs, Parmesan, salt and pepper.
3. Brush chicken thighs with pesto and roll in bread crumbs, coating evenly. Place in a shallow dish, cover and refrigerate for a minimum of 20 minutes or for up to 1 hour. Discard any excess pesto or crumbs. Meanwhile, preheat contact grill.
4. Spray both sides of contact grill with vegetable cooking spray or oil. Spray chicken thighs using a spray pump filled with olive oil or vegetable oil. Place chicken on grill, close lid and grill for 6 to 7 minutes, or until juices run clear when chicken is pierced, chicken reaches an internal temperature of 170°F (75°C) and coating is crispy.

Variation

Use 4 boneless skinless chicken breasts in place of chicken thighs. Grill for same amount of time.

NUTRITIONAL ANALYSIS PER SERVING (WITH PESTO)			
Energy: 372 kcal	Fat: 22 g	Fiber: 1.5 g	Iron: 2.9 mg
Protein: 32 g	Carbohydrate: 11 g	Calcium: 70 mg	Folate: 26 mcg

Pesto

2 to 3	cloves garlic	2 to 3
1¼ cups	fresh basil leaves	300 mL
⅔ cup	pine nuts, toasted (see tip, at left)	150 mL
⅔ cup	olive oil	150 mL

1. In a food processor, finely mince garlic. Add basil leaves and pine nuts and process until chopped. Pour in olive oil while processor is running. Process until smooth.

Variation

If using as a sauce over pasta, add ⅔ cup (150 mL) freshly grated Parmesan cheese at the end and process with a few on/off pulses just until combined. If you plan on freezing your pesto, do not use Parmesan.

NUTRITIONAL ANALYSIS PER SERVING (1 TBSP/15 ML)

| Energy: 35 kcal | Fat: 4 g | Fiber: 0.3 g | Iron: 0.2 mg |
| Protein: 1 g | Carbohydrate: Trace | Calcium: 2 mg | Folate: 2 mcg |

**MAKES ABOUT
1 CUP (250 ML)**

TIPS

Take advantage of abundant fresh basil in late August.

Toast pine nuts in a nonstick skillet over medium heat for about 2 minutes, turning occasionally until lightly browned.

Make ahead

Spoon pesto into an ice cube tray and freeze. Transfer frozen cubes to resealable freezer bags and store in the freezer for up to 2 months.

Crispy Chicken

- Preheat oven to 375°F (190°C)
- Baking sheet, lightly greased

½ cup	plain low-fat yogurt	125 mL
½ tsp	dried tarragon (optional)	2 mL
¼ tsp	salt	1 mL
¼ tsp	freshly ground black pepper	1 mL
1½ cups	finely crushed corn flakes cereal	375 mL
¼ cup	freshly grated Parmesan cheese	50 mL
12	boneless skinless chicken thighs (about 28 oz/800 g total), rinsed and patted dry	12

1. In a bowl, combine yogurt, tarragon, salt and pepper; stir to mix well. In another bowl, combine corn flakes and Parmesan.

2. Roll chicken in yogurt mixture to coat, then roll in crumb mixture. Place on prepared baking sheet and bake in preheated oven for 45 to 50 minutes or until chicken is no longer pink and juices run clear when pierced with a fork.

NUTRITIONAL ANALYSIS PER SERVING

| Energy: 125 kcal | Fat: 3 g | Fiber: 0.1 g | Iron: 1.9 mg |
| Protein: 15 g | Carbohydrate: 9 g | Calcium: 49 mg | Folate: 13 mcg |

Source of:
- Folate and iron

**MAKES
12 SERVINGS**

This dish is so quick and easy, the kids can help to prepare it!

TIP

Serve plain or with plum sauce for dipping

**MAKES
4 SERVINGS**

These slightly sweet grilled chicken breasts are easy to make and pair well with grilled vegetables and a rice pilaf — or try them on their own with a fresh tossed salad.

Make ahead

Prepare through Step 1, cover and refrigerate for up to 12 hours.

Grilled Honey-Ginger Chicken Breasts

- Preheat barbecue to medium-high

2	cloves garlic, minced	2
2 tbsp	grated gingerroot	25 mL
2 tbsp	sodium-reduced soy sauce	25 mL
1 tbsp	freshly squeezed lime juice	15 mL
1 tsp	liquid honey	5 mL
Dash	hot pepper sauce (optional)	Dash
4	boneless skinless chicken breasts	4

1. In a small bowl, combine garlic, ginger, soy sauce, lime juice, honey and hot pepper sauce (if using). Brush over chicken breasts.

2. Place chicken on preheated barbecue and grill for about 6 minutes per side, or until chicken is no longer pink inside and reaches an internal temperature of 170°F (75°C).

NUTRITIONAL ANALYSIS PER SERVING			
Energy: 145 kcal	Fat: 2 g	Fiber: 0.1 g	Iron: 1.1 mg
Protein: 28 g	Carbohydrate: 3 g	Calcium: 18 mg	Folate: 6 mcg

Health Tip

Chicken without skin has less fat than most beef and is low in saturated fat. It is an excellent source of protein.

Honey Dijon Chicken

- Preheat oven to 350°F (180°C)
- Baking sheet, greased

2 tbsp	all-purpose flour	25 mL
¼ tsp	salt	1 mL
¼ tsp	freshly ground black pepper	1 mL
4	boneless skinless chicken breasts (3 oz/90 g each)	4
2 tbsp	liquid honey	25 mL
2 tbsp	Dijon mustard	25 mL
1 tbsp	olive oil	15 mL

1. On a piece of wax paper, combine flour, salt and pepper; coat chicken with mixture. In a small dish, combine honey and mustard; set aside.

2. In a skillet, heat oil over medium-high heat; quickly brown chicken on both sides. Place on greased baking sheet; spread with honey mixture. Bake in preheated oven for 10 to 15 minutes or until chicken is no longer pink inside.

NUTRITIONAL ANALYSIS PER SERVING

Energy: 174 kcal	Fat: 5 g	Fiber: 0.1 g	Iron: 0.9 mg
Protein: 22 g	Carbohydrate: 10 g	Calcium: 20 mg	Folate: 4 mcg

MAKES 4 SERVINGS

To add flavor without adding fat, honey and mustard are a superb combination. For a quickly prepared dinner, this chicken dish has it all: it's easy, nutritious and has a great, zippy taste.

TIP

When sautéing, make sure your pan is large enough to hold the ingredients comfortably. If not, cook ingredients in batches. If food is jammed together, it will steam, which causes it to lose flavor.

**MAKES
4 SERVINGS**

*Fresh lemon juice stars
in this Greek-inspired
chicken recipe. Serve
with rice and Greek
salad.*

TIP

If your contact grill has
more than one temperature
setting, set it to high for this
recipe.

Make ahead

Prepare marinade, cover
and store in the refrigerator
for up to 1 day.

Greek Lemon Chicken

• Contact grill

2	cloves garlic, minced	2
½ cup	chopped fresh oregano (or 1 tbsp/15 mL dried)	125 mL
¼ cup	chopped fresh parsley	50 mL
¼ cup	freshly squeezed lemon juice	50 mL
1 tbsp	olive oil	15 mL
½ tsp	kosher salt	2 mL
¼ tsp	freshly ground black pepper	1 mL
4	boneless skinless chicken breasts	4

1. In a small bowl, whisk together garlic, oregano, parsley, lemon juice, olive oil, salt and pepper.

2. Place chicken breasts in a shallow dish. Brush marinade on chicken, coating evenly. Cover and refrigerate for a minimum of 20 minutes or for up to 1 day. Meanwhile, preheat contact grill.

3. Spray both sides of contact grill with vegetable cooking spray or oil. Place chicken on grill, close lid and grill for 5 to 6 minutes, or until chicken is no longer pink inside and reaches an internal temperature of 170°F (75°C).

Variation

This dish can easily be transformed into chicken souvlaki by slicing the chicken into 1-inch (2.5 cm) chunks and threading onto soaked 9-inch (23 cm) bamboo skewers before grilling. Grill for 5 to 6 minutes, or until chicken is no longer pink inside.

NUTRITIONAL ANALYSIS PER SERVING			
Energy: 170 kcal	Fat: 5 g	Fiber: 0.4 g	Iron: 1.6 mg
Protein: 28 g	Carbohydrate: 3 g	Calcium: 41 mg	Folate: 12 mcg

Sticky Sesame Chicken

- Contact grill

2	cloves garlic, minced	2
1/4 cup	oyster sauce	50 mL
1 tbsp	freshly squeezed lemon juice	15 mL
1 tbsp	liquid honey	15 mL
1 tsp	sesame oil	5 mL
1/4 tsp	freshly ground black pepper	1 mL
4	boneless skinless chicken breasts	4
2 tbsp	sesame seeds	25 mL

1. In a small bowl, whisk together garlic, oyster sauce, lemon juice, honey, sesame oil and pepper.

2. Place chicken breasts in a shallow dish. Brush marinade on chicken, coating evenly. Cover and refrigerate for a minimum of 20 minutes or for up to 1 hour. Meanwhile, preheat contact grill.

3. Spray both sides of contact grill with vegetable cooking spray or oil. Sprinkle sesame seeds on both sides of chicken. Place chicken on grill, close lid and grill for 5 to 6 minutes, or until chicken is no longer pink inside and reaches an internal temperature of 170°F (75°C).

Variations

Use 8 boneless skinless chicken thighs in place of chicken breasts. Grill for same amount of time.

Add 1 tsp (5 mL) minced gingerroot or 1/4 tsp (1 mL) ground ginger to marinade.

NUTRITIONAL ANALYSIS PER SERVING			
Energy: 191 kcal	Fat: 5 g	Fiber: 0.4 g	Iron: 1.5 mg
Protein: 28 g	Carbohydrate: 8 g	Calcium: 60 mg	Folate: 9 mcg

MAKES 4 SERVINGS

Kids are drawn to this "sticky chicky" recipe, another quick weekday meal.

TIP

If your contact grill has more than one temperature setting, set it to high for this recipe.

Make ahead

Prepare marinade, cover and store in the refrigerator for up to 1 day.

**MAKES
4 SERVINGS**

*A quick and easy
supper item. Serve
over plain rice or
noodles.*

TIPS

For a less strong curry
taste, reduce the amount of
curry powder to ½ to
1 tsp (2 to 5 mL).

Add the remaining coconut
milk to any leftovers and
heat gently for a nice
soup-like dish.

Curried Chicken

2 tbsp	vegetable oil	25 mL
2	large onions, sliced	2
¼ tsp	salt	1 mL
¼ tsp	freshly ground black pepper	1 mL
2 tsp	curry powder	10 mL
2 cups	unsweetened coconut milk	500 mL
1½ lbs	boneless skinless chicken (breast or thigh), cut into 1-inch (2.5 cm) pieces	750 g
1 cup	diced tomato (drained if canned)	250 mL
2 tbsp	chopped fresh basil	25 mL

1. In a large nonstick skillet, heat oil over medium-high for about 1 minute. Add onions, salt and pepper; reduce heat to medium. Cook, stirring, until onions are soft. Stir in curry powder and cook for 1 minute. Reduce heat to medium and add coconut milk; cook, stirring, for 3 to 4 minutes, or until thickened. Add chicken and cook, stirring, for about 6 minutes, or until no longer pink inside. Add tomatoes and cook for 2 minutes. Sprinkle with basil and serve.

NUTRITIONAL ANALYSIS PER SERVING

Energy: 582 kcal	Fat: 39 g	Fiber: 4.5 g	Iron: 5.1 mg
Protein: 48 g	Carbohydrate: 14 g	Calcium: 109 mg	Folate: 41 mcg

Health Tip

Although skinless chicken thighs have more fat than skinless chicken breasts, they are higher in iron, which is important for oxygen transport in the body.

Chicken Tacos

1 tbsp	vegetable oil	15 mL
8 oz	skinless boneless chicken breasts, cut into ½-inch (1 cm) cubes (see tip, at left)	250 g
½ tsp	chili powder	2 mL
	Freshly ground black pepper	
1	roasted red bell pepper, finely chopped	1
1	can (14 oz/398 mL) refried beans (see tip, at left)	1
1 cup	corn kernels, drained if canned or thawed if frozen	250 mL
1 cup	shredded Tex-Mex cheese mix or Monterey Jack cheese	250 mL
12	taco shells	12
	Salsa	
	Shredded lettuce	
	Chopped tomato	
	Finely chopped red or green onion	
	Cubed avocado	
	Sour cream	

MAKES 4 SERVINGS

The heat of this Tex-Mex dish is easily bumped up with the addition of a jalapeño or chipotle pepper, or spicy salsa as a garnish.

TIPS

If desired, use 8 oz (250 g) precooked sliced chicken breast or 1 can (10 oz/300 g) cut-up chicken in this recipe. Chop and add to the pan along with the beans.

The consistency of refried beans varies among brands. If yours are almost solid when removed from the can, you may need to add as much as ¼ cup (50 mL) water along with the beans to facilitate integration of the ingredients.

1. In a skillet, heat oil over medium heat. Add chicken and cook, stirring, until lightly browned and no longer pink inside, about 5 minutes. Sprinkle with chili powder and pepper to taste. Cook, stirring, for 1 minute. Add red pepper, beans and corn and bring to a boil.

2. Reduce heat to low and simmer for 2 to 3 minutes. Add cheese and stir until melted.

3. Warm taco shells according to package directions. Fill with bean mixture and garnish with any combination of salsa, lettuce, tomato, onion, avocado and/or sour cream.

NUTRITIONAL ANALYSIS PER SERVING			
Energy: 669 kcal	Fat: 35 g	Fiber: 9.6 g	Iron: 4.0 mg
Protein: 40 g	Carbohydrate: 51 g	Calcium: 599 mg	Folate: 96 mcg

**MAKES
4 SERVINGS**

Chicken thighs grill beautifully on the indoor grill and make for an agreeable change from the usual chicken breasts.

TIPS

If your contact grill has more than one temperature setting, set it to high for this recipe.

For a subtle tartness, dip chicken nuggets in ½ cup (125 mL) buttermilk in place of egg yolks before coating in breading.

Chicken Nuggets

- Contact grill

1¼ cups	corn flakes crumbs	300 mL
⅔ cup	freshly grated Parmesan cheese	150 mL
1 tsp	dried thyme	5 mL
1 tsp	dried parsley	5 mL
1 tsp	garlic powder	5 mL
½ tsp	kosher salt	2 mL
½ tsp	freshly ground black pepper	2 mL
2	egg yolks	2
8	boneless skinless chicken thighs	8

1. In a shallow dish, mix together corn flakes crumbs, Parmesan, thyme, parsley, garlic powder, salt and pepper. In another shallow dish, lightly beat egg yolks.

2. Cut chicken into 1-inch (2.5 cm) pieces. Dip pieces in egg yolk and then in coating. Place in a shallow dish, cover and refrigerate for 15 minutes. Discard any excess egg and crumbs. Meanwhile, preheat contact grill.

3. Spray both sides of contact grill with vegetable cooking spray or oil. Place chicken on grill, close lid and grill for 5 to 6 minutes, or until juices run clear when chicken is pierced and coating is crisp.

NUTRITIONAL ANALYSIS PER SERVING			
Energy: 337 kcal	Fat: 12 g	Fiber: 0.3 g	Iron: 5.4 mg
Protein: 35 g	Carbohydrate: 20 g	Calcium: 212 mg	Folate: 41 mcg

Turkiaki Fiesta

2 tsp	vegetable oil	10 mL
1 lb	ground or slivered turkey or chicken	500 g
1 cup	diagonally sliced celery	250 mL
¾ cup	chopped green onions	175 mL
2 tbsp	teriyaki sauce	25 mL
Pinch	salt	Pinch
Pinch	freshly ground black pepper	Pinch
1	large red bell pepper, cubed	1
1	can (10 oz/284 mL) water chestnuts, drained	1
2 cups	snow peas, trimmed	500 mL
1 tbsp	sesame seeds (optional)	15 mL

1. In a wok or nonstick skillet, heat oil over high heat. Add turkey and stir-fry for about 4 minutes or until lightly browned and no longer pink inside. Add celery, green onions, teriyaki sauce, salt and pepper. Cover and steam for 4 minutes. Add red pepper, water chestnuts and snow peas; cover and cook for 6 minutes, stirring occasionally. Serve sprinkled with sesame seeds (if using).

NUTRITIONAL ANALYSIS PER SERVING

Energy: 238 kcal	Fat: 6 g	Fiber: 4.6 g	Iron: 3.1 mg
Protein: 34 g	Carbohydrate: 12 g	Calcium: 60 mg	Folate: 38 mcg

Good source of:
• Iron and fiber

Source of:
• Calcium and folate

MAKES 5 SERVINGS

This recipe combines either ground or slivered poultry with Asian seasonings and vegetables. Add extra teriyaki sauce if a stronger flavor is desired. Serve with cooked rice.

TIPS

If using ground turkey or chicken in this recipe, ensure that the meat is cooked through and no longer pink. Ground meat is considered a high-risk food as bacteria can spread during the grinding process.

If you don't have any sesame seeds in your cupboard, stir ½ tsp (2 mL) sesame oil into the dish just before serving.

**MAKES
6 SERVINGS**

This is a terrific alternative to traditional beef chili, and it's light on spices, which some pregnant women have difficulty digesting.

TIP

This recipe freezes well. Make a batch during pregnancy and freeze leftovers for a quick healthy meal after the baby arrives.

Make ahead

Spoon into an airtight container and store in the refrigerator for up to 3 days or in the freezer for up to 3 months.

Turkey Chili

1 tbsp	olive oil	15 mL
½	green bell pepper, chopped	½
½	red bell pepper, chopped	½
1 lb	lean ground turkey	500 g
1	can (28 oz/796 mL) crushed tomatoes	1
1	can (5½ oz/156 mL) tomato paste	1
1 cup	frozen corn kernels	250 mL
1 tbsp	ground cumin	15 mL
1 tbsp	chili powder	15 mL
1 tsp	salt	5 mL
½ tsp	freshly ground black pepper	2 mL
¼ tsp	ground cinnamon	1 mL
1	can (19 oz/540 mL) red kidney beans, drained and rinsed	1
1	can (19 oz/540 mL) white kidney beans, drained and rinsed	1

1. In a large saucepan, heat oil over medium-high heat. Sauté green pepper and red pepper until tender, about 5 minutes. Transfer to a plate and set aside.

2. In the same saucepan, brown turkey over medium-high heat. Drain any excess fat. Add peppers, tomatoes, tomato paste, corn, cumin, chili powder, salt, pepper and cinnamon; stir well. Gently stir in red and white kidney beans; bring to a boil. Cover, reduce heat and simmer, stirring occasionally, for 20 minutes to let flavors blend.

NUTRITIONAL ANALYSIS PER SERVING			
Energy: 405 kcal	Fat: 11 g	Fiber: 11.6 g	Iron: 7.5 mg
Protein: 29 g	Carbohydrate: 52 g	Calcium: 114 mg	Folate: 199 mcg

Fish and Seafood

Parmesan Herb-Baked Fish Fillets 216

Baked Fish with Tomatoes and
Roasted Red Pepper 217

South Side Halibut 218

Salmon with Roasted Vegetables 219

Honey Dill Salmon with Dijon 220

Baked Lemon Salmon with Mango Salsa 221

Soy-Glazed Salmon 222

Salmon Burgers 223

Sole and Spinach Casserole 224

Parmesan-Crusted Snapper with
Tomato Olive Sauce 226

The Narrows Crab Cakes 227

Sweet and Spicy Shrimp with Broccoli 228

Garlic Chili Shrimp 229

Coconut Shrimp Curry 230

**MAKES
4 SERVINGS**

This elegant entrée is a great dish for entertaining.

TIPS

For convenience and speed, this recipe uses frozen fish fillets, but fresh fish may also be used. If you prefer a thicker fish fillet such as salmon or halibut, increase the cooking time by about 5 minutes.

If available, substitute 1 to 2 tbsp (15 to 25 mL) chopped fresh basil for the dried basil.

Remember to use dry bread crumbs in this recipe; fresh bread crumbs will make the dish too soggy.

Parmesan Herb-Baked Fish Fillets

- Preheat oven to 400°F (200°C)
- 11- by 7-inch (2 L) baking dish, greased

1	package (1 lb/500 g) frozen fish fillets, thawed and patted dry	1
¼ cup	freshly grated Parmesan cheese	50 mL
¼ cup	light mayonnaise	50 mL
2 tbsp	chopped green onions	25 mL
1 tbsp	chopped pimiento or red bell pepper	15 mL
	Cayenne pepper	
½ cup	dry bread crumbs	125 mL
½ tsp	dried basil	2 mL
	Freshly ground black pepper	

1. Place fish fillets in a single layer in bottom of prepared baking dish. Set aside.

2. In a small bowl, stir together cheese, mayonnaise, onions, pimiento and cayenne to taste. Spread mixture evenly over fish fillets.

3. In a separate bowl, combine bread crumbs, basil and pepper to taste; sprinkle over top of fish. Bake in preheated oven for 10 to 12 minutes or until fish is opaque and flakes easily with fork.

NUTRITIONAL ANALYSIS PER SERVING			
Energy: 203 kcal	Fat: 6 g	Fiber: 0.3 g	Iron: 1.1 mg
Protein: 26 g	Carbohydrate: 11 g	Calcium: 91 mg	Folate: 29 mcg

Baked Fish with Tomatoes and Roasted Red Pepper

Good source of:
• Iron

Source of:
• Calcium and folate

• Preheat oven to 375°F (190°C)
• 6-cup (1.5 L) shallow baking dish, lightly greased

MAKES 4 SERVINGS

This tasty bake is particularly delicious accompanied by fluffy mashed potatoes. Serve with a simple green salad for a complete meal.

1 lb	sole fillets or other firm white fish, such as snapper or halibut	500 g
20	cherry or grape tomatoes	20
½ cup	sliced roasted red bell pepper (see tip, page 167)	125 mL
⅓ cup	mayonnaise	75 mL
1 tbsp	Dijon mustard	15 mL
1 tbsp	Worcestershire sauce	15 mL
¼ tsp	salt	1 mL
	Freshly ground black pepper	
1 cup	dry bread crumbs	250 mL
2 tbsp	butter, melted	25 mL

TIP

If using frozen fish fillets in this recipe, thaw in the refrigerator during the day or in the microwave for about 6 minutes on Defrost.

1. In a microwave-safe dish, combine fish fillets with 2 tbsp (25 mL) water. Cover tightly with plastic wrap and microwave on High until fish flakes easily, about 3 minutes. (Or, in a skillet over medium heat, combine fish fillets with water to cover. Bring to a boil. Reduce heat to low and simmer until fish is just cooked through and flakes easily, about 5 minutes.) Using two forks, flake fish.

2. In prepared baking dish, combine fish, tomatoes and red pepper.

3. In a small bowl, whisk together mayonnaise, mustard, Worcestershire sauce, salt and pepper to taste. Spoon over fish mixture and stir to combine.

4. In a separate bowl, combine bread crumbs and butter. Sprinkle evenly over sauce. Bake in preheated oven until top is golden, about 15 minutes.

NUTRITIONAL ANALYSIS PER SERVING			
Energy: 394 kcal	Fat: 21 g	Fiber: 1.5 g	Iron: 2.8 mg
Protein: 26 g	Carbohydrate: 24 g	Calcium: 66 mg	Folate: 34 mcg

South Side Halibut

MAKES
4 SERVINGS

Nothing could be easier than this citrus-flavored fish dish, which is ready in less than 15 minutes. Use snapper, sole or any firm white fish if halibut isn't available.

TIP

You can use frozen fish for this recipe, if desired. To cook from its frozen state, double the cooking time to 20 minutes per inch (2.5 cm) of thickness, measuring the fish from its thickest point.

• Preheat oven to 400°F (200°C)
• Baking dish

1 tsp	vegetable oil	5 mL
1	clove garlic, minced	1
⅓ cup	finely chopped onion	75 mL
2 tbsp	chopped fresh parsley	25 mL
½ tsp	grated orange zest	2 mL
Pinch	freshly ground black pepper	Pinch
¼ cup	freshly squeezed orange juice	50 mL
1 tbsp	freshly squeezed lemon juice	15 mL
4	halibut steaks (4 oz/125 g each) or 1 lb (500 g) halibut or Pacific snapper fillets	4

1. In a small skillet, heat oil over medium heat. Sauté garlic and onion until tender. Remove from heat; stir in parsley, orange zest and pepper. Combine orange juice and lemon juice.

2. Arrange fish in baking dish. Spread onion mixture over fish; pour juice over top. Cover tightly with foil. Bake in preheated oven for 8 to 10 minutes or until fish flakes easily when tested with fork.

NUTRITIONAL ANALYSIS PER SERVING			
Energy: 148 kcal	Fat: 3 g	Fiber: 0.3 g	Iron: 1.0 mg
Protein: 26 g	Carbohydrate: 3 g	Calcium: 25 mg	Folate: 27 mcg

Health Tip

Fish is a terrific source of high-quality protein and is low in saturated fat. It also contains omega 3 fatty acids, which contribute to heart health.

Salmon with Roasted Vegetables

- Preheat oven to 425°F (220°C)
- 11- by 7-inch (2 L) baking dish

1 tbsp	olive oil	15 mL
2 tsp	minced garlic	10 mL
2 tsp	dried thyme, divided	10 mL
1 cup	diced peeled sweet potatoes	250 mL
1 cup	diced zucchini or red bell peppers	250 mL
1 cup	diced peeled parsnips or potatoes	250 mL
2 tbsp	freshly squeezed lemon juice	25 mL
¼ tsp	freshly ground black pepper	1 mL
1	salmon tail (8 to 12 oz/250 to 375 g), patted dry	1

1. In a small bowl, stir together olive oil, garlic and 1 tsp (5 mL) of the thyme. Place sweet potatoes, zucchini and parsnips in baking dish and sprinkle with oil mixture; toss to coat. Spread out vegetables in a single layer and roast in preheated oven for 15 minutes.

2. In the bowl used for oil mixture, combine remaining thyme, lemon juice and pepper. Brush mixture over salmon tail.

3. Remove vegetables from oven and stir. Place salmon, skin side down, on top of vegetables. Bake for 10 to 15 minutes or until fish is opaque and flakes easily with a fork. Remove skin from salmon before serving.

NUTRITIONAL ANALYSIS PER SERVING			
Energy: 568 kcal	Fat: 28 g	Fiber: 4.7 g	Iron: 5.4 mg
Protein: 42 g	Carbohydrate: 36 g	Calcium: 303 mg	Folate: 89 mcg

Excellent source of:
- Calcium, folate and iron

Good source of:
- Fiber

MAKES 2 SERVINGS

Here's a great dish for parents who want to savor a quiet meal together after the children have been fed and put to bed. With or without the kids, it's a perfect meal for 2.

TIP

The tail end of the salmon, which contains the fewest bones, is used in this recipe. However, you can substitute two 4-oz (125 g) salmon fillets, if desired.

The indoor grill might have been created with salmon fillets in mind — they turn out that scrumptious.

TIP

If your contact grill has more than one temperature setting, set it to medium-high for this recipe.

Make ahead

Prepare marinade, cover and store in the refrigerator for up to 1 day.

Honey Dill Salmon with Dijon

• Contact grill

2 tbsp	chopped fresh dill	25 mL
2 tbsp	mayonnaise	25 mL
2 tbsp	Dijon mustard	25 mL
1 tbsp	liquid honey	15 mL
1/2 tsp	salt	2 mL
1/4 tsp	freshly ground black pepper	1 mL
1 lb	salmon fillet, cut into 4 pieces	500 g
	Additional freshly squeezed lemon juice	

1. In a small bowl, whisk together dill, mayonnaise, mustard, honey, salt and pepper.

2. Place salmon fillets in a shallow dish and brush with marinade, coating evenly. Cover and refrigerate for a minimum of 20 minutes or for up to 1 hour. Meanwhile, preheat contact grill.

3. Spray both sides of contact grill with vegetable cooking spray or oil. Place salmon on grill, close lid and grill for 4 to 6 minutes, or until fish is opaque and flakes easily with a fork. Sprinkle with freshly squeezed lemon juice.

Variations

Use other firm fillets, such as steelhead trout, in place of salmon and grill for 4 to 6 minutes, or until fish is opaque and flakes easily with a fork.

Use 2 tsp (10 mL) dried dillweed in place of fresh dill.

NUTRITIONAL ANALYSIS PER SERVING			
Energy: 335 kcal	Fat: 22 g	Fiber: Trace	Iron: 1.3 mg
Protein: 29 g	Carbohydrate: 5 g	Calcium: 110 mg	Folate: 34 mcg

Baked Lemon Salmon with Mango Salsa

Good source of:
- Folate

Source of:
- Calcium and iron

- Preheat toaster oven to 400°F (200°C)
- 8-inch (2 L) square baking dish

1 tbsp	grated lemon zest	15 mL
2 tbsp	freshly squeezed lemon juice	25 mL
1 tbsp	olive oil	15 mL
2 tsp	Russian-style mustard	10 mL
½ tsp	freshly ground black pepper	2 mL
4	salmon fillets (about 6 oz/175 g each), skin removed	4

Mango Salsa

2	green onions, finely chopped	2
1	ripe mango, peeled and diced	1
¼ cup	chopped red bell pepper	50 mL
2 tbsp	chopped fresh cilantro	25 mL
2 tbsp	freshly squeezed lime juice	25 mL

1. In a small bowl, whisk together lemon zest, lemon juice, oil, mustard and pepper.

2. Place salmon in a single layer in baking dish. Pour marinade over fish. Marinate for 20 minutes.

3. Bake in preheated toaster oven for 12 to 15 minutes, or until salmon is just cooked in center.

4. *Meanwhile, prepare mango salsa:* In a bowl, combine green onions, mango, red pepper, cilantro and lime juice. Serve salsa with salmon.

MAKES 4 SERVINGS

MAKES ABOUT 1¼ CUPS (300 ML) SALSA

This is perfect for a quick weeknight meal, yet elegant enough for entertaining. Papaya or pineapple could be used in place of mango. Serve the salmon hot or cold.

NUTRITIONAL ANALYSIS PER SERVING			
Energy: 489 kcal	Fat: 27 g	Fiber: 1.5 g	Iron: 1.9 mg
Protein: 40 g	Carbohydrate: 11 g	Calcium: 152 mg	Folate: 49 mcg

**MAKES
4 SERVINGS**

The flavors here are similar to teriyaki sauce.

Soy-Glazed Salmon

- Preheat toaster oven to 400°F (200°C)
- 8-inch (2 L) square baking dish, lightly greased

2 tbsp	packed brown sugar	25 mL
2 tbsp	soy sauce	25 mL
2 tbsp	rice vinegar or freshly squeezed lemon juice	25 mL
1 tbsp	vegetable oil	15 mL
4	salmon fillets (about 6 oz/175 g each), skin removed	4

1. In a small bowl or measuring cup, combine brown sugar, soy sauce, vinegar and oil. Stir to dissolve sugar.

2. Arrange salmon fillets in a single layer in prepared baking dish. Spoon sauce over salmon.

3. Bake in preheated toaster oven for 12 to 15 minutes, or until salmon is just cooked in center. Spoon glaze over salmon before serving.

Variation

Honey Mustard Salmon: In a small bowl, combine 2 tbsp (25 mL) liquid honey, 2 tbsp (25 mL) freshly squeezed lemon juice, 1 tbsp (15 mL) Dijon mustard and 1 tbsp (15 mL) olive oil. Spoon over salmon in place of soy glaze.

NUTRITIONAL ANALYSIS PER SERVING			
Energy: 438 kcal	Fat: 27 g	Fiber: Trace	Iron: 2.0 mg
Protein: 40 g	Carbohydrate: 7 g	Calcium: 145 mg	Folate: 48 mcg

Salmon Burgers

1	can (7½ oz/213 g) salmon, drained	1
1	egg, beaten	1
½ cup	fine dry bread crumbs, divided	125 mL
1 tsp	dried Italian seasoning	5 mL
¼ tsp	salt	1 mL
	Freshly ground black pepper	
2 tbsp	vegetable oil	25 mL
2	onion or whole wheat buns, split and toasted	2
	Tartar sauce	

1. In a bowl, combine salmon, egg, ¼ cup (50 mL) of the bread crumbs, Italian seasoning, salt and pepper to taste. Mix well. Form mixture into 2 patties, about ½ inch (1 cm) thick. Spread remaining bread crumbs on a plate. Dip each patty into crumbs, covering both sides.

2. In a nonstick skillet, heat oil over medium heat. Add patties and cook, turning once, until hot and golden, about 3 minutes per side.

3. Serve on warm buns slathered with tartar sauce and add your favorite toppings.

NUTRITIONAL ANALYSIS PER SERVING

Energy: 502 kcal	Fat: 24 g	Fiber: 2.4 g	Iron: 3.4 mg
Protein: 32 g	Carbohydrate: 39 g	Calcium: 339 mg	Folate: 55 mcg

Health Tip

Salmon has the highest levels of any fish of omega 3 fatty acids. Omega 3 fats contribute to heart health by lowering LDL cholesterol and triglycerides, among other heart-protective effects.

Excellent source of:
- Calcium

Good source of:
- Folate and iron

Source of:
- Fiber

**MAKES
2 SERVINGS**

Nothing says lunch or a quick dinner better than a good burger. Here's a yummy fish-based version that can easily be varied by changing the toppings. To serve more, simply double or triple the recipe.

**MAKES
4 SERVINGS**

Don't be discouraged by the number of steps in this recipe — it is really very simple to prepare!

Sole and Spinach Casserole

• Preheat broiler
• Casserole

14 oz	fillets of sole or other white fish	400 g

Seasoned Spinach

1½ cups	spinach, trimmed and washed, but not dried	375 mL
1 tsp	soy sauce (low sodium)	5 mL
1 tsp	butter or margarine	5 mL
½ tsp	salt	2 mL
¼ tsp	freshly ground black pepper	1 mL
1 tbsp	all-purpose flour	15 mL

White Sauce

1 tbsp	butter or margarine	15 mL
1½ tbsp	all-purpose flour	22 mL
1 cup	whole milk	250 mL
½ tsp	salt	2 mL
½ tsp	freshly ground black pepper	2 mL

Mushrooms

1 tbsp	butter or margarine	15 mL
1 tbsp	olive oil	15 mL
2 cups	sliced mushrooms	500 mL
¼ cup	freshly grated Parmesan cheese	50 mL

1. In a skillet or poacher or steamer, poach sole until it flakes with a fork. Drain.

2. *Prepare the seasoned spinach:* In a large saucepan, over high heat, cook spinach (with no more water than is clinging to the leaves) until soft. Add soy sauce, butter, salt and pepper. Sprinkle flour over spinach and stir thoroughly to absorb any excess liquid.

3. *Prepare the white sauce:* In a large skillet, melt butter over low heat. Stir in flour; cook, stirring, for 3 to 5 minutes. Slowly whisk in milk; cook, whisking constantly, until sauce is thickened and smooth. Add salt and pepper.

4. *Prepare the mushrooms:* In a small skillet, over medium-high heat, melt butter and olive oil. Add mushrooms and cook for about 5 minutes or until softened. Set aside.

5. Spread seasoned spinach in a layer on bottom of casserole. Arrange poached sole fillets on top of spinach. Sprinkle mushrooms over sole. Pour white sauce over. Sprinkle with cheese. Broil until white sauce starts to bubble.

NUTRITIONAL ANALYSIS PER SERVING

Energy: 261 kcal	Fat: 15 g	Fiber: 2.0 g	Iron: 2.2 mg
Protein: 23 g	Carbohydrate: 10 g	Calcium: 178 mg	Folate: 68 mcg

Health Tip

Spinach is one of nature's nutrient giants. This dark green veggie is quick to prepare and is chock full of vitamins, including folate and vitamins A and K, as well as minerals such as iron and magnesium.

**MAKES
4 SERVINGS**

Here's a quick and easy dish that takes advantage of the rich Mediterranean flavors of bottled antipasto sauce.

TIPS

The preferred bread crumbs are Japanese panko, which are quite coarse and produce a particularly crunchy crust. However, they can be a bit tricky to find as they are not always identified as such. They keep well; just store in a resealable bag after opening and use before the expiration date.

There are many kinds of antipasto sauce on the market. When making this recipe, check the label to ensure that it contains tomato and black olives.

For a hint of spice, add a pinch of cayenne pepper to the bread crumb mixture.

Stir 1 tbsp (15 mL) drained capers into antipasto sauce before serving.

Parmesan-Crusted Snapper with Tomato Olive Sauce

1 cup	coarse dry bread crumbs, such as panko (see tip, at left)	250 mL
½ cup	freshly grated Parmesan cheese	125 mL
½ tsp	salt	2 mL
	Freshly ground black pepper	
1 lb	snapper or other firm white fish fillets, patted dry, cut into 4 pieces	500 g
2 tbsp	mayonnaise	25 mL
1 tbsp	vegetable oil	15 mL
½ cup	bottled antipasto sauce (see tip, at left)	125 mL

1. In a bowl, combine bread crumbs, cheese, salt and pepper to taste. Spread mixture on a plate.

2. Brush fish evenly with mayonnaise, then dip in crumb mixture.

3. In a skillet, heat oil over medium heat. Add fish and cook, turning once, until it flakes easily when tested with a knife and outside is crisp and golden, about 3 minutes per side. Serve immediately topped with antipasto sauce.

NUTRITIONAL ANALYSIS PER SERVING

Energy: 360 kcal	Fat: 14 g	Fiber: 0.9 g	Iron: 2.0 mg
Protein: 33 g	Carbohydrate: 24 g	Calcium: 220 mg	Folate: 26 mcg

The Narrows Crab Cakes

MAKES 6 SERVINGS

1	stalk celery, finely chopped	1
¼ cup	finely chopped onion	50 mL
1 tbsp	chopped fresh parsley	15 mL
4	egg whites, lightly beaten	4
1 cup	fine dry bread crumbs, divided	250 mL
2 tsp	Worcestershire sauce	10 mL
1 tsp	dry mustard	5 mL
½ tsp	salt	2 mL
2	cans (6 oz/170 g each) crabmeat, drained and flaked	2
	Lemon wedges	

1. In a skillet sprayed with nonstick cooking spray, cook celery, onion and parsley over medium heat, stirring, until tender, about 5 minutes.

2. In a bowl, stir together egg whites, ¾ cup (175 mL) of the bread crumbs, Worcestershire sauce, mustard and salt. Stir in celery mixture and crabmeat, mixing well. Using about ⅓ cup (75 mL) crab mixture for each, shape into ½-inch (1 cm) thick patties. Coat with remaining bread crumbs.

3. Spray skillet again with cooking spray. Cook patties over medium heat for about 3 minutes per side or until golden. Serve with lemon wedges.

Crab cakes are a traditional favorite at seaside restaurants, where the ambience and the presentation can range from casual to elegant. This version can be served as a dinner entrée or, if you prefer, you can reduce the size of the cakes to serve as a great finger-food appetizer.

TIP

These crab cakes will freeze well, so use what you need and freeze the remainder for another meal.

NUTRITIONAL ANALYSIS PER SERVING			
Energy: 143 kcal	Fat: 2 g	Fiber: 0.4 g	Iron: 1.3 mg
Protein: 16 g	Carbohydrate: 14 g	Calcium: 88 mg	Folate: 19 mcg

**MAKES
4 SERVINGS AS A
MAIN MEAL, 8 AS
AN APPETIZER**

*You may want to double
up on this recipe, as it
is truly delicious. We
suggest serving it over
flavorful jasmine rice.*

TIP

You can find garlic chili
sauce in the specialty
section or Thai section of
most large supermarkets.

Sweet and Spicy Shrimp with Broccoli

Sauce

1 tbsp	granulated sugar	15 mL
1 tbsp	garlic chili sauce	15 mL
1 tbsp	ketchup	15 mL
1 tsp	soy sauce	5 mL
1 tsp	cornstarch	5 mL
1 lb	large shrimp, thawed, peeled and deveined	500 g
3 tbsp	vegetable oil, divided	45 mL
½ tsp	salt	2 mL
Pinch	freshly ground white pepper	Pinch
2 tbsp	chopped onion	25 mL
1 tsp	minced garlic	5 mL
2 cups	broccoli florets, cooked and drained	500 mL
¼ cup	chopped fresh cilantro	50 mL

1. *Prepare the sauce:* In a small bowl, combine ¼ cup (50 mL) water, sugar, chili sauce, ketchup, soy sauce and cornstarch.

2. Pat shrimp dry with paper towels and place in a shallow dish. Drizzle with 1 tbsp (15 mL) of the oil and sprinkle with salt and pepper. Cover and refrigerate for 15 minutes.

3. In a wok or nonstick skillet, heat the remaining oil over medium-high heat. Add onion and garlic; cook, stirring, for about 30 seconds, until onion is softened. Add shrimp and cook, stirring, until bright pink and opaque, about 4 minutes. Pour sauce over shrimp and cook, stirring, until sauce begins to bubble. Stir in broccoli and cilantro and heat through for about 1 minute.

NUTRITIONAL ANALYSIS PER SERVING (1 OF 4 SERVINGS)			
Energy: 296 kcal	Fat: 13 g	Fiber: 1.7 g	Iron: 2.5 mg
Protein: 23 g	Carbohydrate: 22 g	Calcium: 109 mg	Folate: 62 mcg

Garlic Chili Shrimp

1 tbsp	vegetable oil	15 mL
1 lb	peeled and deveined shrimp, thawed if frozen	500 g
1 tbsp	minced garlic	15 mL
2 tbsp	sweet sherry, sake or vodka	25 mL
2 tbsp	soy sauce	25 mL
1 to 2 tsp	Asian chili sauce	5 to 10 mL
2 tbsp	chopped green onion	25 mL

1. In a skillet, heat oil over medium-high heat. Add shrimp and cook, stirring, until they firm up and turn pink, 3 to 5 minutes. Using a slotted spoon, transfer to a platter or serving plate.

2. Add garlic to pan and cook, stirring, for 30 seconds. Add sherry, soy sauce and Asian chili sauce and stir until mixture boils, about 30 seconds. Pour over shrimp. Garnish with green onion and serve immediately.

NUTRITIONAL ANALYSIS PER SERVING

Energy: 162 kcal	Fat: 4 g	Fiber: 0.1 g	Iron: 2.2 mg
Protein: 23 g	Carbohydrate: 4 g	Calcium: 85 mg	Folate: 26 mcg

Good source of:
• Iron

Source of:
• Calcium and folate

MAKES 4 SERVINGS

With a bag of shrimp in the freezer and two basic bottled Asian sauces, you can make this zesty Chinese-inspired dish at a moment's notice. Serve on a small white oval platter to emphasize its simplicity. For a more colorful presentation, spread over a bed of lettuce leaves or sliced cucumber spiked with hot pepper flakes. Accompany with hot white rice.

TIP

Virtually all shrimp sold today has been previously frozen, so there are few benefits to purchasing shrimp from a fish market. Bags of frozen shelled, cleaned shrimp, which can be kept in the freezer for as long as 2 months, are an indispensable convenience food. They should be thawed before cooking and not refrozen after thawing. Cook shrimp quickly over high heat for about 3 minutes. Cooking at too low a temperature produces a mushy texture, and overcooking makes them tough.

**MAKES
4 SERVINGS**

If you're lucky enough to have traveled to Thailand, you'll know that this is a version of the basic coconut milk curry that is served all over the country, but particularly in the south, where coconuts and shrimp are abundant. This quick and easy recipe is delicious over hot white rice.

TIPS

Many Thai cooks make their own curry paste, but bottled versions are now available in supermarkets with a well-stocked Asian foods section.

For a spicier version, increase the amount of curry paste. But be careful — a little goes a long way.

Coconut Shrimp Curry

1 tbsp	vegetable oil	15 mL
1 lb	peeled and deveined shrimp, thawed if frozen	500 g
	Freshly ground black pepper	
1 tbsp	red curry paste (see tip, at left)	15 mL
1 cup	coconut milk	250 mL
2 tbsp	fish sauce	25 mL
2 tbsp	freshly squeezed lime juice	25 mL
1 tbsp	granulated sugar	15 mL
	Cooked white rice	

1. In a skillet, heat oil over medium-high heat. Add shrimp and cook, stirring, until they firm up and turn pink, 3 to 5 minutes. Season with pepper to taste. Using a slotted spoon, transfer to a deep platter and keep warm. Return pan to element.

2. Add red curry paste and cook, stirring, until it releases its aroma, 1 to 2 minutes. Stir in coconut milk, fish sauce, lime juice and sugar. Bring to a boil. Simmer for 1 to 2 minutes to combine flavors. Pour over shrimp. Serve immediately over hot white rice.

NUTRITIONAL ANALYSIS PER SERVING			
Energy: 310 kcal	Fat: 20 g	Fiber: 1.4 g	Iron: 3.1 mg
Protein: 24 g	Carbohydrate: 10 g	Calcium: 93 mg	Folate: 35 mcg

Health Tip

Many people believe that, to lower blood cholesterol, seafood should be avoided. However, dietary cholesterol, such as the cholesterol found in shrimp, has very little effect on blood cholesterol levels. It is saturated fats and trans fatty acids that are more influential on blood cholesterol levels.

Meat

Beef Fajitas 232

Beef Stroganoff 233

Beef Souvlaki 234

20-Minute Chili 235

Meatballs with Teriyaki Sauce 236

Meatball Pasta Sauce 237

Homestyle Meatloaf 238

Meatloaf "Muffins" with Barbecue Sauce 239

Beef Lettuce Wraps 240

Quick and Easy Cabbage Rolls 241

Spiced Veal Stir-fry 242

Just Peachy Pork 243

Orange Ginger Pork and Vegetables 244

Teriyaki Pork Chops 245

Savory Lamb Chops 246

**MAKES
5 SERVINGS**

Fajitas have become popular, in part because they are fun to put together as well as to eat. This version is assembled, then baked.

Make ahead

For convenience, assemble fajitas early in the day, cover and refrigerate. Bake just before serving.

Beef Fajitas

- Preheat oven to 350°F (180°C)
- 13- by 9-inch (3 L) baking dish, greased

1 tbsp	vegetable oil	15 mL
2	onions, thinly sliced	2
1	green bell pepper, cut into thin strips	1
1	red bell pepper, cut into thin strips	1
1 lb	beef steak (round, flank or sirloin), trimmed and thinly sliced across the grain	500 g
2	tomatoes, diced	2
2	cloves garlic, minced	2
2 tsp	chili powder	10 mL
1 tsp	hot pepper sauce	5 mL
½ tsp	freshly ground black pepper	2 mL
½ tsp	dry mustard	2 mL
½ tsp	ground ginger	2 mL
10	8-inch (20 cm) soft flour tortillas	10
⅔ cup	shredded light Cheddar cheese	150 mL

1. In a large nonstick skillet, heat oil over medium-high heat; cook onions, green pepper and red pepper, stirring, for 4 to 5 minutes. Remove from pan.

2. Add beef to pan; brown for 2 minutes. Stir in tomatoes, garlic, chili powder, hot pepper sauce, pepper, mustard and ginger; heat through. Return vegetables to skillet; heat through.

3. Divide mixture among tortillas; sprinkle mixture with 1 tbsp (15 mL) cheese and roll up. Place in prepared baking dish. Bake in preheated oven for about 10 minutes to heat through.

NUTRITIONAL ANALYSIS PER SERVING			
Energy: 647 kcal	Fat: 22 g	Fiber: 1.7 g	Iron: 5.3 mg
Protein: 36 g	Carbohydrate: 74 g	Calcium: 107 mg	Folate: 25 mcg

Beef Stroganoff

- Preheat oven to 250°F (120°C)

1 tbsp	vegetable oil	15 mL
2 tbsp	butter, divided	25 mL
8 oz	sliced mushrooms	250 g
1 lb	sirloin steak, cut into ½-inch (1 cm) strips	500 g
¼ tsp	salt	1 mL
	Freshly ground black pepper	
2 tbsp	minced shallots or finely chopped green onion (white parts only)	25 mL
1 tbsp	all-purpose flour	15 mL
1 cup	beef stock	250 mL
1 tbsp	Dijon mustard	15 mL
½ cup	sour cream	125 mL
1	dill pickle, finely chopped	1
	Hot buttered egg noodles	

1. In a skillet, heat oil and 1 tbsp (15 mL) of the butter over medium-high heat. Add mushrooms and cook, stirring, until they begin to lose their liquid, about 7 minutes. Using a slotted spoon, transfer to a plate and keep warm in preheated oven.

2. Add remaining butter to pan. Add steak strips and sauté until desired degree of doneness, about 1½ minutes per side for medium. Season with salt and pepper to taste. Transfer to a warm platter and keep warm in oven.

3. Reduce heat to medium. Add shallots to pan and cook, stirring, for 1 minute. Add flour and cook, stirring, for 1 minute. Add stock. Bring to a boil. Cook, stirring, until thickened, about 3 minutes. Stir in mustard.

4. Return mushrooms to pan. Add sour cream and chopped dill pickle and cook, stirring, just until cream is heated through, about 1 minute. (Do not let mixture boil or it will curdle.) Pour over steak and serve with hot noodles.

NUTRITIONAL ANALYSIS PER SERVING			
Energy: 315 kcal	Fat: 18 g	Fiber: 1.8 g	Iron: 4.0 mg
Protein: 30 g	Carbohydrate: 7 g	Calcium: 76 mg	Folate: 30 mcg

Excellent source of:
- Iron

Source of:
- Calcium and folate

MAKES 4 SERVINGS

Here's a dish that is quick to make yet elegant enough for special occasions. The sauce is delicious over hot buttered egg noodles. Just add a bottle of robust red wine and a crisp green salad.

**MAKES
4 SERVINGS**

Skewered marinated meat is a breeze on the grill and lends itself to advance preparation. Serve this Greek-inspired dish with Tzatziki Sauce (see recipe, page 159) and Greek Summer Salad (see recipe, page 184).

TIP

If your contact grill has more than one temperature setting, set it to high for this recipe.

Beef Souvlaki

• Contact grill
• Eight 9-inch (23 cm) bamboo skewers

2	cloves garlic, minced	2
1 tbsp	chopped fresh oregano (or 1 tsp/5 mL dried oregano)	15 mL
1 tbsp	olive oil	15 mL
2 tsp	freshly squeezed lemon juice	10 mL
½ tsp	kosher salt	2 mL
¼ tsp	freshly ground black pepper	1 mL
1 lb	top sirloin steak, cut into 1-inch (2.5 cm) cubes	500 g
8	Greek pitas	8
4	small tomatoes, quartered	4
1	red onion, quartered	1

1. Soak bamboo skewers in hot water for 30 minutes.

2. In a small bowl, whisk together garlic, oregano, olive oil, lemon juice, salt and pepper.

3. Thread cubes of beef on soaked bamboo skewers and place in a shallow dish. Brush marinade on steak, coating evenly. Cover and refrigerate for a minimum of 20 minutes or for up to 1 day. Meanwhile, preheat contact grill.

4. Spray both sides of contact grill with vegetable cooking spray or oil. Separate onion quarters into slices, place on grill, close lid and grill for 4 minutes. Place tomato quarters on grill, close lid and grill for 1 minute. Transfer to a bowl, cover and keep warm.

5. Place skewers on grill, close lid and grill for 5 to 6 minutes, or until steak reaches an internal temperature of 160°F (71°C) for medium or 170°F (75°C) for well done.

6. Reduce grill to medium heat, if possible. Just before serving, place pitas on grill and, with lid open, heat pitas for 1 minute.

7. Remove meat from skewers. On each pita, place meat, tomatoes and onion. Roll up.

NUTRITIONAL ANALYSIS PER SERVING			
Energy: 658 kcal	Fat: 9 g	Fiber: 2.1 g	Iron: 3.7 mg
Protein: 49 g	Carbohydrate: 103 g	Calcium: 51 mg	Folate: 29 mcg

20-Minute Chili

1 lb	lean ground beef or turkey	500 g
2	large cloves garlic, finely chopped	2
1	large onion, chopped	1
1	large green bell pepper, chopped	1
4 tsp	chili powder	20 mL
1 tbsp	all-purpose flour	15 mL
1 tsp	dried basil	5 mL
1 tsp	dried oregano	5 mL
¼ to ½ tsp	hot pepper flakes	1 to 2 mL
2 cups	tomato pasta sauce	500 mL
1⅓ cups	beef stock	325 mL
1	can (19 oz/540 mL) kidney beans or pinto beans, rinsed and drained	1
	Salt and freshly ground black pepper	

1. In a Dutch oven or large saucepan, over medium-high heat, cook beef, breaking up with a wooden spoon, for 5 minutes or until no longer pink.

2. Reduce heat to medium. Add garlic, onion, green pepper, chili powder, flour, basil, oregano and hot pepper flakes; cook, stirring, for 4 minutes or until vegetables are softened. Stir in tomato sauce and beef stock. Bring to a boil; cook, stirring, until thickened. Add beans; season with salt and pepper to taste. Reduce heat and simmer, covered, for 10 minutes.

NUTRITIONAL ANALYSIS PER SERVING (1 OF 6)			
Energy: 315 kcal	Fat: 14 g	Fiber: 7.0 g	Iron: 5.0 mg
Protein: 24 g	Carbohydrate: 26 g	Calcium: 62 mg	Folate: 106 mcg

Health Tip

The beans in any chili recipe give the fiber content a real boost.

MAKES 4 TO 6 SERVINGS

Here's a streamlined version of chili that's a snap. Make a double batch and have containers stashed away in the freezer for quick microwave meals. Just ladle into bowls and, if desired, top with shredded Monterey Jack cheese. Set out a basket of crusty bread — supper is that easy.

TIP

Add just a pinch of hot pepper flakes for a mild chili; but if you want to turn up the heat, use amount specified in the recipe.

**MAKES
4 SERVINGS**

**MAKES ABOUT
1 CUP (250 ML)
SAUCE**

*Serve the humble
meatball with pasta,
mashed potatoes,
stir-fried rice, in
sandwiches or as
appetizers. Try one
of the other suggested
sauces or use your
own family recipe.*

Meatballs with Teriyaki Sauce

- Preheat toaster oven to 375°F (190°C)
- 8-inch (2 L) square baking dish, lightly greased

Meatballs

1 lb	lean ground beef, chicken or turkey	500 g
½ cup	fresh bread crumbs	125 mL
1	egg, beaten	1
¼ cup	finely chopped green onion	50 mL
2 tbsp	Worcestershire sauce	25 mL
½ tsp	salt	2 mL
½ tsp	freshly ground black pepper	2 mL

Teriyaki Sauce

½ cup	chicken stock	125 mL
¼ cup	soy sauce	50 mL
¼ cup	rice wine (mirin) or orange juice	50 mL
2 tbsp	granulated sugar	25 mL
1 tbsp	chopped gingerroot	15 mL

1. *Prepare the meatballs:* In a large bowl, combine ground meat, bread crumbs, egg, green onion, Worcestershire sauce, salt and pepper. Shape mixture into about 25 meatballs (about 1 inch/2.5 cm in diameter). Arrange in prepared baking dish.

2. *Prepare the sauce:* In a medium bowl, combine chicken stock, soy sauce, rice wine, sugar and ginger. Pour sauce over meatballs.

3. Bake in preheated toaster oven for 40 minutes, carefully stirring occasionally.

Variations

Meatballs with Sweet and Sour Sauce: For sauce, combine ¾ cup (175 mL) ketchup, ½ cup (125 mL) pineapple juice, ¼ cup (50 mL) white vinegar, 2 tbsp (25 mL) packed brown sugar and 1 tbsp (15 mL) soy sauce.

Meatballs with Tomato Sauce: For sauce, combine 1½ cups (375 mL) tomato sauce, 2 minced cloves garlic, 1 chopped small onion and ¼ cup (50 mL) freshly grated Parmesan cheese.

NUTRITIONAL ANALYSIS PER SERVING			
Energy: 432 kcal	Fat: 21 g	Fiber: 0.4 g	Iron: 4.6 mg
Protein: 31 g	Carbohydrate: 28 g	Calcium: 54 mg	Folate: 40 mcg

Meatball Pasta Sauce

1	egg, lightly beaten	1
½	onion, diced	½
18 oz	lean ground beef, divided	540 g
2 tbsp	freshly grated Parmesan cheese	25 mL
2 tbsp	dry bread crumbs	25 mL
1 tsp	dried savory	5 mL
1 tsp	dried oregano	5 mL
½ tsp	salt	2 mL
½ tsp	freshly ground black pepper	2 mL
2 tbsp	vegetable oil, divided	25 mL
1	jar (24 oz/700 mL) pasta sauce	1
1 tbsp	granulated sugar	15 mL
1 tbsp	dried basil	15 mL
1 tbsp	garlic powder	15 mL

1. In a medium bowl, combine egg, onion, 1 lb (500 g) of the beef, Parmesan, bread crumbs, savory, oregano, salt and pepper; mix well. Shape into meatballs, using approximately 1 tsp (5 mL) beef mixture for each meatball. (Makes about 48 meatballs.)

2. In a large nonstick skillet, heat 1 tbsp (15 mL) of the oil over medium-high heat. Add meatballs, in batches as necessary, and cook for 10 to 15 minutes, or until no longer pink inside. Set aside.

3. In a large saucepan, heat the remaining oil over medium-high heat. Add the remaining beef and cook, breaking up with a spoon, until browned, about 5 minutes. Add pasta sauce, sugar, basil and garlic powder; cook for 15 minutes. Add meatballs; reduce heat to medium and cook until meatballs are heated through, about 15 minutes.

NUTRITIONAL ANALYSIS PER SERVING (1 CUP/250 ML)			
Energy: 232 kcal	Fat: 14 g	Fiber: 1.6 g	Iron: 2.7 mg
Protein: 16 g	Carbohydrate: 11 g	Calcium: 59 mg	Folate: 20 mcg

Good source of:
• Iron

Source of:
• Calcium and folate

MAKES 8 CUPS (2 L)

A great source of iron, and very tasty. It's also a good recipe for older infants and toddlers! Serve over noodles or plain rice.

TIP

Freeze in single or double portions.

Make ahead

Place in an airtight container and store in the freezer for up to 3 months.

**MAKES
6 SERVINGS**

*This old standby is still
a big favorite. Instead
of ground beef you
can use a combination
of ground meats such
as pork, veal, turkey
or chicken. Slice
leftovers to serve in
sandwiches.*

Homestyle Meatloaf

• Preheat toaster oven to 350°F (180°C)
• 8- by 4-inch (1.5 L) loaf pan

1 tbsp	olive oil	15 mL
3	cloves garlic, finely chopped	3
1	onion, chopped	1
1	egg	1
1½ lbs	lean ground beef	750 g
½ cup	fresh bread crumbs	125 mL
½ cup	ketchup or chili sauce	125 mL
1 tbsp	prepared horseradish	15 mL
1 tbsp	Worcestershire sauce	15 mL
1 tbsp	Dijon mustard	15 mL
½ tsp	dried sage	2 mL
½ tsp	salt	2 mL
¼ tsp	freshly ground black pepper	1 mL

Topping

¼ cup	ketchup	50 mL
1 tsp	prepared horseradish	5 mL
1 tsp	Dijon mustard	5 mL

1. In a small skillet, heat oil over medium-high heat. Add garlic and onion. Cook, stirring occasionally, for 3 minutes, or until softened.

2. In a large bowl, beat egg. Add ground beef, cooked onion mixture, bread crumbs, ketchup, horseradish, Worcestershire sauce, mustard, sage, salt and pepper. Mix together thoroughly. Pack into loaf pan.

3. *Prepare the topping:* In a small bowl, combine ketchup, horseradish and mustard. Spread over top of meatloaf.

4. Bake in preheated toaster oven for 70 to 75 minutes, or until a meat thermometer registers 170°F (75°C). Let stand for 10 to 15 minutes. Pour off any accumulated fat before slicing.

NUTRITIONAL ANALYSIS PER SERVING			
Energy: 387 kcal	Fat: 23 g	Fiber: 1.0 g	Iron: 3.5 mg
Protein: 27 g	Carbohydrate: 18 g	Calcium: 49 mg	Folate: 26 mcg

Meatloaf "Muffins" with Barbecue Sauce

- Preheat oven to 375°F (190°C)
- 12-cup muffin tin, greased

Meatloaf "Muffins"

1½ lb	lean ground beef	750 g
¾ cup	oatmeal, dry bread crumbs or cracker crumbs	175 mL
¼ cup	wheat bran	50 mL
1	can (5.4 oz/160 mL) 2% evaporated milk	1
1	egg	1
1 tsp	chili powder	5 mL
½ tsp	garlic powder	2 mL
¼ tsp	salt	1 mL
¼ tsp	freshly ground black pepper	1 mL

Barbecue Sauce

1 cup	ketchup	250 mL
¼ cup	finely chopped onion	50 mL
2 tbsp	packed brown sugar	25 mL
½ tsp	hot pepper sauce (optional)	2 mL

1. *Prepare the meatloaf "muffins":* In a large bowl, combine ground beef, oatmeal, bran, milk, egg, chili powder, garlic powder, salt and pepper. Divide mixture evenly among muffin cups, pressing down lightly.

2. *Prepare the barbecue sauce:* In another bowl, combine ketchup, onion, sugar and hot pepper sauce (if using). Spoon about 1 tbsp (15 mL) sauce over each muffin.

3. Bake in preheated oven for 25 to 30 minutes or until meat is no longer pink in center.

NUTRITIONAL ANALYSIS PER SERVING			
Energy: 418 kcal	Fat: 21 g	Fiber: 2.0 g	Iron: 3.9 mg
Protein: 29 g	Carbohydrate: 27 g	Calcium: 116 mg	Folate: 32 mcg

Excellent source of:
- Iron

Source of:
- Calcium, folate and fiber

MAKES 6 SERVINGS

MAKES ABOUT 1 CUP (250 ML) SAUCE

These meaty "muffins" are a favorite of kids and adults. Instead of making the sauce, you can substitute 1 cup (250 mL) of your favorite prepared barbecue sauce.

TIPS

If you don't like onion pieces in the sauce, substitute ¼ tsp (1 mL) onion or garlic powder. Limit use of onion and garlic salt, as they add unnecessary sodium.

Adding wheat bran is a great way to boost the fiber content of meat loaf, meatballs and hamburgers. Use about ¼ cup (50 mL) per 1½ lb (750 g) ground meat. Adding canned evaporated milk or skim-milk powder helps to increase calcium.

MAKES 8 WRAPS

You can serve this fresh, simple recipe as either an appetizer or an easy supper item.

TIP

You'll need ½ cup (125 mL) uncooked jasmine rice to make 1 cup (250 mL) cooked.

Beef Lettuce Wraps

Sauce

3 tbsp	soy sauce	45 mL
3 tbsp	garlic chili sauce (see tip, page 228)	45 mL
2	green onions, finely chopped	2
1	clove garlic, finely chopped or crushed	1
3 tbsp	soy sauce	45 mL
2 tbsp	granulated sugar	25 mL
2 tbsp	rice wine or rice vinegar	25 mL
1 tbsp	grated gingerroot	15 mL
1 tbsp	sesame oil	15 mL
1 tsp	freshly ground black pepper	5 mL
1 lb	boneless beef sirloin steak, thinly sliced	500 g
1 tbsp	sesame seeds	15 mL
8	iceberg lettuce leaves, washed and dried	8
1 cup	cooked jasmine rice	250 mL

1. *Prepare the sauce:* In a small bowl, combine soy sauce and chili sauce.

2. In another small bowl, combine green onions, garlic, soy sauce, sugar, rice wine, ginger, sesame oil, 1 tbsp (15 mL) of the sauce and pepper.

3. Place steak pieces in a shallow dish. Brush with marinade, coating evenly. Cover and refrigerate for 1 to 2 hours.

4. Heat a large nonstick skillet over high heat for 1 minute. Cook steak, stirring, for 3 to 4 minutes, or to desired doneness. Sprinkle with sesame seeds. Set aside. Discard any excess marinade.

5. Spread about 2 tsp (10 mL) sauce on each lettuce leaf. Add 2 tbsp (30 mL) rice and top with a few pieces of steak. Wrap the lettuce around the mixture and serve.

NUTRITIONAL ANALYSIS PER SERVING (1 WRAP)			
Energy: 164 kcal	Fat: 5 g	Fiber: 1.1 g	Iron: 2.3 mg
Protein: 16 g	Carbohydrate: 13 g	Calcium: 38 mg	Folate: 23 mcg

Quick and Easy Cabbage Rolls

1	large head cabbage (3 to 4 lbs/ 1.5 to 2 kg), frozen overnight	1
1	onion, finely chopped	1
1	clove garlic, minced	1
12 oz	lean ground pork	375 g
12 oz	lean or extra-lean ground beef	375 g
¾ cup	white rice	175 mL
1 tsp	salt	5 mL
½ tsp	freshly ground black pepper	2 mL
1	can (10 oz/284 mL) condensed tomato soup, undiluted	1
1	can (5½ oz/156 mL) tomato paste	1
1 tsp	granulated sugar	5 mL

1. In a large bowl, run lukewarm water over frozen head of cabbage to defrost. Drain and set aside.

2. In another large bowl, using your hands or a fork, combine onion, garlic, ground pork, ground beef, rice, salt and pepper; mix well.

3. Carefully peel leaves off cabbage, one at a time. Cut out the hard center piece of each cabbage leaf in the shape of a triangle. Add about ½ cup (125 mL) meat mixture just above the tip of the triangle. (The amount of meat needed for each roll will vary depending on the size of the cabbage leaf.) Fold leaves over meat and roll up. Use toothpicks to hold rolls together, if necessary.

4. Place cabbage rolls in a large stockpot. Cover with water and bring to a boil over high heat. Add tomato soup, tomato paste and sugar, stirring gently to incorporate. Reduce heat, cover and simmer for 1½ hours, until cabbage is tender and pork and beef are no longer pink.

NUTRITIONAL ANALYSIS PER SERVING (1 ROLL)

Energy: 370 kcal	Fat: 23 g	Fiber: 3.3 g	Iron: 3.2 mg
Protein: 25 g	Carbohydrate: 16 g	Calcium: 75 mg	Folate: 62 mcg

Good source of:
- Folate and iron

Source of:
- Calcium and fiber

MAKES ABOUT 12 ROLLS

The quick and easy part of this recipe comes from using a frozen head of cabbage. This differs from the traditional method of boiling and draining cabbage leaves before adding meat. Just defrost, and the leaves of the cabbage are ready to roll!

TIP

This recipe freezes wonderfully. Make it while you're pregnant and freeze the leftovers in small batches for a fast, healthy meal once your new bundle of joy arrives and there is very little time in the day for cooking!

Make ahead

Place in an airtight container and store in the freezer for up to 3 months.

Spiced Veal Stir-fry

This delicious stir-fry recipe uses veal seasoned with ginger, garlic, hot pepper flakes — and cinnamon! Serve over rice.

TIPS

Stir-frying and sautéing are basically the same method of cooking: food is cooked quickly in a pan with sloping sides.

If desired, replace the white wine in this recipe with additional chicken stock.

1 tsp	ground ginger	5 mL
½ tsp	garlic powder	2 mL
¼ tsp	hot pepper flakes	1 mL
Pinch	ground cinnamon	Pinch
Pinch	allspice	Pinch
Pinch	ground cloves	Pinch
1¼ lb	veal scaloppine, cut into thin strips	625 g
1 cup	chicken stock	250 mL
¼ cup	dry white wine (optional)	50 mL
3 tbsp	soy sauce	45 mL
2 tbsp	cornstarch	25 mL
2 tbsp	vegetable oil, divided	25 mL
3	carrots, sliced	3
3	stalks celery, diagonally sliced	3
1	green bell pepper, chopped	1
1	onion, chopped	1
2 cups	mushrooms, quartered	500 mL

1. Combine ginger, garlic powder, hot pepper flakes, cinnamon, allspice and cloves. Transfer one-third of the spice mixture to bowl; add veal and toss to coat. Chill for 1 to 2 hours.

2. Combine remaining spice mixture, chicken stock, wine (if using), soy sauce and cornstarch; set sauce aside.

3. In a large skillet, heat 1 tbsp (15 mL) of the oil over medium-high heat; sauté carrots, celery, green pepper, onion and mushrooms for 5 minutes or until tender. Remove from pan. Add remaining oil to skillet; brown veal for about 2 minutes. Add sauce and bring to a boil; cook, stirring, until thickened. Return vegetables to skillet and heat through.

NUTRITIONAL ANALYSIS PER SERVING			
Energy: 206 kcal	Fat: 7 g	Fiber: 2.3 g	Iron: 2.0 mg
Protein: 24 g	Carbohydrate: 11 g	Calcium: 39 mg	Folate: 34 mcg

Just Peachy Pork

- Preheat oven to 350°F (180°C)
- 8-cup (2 L) baking or gratin dish

1	can (14 oz/398 mL) sliced peaches, drained, ¼ cup (50 mL) syrup reserved	1
1 cup	diced green bell pepper or 1½ cups (375 mL) frozen mixed bell pepper strips	250 mL
½ cup	barbecue sauce	125 mL
1 tbsp	Dijon mustard	15 mL
1 lb	pork tenderloin, cut into ½-inch (1 cm) thick slices	500 g

1. In a saucepan, over medium heat, combine peaches, reserved syrup, green pepper, barbecue sauce and mustard. Bring to a boil.

2. Reduce heat to low and simmer for 3 minutes. Place pork slices in a single layer in baking dish. Pour sauce over meat.

3. Bake in preheated oven until just a hint of pink remains, about 30 minutes.

NUTRITIONAL ANALYSIS PER SERVING

Energy: 231 kcal	Fat: 4 g	Fiber: 3.6 g	Iron: 2.7 mg
Protein: 28 g	Carbohydrate: 21 g	Calcium: 23 mg	Folate: 16 mcg

Health Tip

A serving of pork tenderloin has less saturated fat than the same size serving of a chicken leg with the skin left on.

MAKES 4 SERVINGS

Loaded with peaches, this sweet and tangy sauce is a great accompaniment for pork. Serve over hot white rice and add an assortment of steamed vegetables in season for a delightfully different meal. Although it bakes for 30 minutes, it takes almost no time to prepare.

TIP

Pork tenderloin is the most tender and juicy cut of pork. It is a great boon to convenience as it cooks quickly and produces excellent results. Widely available, fresh pork tenderloin will keep for 3 days in the refrigerator. If freezing, place in a resealable freezer bag and use within 3 months. Thaw before cooking.

**MAKES
4 SERVINGS**

In Chinese cooking, gingerroot is valued as much for its healthful properties — it is believed to have stimulating and cleansing benefits — as its zesty flavor. Here, it brings out the best of both the pork and vegetables in this easy stir-fry. Serve with brown rice for additional fiber.

TIPS

Adjust the quantity of hot pepper flakes to suit your taste. Or, for a more Asian version of this dish, omit the hot pepper flakes and substitute an Asian chili paste instead. Sambal oelek, a bottled chili paste, easily identified by its bright red color, is readily available in Asian markets. Try adding ½ tsp (2 mL) of this zesty mix to the pan after the pork is browned.

Bok choy is a Chinese green frequently used in stir-fries. Use both stalks and leaves.

Orange Ginger Pork and Vegetables

2 tbsp	vegetable oil, divided	25 mL
2	carrots, sliced	2
1	onion, sliced	1
1	green bell pepper, cut into thin strips	1
1	red bell pepper, cut into thin strips	1
1 cup	sliced celery	250 mL
1 lb	well-trimmed boneless pork loin, cut into thin strips	500 g
1	clove garlic, minced	1
2 tsp	grated gingerroot	10 mL
¼ tsp	hot pepper flakes	1 mL
2 cups	shredded bok choy	500 mL
½ cup	orange juice	125 mL
	Salt	

1. In a large skillet, heat 1 tbsp (15 mL) of the oil over medium-high heat; sauté carrots, onion, green pepper, red pepper and celery for about 5 minutes or until tender. Remove from pan.

2. Add the remaining oil to skillet. Brown pork with garlic, ginger and hot pepper flakes until pork is no longer pink. Return vegetables to skillet; add bok choy. Add orange juice; heat through, 2 to 3 minutes. Season with salt to taste.

NUTRITIONAL ANALYSIS PER SERVING			
Energy: 294 kcal	Fat: 14 g	Fiber: 3.6 g	Iron: 2.2 mg
Protein: 29 g	Carbohydrate: 14 g	Calcium: 97 mg	Folate: 65 mcg

Teriyaki Pork Chops

- Contact grill

1 tsp	vegetable oil	5 mL
2	cloves garlic, minced	2
1 tsp	minced gingerroot	5 mL
1/4 cup	soy sauce	50 mL
2 tbsp	packed brown sugar	25 mL
1 tbsp	freshly squeezed lemon juice	15 mL
1 tbsp	sherry	15 mL
8	boneless pork loin chops	8

1. In a small saucepan, heat oil over medium heat. Sauté garlic and gingerroot for 1 minute. Stir in soy sauce, brown sugar, lemon juice and sherry and bring to a boil. Reduce heat to medium-low and simmer for 5 minutes, stirring, until marinade has thickened. Let cool completely.

2. Place pork in a shallow dish and brush with marinade, coating evenly. Cover and refrigerate for a minimum of 20 minutes or for up to 1 hour. Meanwhile, preheat contact grill.

3. Spray both sides of contact grill with vegetable cooking spray or oil. Place pork on grill, close lid and grill for 5 to 8 minutes, or until just a hint of pink remains in pork and internal temperature reaches 160°F (71°C).

Variation

Use 4 boneless skinless chicken breasts in place of pork chops. Grill on high for 5 to 6 minutes, or until chicken is no longer pink inside and reaches an internal temperature of 170°F (75°C).

MAKES 4 SERVINGS

Serve this Asian-inspired recipe with sticky rice and grilled or stir-fried vegetables for a palate-pleasing dinner.

TIPS

If your contact grill has more than one temperature setting, set it to high for this recipe.

For a mellower taste, use an equal amount of liquid honey in place of brown sugar.

Make ahead

Prepare marinade, cover and store in the refrigerator for up to 1 day.

NUTRITIONAL ANALYSIS PER SERVING			
Energy: 336 kcal	Fat: 12 g	Fiber: 0.1 g	Iron: 2.1 mg
Protein: 44 g	Carbohydrate: 8 g	Calcium: 48 mg	Folate: 12 mcg

**MAKES
4 SERVINGS**

*Tasty, elegant, simple
and quick to make,
this recipe is a keeper.
Serve with mashed
potatoes and steamed
green beans.*

Savory Lamb Chops

• Preheat broiler or grill

2 tbsp	bottled oil and vinegar dressing	25 mL
1 tbsp	Dijon mustard	15 mL
1½ lbs	lamb chops, thawed if frozen	750 g
2 tbsp	prepared sun-dried tomato pesto	25 mL

1. In a bowl, combine dressing and mustard.
2. Pat lamb chops dry. Brush both sides with mixture.
3. Place on broiling pan about 6 inches (15 cm) from heat. Cook, turning once, until desired degree of doneness, 8 to 10 minutes. Serve topped with a dollop of pesto.

NUTRITIONAL ANALYSIS PER SERVING			
Energy: 306 kcal	Fat: 15 g	Fiber: 0 g	Iron: 3.5 mg
Protein: 38 g	Carbohydrate: 2 g	Calcium: 36 mg	Folate: 4 mcg

Health Tip

Iron deficiency anemia is a common problem in pregnancy. Red meat, including lamb, is a good source of dietary iron.

Vegetarian

Mixed Winter Beans 248

Stir-fried Vegetables with Tofu 249

Grilled Tofu 250

Sweet and Tasty Tofu 250

Chickpea Tofu Stew 251

Vegetarian Chili. 252

Chickpea-Herb Burgers 253

Spaghetti with Zucchini Balls
    and Tomato Sauce. 254

Lentil Spaghetti Sauce. 255

Vegetarian Shepherd's Pie with
    Peppered Potato Topping 256

Zucchini, Mushroom and Bean Loaf
    with Tomato Sauce 257

Roasted Yam Fajitas 258

Falafel in Pita 260

Spinach Risotto. 261

Egg and Mushroom Fried Rice 262

Swiss Chard Frittata in a Pita 263

Spinach Frittata 264

**MAKES
6 SERVINGS**

You need only one pot to prepare this economical meatless dish. It uses an assortment of dried beans with lots of winter produce to produce a tasty pot of old-fashioned baked beans, chock full of protein, fiber, vitamins and antioxidants.

TIP

Keep single servings on hand in the freezer for quick microwave meals.

Mixed Winter Beans

2 cups	assorted dried beans (romano, white, kidney, pinto)	500 mL
1	can (28 oz/796 mL) tomatoes	1
1	can (19 oz/540 mL) chickpeas, drained and rinsed	1
2	carrots, sliced	2
1	onion, chopped	1
1	clove garlic, minced	1
1 cup	shredded cabbage	250 mL
½ cup	diced peeled turnip	125 mL
1 tbsp	chili powder	15 mL
1 tsp	Worcestershire sauce	5 mL
½ tsp	salt	2 mL
¼ tsp	freshly ground black pepper	1 mL
	Chopped fresh parsley	

1. Cover beans with water and soak overnight; drain and rinse. In a 4-quart (4 L) saucepan, cover beans with fresh water; bring to a boil. Reduce heat and simmer, covered, for 40 to 50 minutes or until tender. Drain and rinse; return to saucepan.

2. Add tomatoes, chickpeas, carrots, onion, garlic, cabbage, turnip, chili powder, Worcestershire sauce, salt and pepper. Add water to cover; bring to a boil. Reduce heat and simmer, uncovered, for 30 to 40 minutes or until vegetables are tender. Garnish with parsley.

NUTRITIONAL ANALYSIS PER SERVING			
Energy: 392 kcal	Fat: 3 g	Fiber: 17.1 g	Iron: 9.1 mg
Protein: 24 g	Carbohydrate: 72 g	Calcium: 235 mg	Folate: 410 mcg

Stir-fried Vegetables with Tofu

2 tbsp	vegetable oil	25 mL
3	carrots, sliced diagonally	3
3	stalks celery, sliced diagonally	3
1	large onion, cut into wedges	1
¼	small cabbage, sliced thinly	¼
1 cup	snow peas, trimmed	250 mL
1 cup	sliced mushrooms	250 mL
1 cup	firm tofu, cubed (see tips, at right)	250 mL
½ cup	vegetable stock, tomato juice or vegetable juice cocktail	125 mL
1 tbsp	cornstarch	15 mL
1 tsp	finely chopped gingerroot (or ½ tsp/2 mL ground ginger)	5 mL
¼ tsp	freshly ground black pepper	1 mL

1. In a wok or large heavy skillet, heat oil over high heat. When oil is very hot, add carrots, celery and onion; cover and steam for 5 minutes. Add cabbage, snow peas, mushrooms and tofu; steam, covered, for 5 minutes longer.

2. Mix together vegetable stock, cornstarch, ginger and pepper; pour over vegetable mixture. Stir-fry for 1 minute or until sauce thickens. Serve over hot rice.

NUTRITIONAL ANALYSIS PER SERVING

| Energy: 157 kcal | Fat: 8 g | Fiber: 3.7 g | Iron: 5.9 mg |
| Protein: 10 g | Carbohydrate: 14 g | Calcium: 145 mg | Folate: 60 mcg |

Health Tip

Even non-vegetarians can include meatless meals in their diets. Vegetarianism has many health benefits, and vegetarian meals are often higher in vitamins, minerals and fiber while being lower in total calories.

Excellent source of:
• Iron

Good source of:
• Folate

Source of:
• Calcium and fiber

MAKES 6 SERVINGS

Gingerroot adds zest to this tasty dish.

TIPS

Make sure to buy tofu that has been coagulated with calcium sulfate or calcium chloride. Read the ingredient list on the label for the coagulant. Otherwise, you won't get nearly as much calcium out of this recipe.

Tofu is best stored in water in a covered container in the refrigerator. Change the water daily to keep tofu fresh for 1 week.

MAKES 4 SERVINGS

Tofu cubes acquire a delectable crispy exterior in this grilled wonder.

TIPS

Firm or extra-firm tofu is best for the indoor grill.

Make sure to buy tofu that has been coagulated with calcium sulfate or calcium chloride. Read the ingredient list on the label for the coagulant. Otherwise, you won't get nearly as much calcium out of this recipe.

Grilled Tofu

- Preheat contact grill to high

2	cloves garlic, minced	2
¼ cup	tamari	50 mL
1 tbsp	minced gingerroot	15 mL
1 tsp	sesame oil	5 mL
1 tsp	chili garlic sauce	5 mL
1	package (12 oz/375 g) extra-firm tofu (see tip, at left), cut into 1-inch (2.5 cm) cubes	1

1. In a small bowl, whisk together garlic, tamari, ginger, sesame oil and chili garlic sauce.

2. Place tofu cubes in a shallow dish. Pour marinade over tofu and toss to coat. Cover and refrigerate for a minimum of 20 minutes or for up to 1 day. Meanwhile, preheat contact grill to high.

3. Spray both sides of contact grill with vegetable cooking spray or oil. Place tofu on grill, close lid and grill for 6 to 7 minutes, or until tofu is crisp and grill-marked.

NUTRITIONAL ANALYSIS PER SERVING			
Energy: 158 kcal	Fat: 9 g	Fiber: 0.1 g	Iron: 10.1 mg
Protein: 16 g	Carbohydrate: 6 g	Calcium: 646 mg	Folate: 30 mcg

MAKES 4 SERVINGS

A very light lunch or supper. Serve with rice or rice noodles.

TIP

Place any leftovers in an airtight container and store in the refrigerator for up to 2 days.

Sweet and Tasty Tofu

1 lb	firm tofu, drained (see tip, above left)	500 g
2 tsp	salt	10 mL
2 tbsp	vegetable oil	25 mL
1 tbsp	grated gingerroot	15 mL
¾ cup	chopped fresh cilantro	175 mL
2 tbsp	soy sauce	25 mL
2 tsp	packed brown sugar	10 mL

1. Cut tofu into 4 slices and place in a large saucepan. Add 4 cups (1 L) water and salt; soak for 20 minutes. Bring to a boil over medium heat and cook for 5 minutes. Drain and transfer to a serving dish. Set aside.

2. In a saucepan, heat oil over medium-high heat. Add ginger and cook for 2 minutes. Add cilantro, soy sauce and brown sugar; cook for 2 minutes. Pour sauce over tofu and serve.

NUTRITIONAL ANALYSIS PER SERVING			
Energy: 257 kcal	Fat: 18 g	Fiber: 0.1 g	Iron: 13.4 mg
Protein: 21 g	Carbohydrate: 8 g	Calcium: 868 mg	Folate: 38 mcg

Chickpea Tofu Stew

- Preheat oven to 375°F (190°C)
- 6-cup (1.5 L) casserole dish

1 lb	ripe tomatoes (about 4)	500 g
3 tbsp	olive oil	45 mL
½ tsp	salt	2 mL
½ tsp	paprika	2 mL
½ tsp	cumin seeds	2 mL
½ tsp	chili powder	2 mL
2½ cups	thinly sliced onion	625 mL
½	green bell pepper, thinly sliced	½
4	cloves garlic, thinly sliced	4
2	bay leaves	2
1 cup	hot water	250 mL
2 tsp	freshly squeezed lime juice	10 mL
2 cups	cooked chickpeas	500 mL
8 oz	firm tofu (see tip, at right), cut into ½-inch (1 cm) cubes	250 g
1 tsp	olive oil (optional)	5 mL
¼ cup	finely diced red onion	50 mL
	Few sprigs fresh cilantro, chopped	

MAKES 4 SERVINGS

A filling and flavorful winter dish, this stew is bolstered with the addition of super-nutritious tofu. It is imperative to use firm tofu (often called "pressed tofu"), as the soft variety will disintegrate. For chickpeas, you can either cook your own or use the canned variety.

TIPS

Excellent served with a salad, steamed rice and a yogurt-based sauce.

For a spicier flavor, substitute cayenne pepper for the chili powder.

Make sure to buy tofu that has been coagulated with calcium sulfate or calcium chloride. Read the ingredient list on the label for the coagulant. Otherwise, you won't get nearly as much calcium out of this recipe.

1. Blanch tomatoes in boiling water for 30 seconds. Over a bowl, peel, core and deseed them. Chop tomatoes into chunks and set aside. Strain any accumulated tomato juices from bowl; add the juices to the tomatoes.

2. In a large skillet, heat olive oil over high heat for 30 seconds. Add salt, paprika, cumin seeds and chili powder in quick succession. Stir-fry for 30 seconds. Add onion and stir-fry for 1 minute. Add green pepper and stir-fry for 2 to 3 minutes, until soft. Add garlic and stir-fry for 1 minute. Add tomato flesh and juices. Stir-cook for 3 minutes to break up tomato somewhat. Add bay leaves, hot water and lime juice. Cook, stirring often, for 5 minutes.

3. Transfer sauce to casserole dish. Fold chickpeas into the sauce. Distribute tofu cubes evenly over the surface and gently press them down into the sauce.

4. Bake in preheated oven, uncovered, for 25 to 30 minutes, until bubbling and bright. Drizzle with olive oil (if using) and garnish with red onions and cilantro.

NUTRITIONAL ANALYSIS PER SERVING			
Energy: 399 kcal	Fat: 20 g	Fiber: 9.6 g	Iron: 10.4 mg
Protein: 20 g	Carbohydrate: 41 g	Calcium: 518 mg	Folate: 196 mcg

**MAKES
8 SERVINGS**

Instead of beef chili, why not try this high-fiber vegetarian alternative? If you have never tried a meatless chili before, you may be pleasantly surprised to find it tastes similar to the traditional beef version with significantly less fat and more fiber.

TIP

You can substitute any canned beans you have in the house. Canned lentils, navy beans and white kidney beans will all work equally well in this recipe.

Make ahead

Spoon into an airtight container and store in the refrigerator for up to 3 days or in the freezer for up to 3 months.

Vegetarian Chili

1 tbsp	olive oil	15 mL
1	onion, chopped	1
1	green bell pepper, chopped	1
1	red bell pepper, chopped	1
1	clove garlic, minced	1
1	can (28 oz/796 mL) diced tomatoes, with juice	1
1	can (5½ oz/156 mL) tomato paste	1
1	can (19 oz/540 mL) kidney beans, drained and rinsed	1
1	can (19 oz/540 mL) black beans, drained and rinsed	1
1 cup	bulgur	250 mL
1 tbsp	ground cumin	15 mL
1 tbsp	chili powder	15 mL
1 tsp	salt	5 mL
½ tsp	freshly ground black pepper	2 mL
Pinch	ground allspice	Pinch

1. In a large saucepan, heat oil over medium heat. Sauté onion, green pepper and red pepper until tender, about 5 minutes. Add garlic and sauté for 1 minute. Add tomatoes, tomato paste, kidney beans, black beans, 3 cups (750 mL) water, bulgur, cumin, chili powder, salt, pepper and allspice. Bring to a boil. Cover, reduce heat and simmer, stirring occasionally, until bulgur is tender, about 20 minutes.

NUTRITIONAL ANALYSIS PER SERVING

Energy: 259 kcal	Fat: 3 g	Fiber: 8.6 g	Iron: 5.3 mg
Protein: 13 g	Carbohydrate: 49 g	Calcium: 89 mg	Folate: 146 mcg

Health Tip

Folate has been found to help prevent neural tube defects. The recommended dietary allowance (RDA) for pregnant women is 600 mcg every day from food and supplemental sources.

Chickpea-Herb Burgers

- Preheat oven to 375°F (190°C) or grill to high
- Parchment-lined baking sheet or greased grill

2	cloves garlic, minced	2
1	can (19 oz/540 mL) chickpeas, drained	1
3 cups	shredded carrots	750 mL
½ cup	grated onions	125 mL
1 tbsp	vegetable oil	15 mL
1	egg	1
½ cup	spelt flakes	125 mL
¼ cup	unblanched almonds	50 mL
¼ cup	sunflower seeds	50 mL
2 tbsp	flax seeds	25 mL
2 tbsp	chopped fresh parsley	25 mL
2 tbsp	chopped fresh basil	25 mL
1 tbsp	chopped fresh thyme	15 mL
	Salt and freshly ground black pepper	

1. In a food processor or blender, purée garlic, chickpeas, carrots, onions and oil until well combined.

2. Add egg, spelt flakes, almonds, sunflower seeds, flax seeds, parsley, basil and thyme. Process until finely chopped and holding together. Season to taste with salt and pepper.

3. Form mixture into 6 patties. Arrange patties on prepared baking sheet or grill. Bake in preheated oven or grill for 3 minutes per side, being careful to turn burgers gently.

NUTRITIONAL ANALYSIS PER SERVING			
Energy: 250 kcal	Fat: 10 g	Fiber: 11.6 g	Iron: 3.3 mg
Protein: 10 g	Carbohydrate: 33 g	Calcium: 79 mg	Folate: 9 mcg

Health Tip

A diet high in fiber can help to prevent the constipation and hemorrhoids associated with pregnancy. Aim to get 25 to 35 g of fiber each day.

Excellent source of:
- Fiber

Good source of:
- Iron

Source of:
- Calcium

MAKES 6 SERVINGS

Whether grilled on the barbecue or baked in the oven, these burgers are great with all the trimmings.

**MAKES
4 SERVINGS**

A creative way to serve a vegetarian meal, this recipe is rich in flavor and nutrients. The mild Middle Eastern spicing in both the sauce and the zucchini balls adds enticing taste. The chickpeas are filled with fiber and combine with the eggs to make a complete source of protein.

TIP

This intriguing tomato sauce differs from traditional recipes because of the addition of cumin and cinnamon. You may want to double the recipe and save some for later use.

Spaghetti with Zucchini Balls and Tomato Sauce

- Preheat oven to 400°F (200°C)
- Baking sheet, greased

1 tsp	olive oil	5 mL
1	onion, finely chopped	1
3	cloves garlic, minced	3
1	stick cinnamon (5 inches/12 cm)	1
1	can (28 oz/796 mL) crushed tomatoes	1
1 tsp	crushed dried oregano	5 mL
1 tsp	ground cumin	5 mL
¼ tsp	granulated sugar	1 mL
¼ tsp	salt	1 mL
¼ tsp	freshly ground black pepper	1 mL
12 oz	spaghetti	375 g
	Freshly grated Parmesan cheese (optional)	

Zucchini Balls

3 cups	grated zucchini (2 to 3 medium)	750 mL
1 cup	drained rinsed chickpeas	250 mL
2	eggs, lightly beaten	2
2	cloves garlic, minced	2
1	slice whole wheat bread, crumbled	1
¾ cup	quick-cooking rolled oats	175 mL
½ cup	cornmeal	125 mL
1 tsp	ground cumin	5 mL
½ tsp	ground coriander	2 mL
½ tsp	ground ginger	2 mL
½ tsp	salt	2 mL
½ tsp	freshly ground black pepper	2 mL
¼ tsp	ground cardamom	1 mL

1. In a large skillet, heat oil over medium-high heat; sauté onion for 3 minutes. Add garlic, cinnamon stick, tomatoes, oregano, cumin, sugar, salt and pepper; bring to a boil. Reduce heat and simmer, uncovered, for 30 minutes, stirring occasionally. Remove cinnamon stick.

2. *Prepare the zucchini balls:* Squeeze out excess moisture from zucchini. Purée half of the chickpeas. In a bowl, mix together zucchini, puréed and whole chickpeas, eggs, garlic, bread, oats, cornmeal, cumin, coriander, ginger, salt, pepper and cardamom. Form into 1-inch (2.5 cm) balls; place on prepared baking sheet. Bake in preheated oven for 10 to 15 minutes or until lightly browned.

3. Meanwhile, cook spaghetti according to package directions; drain and arrange on 4 plates. Spoon tomato sauce over spaghetti; top with zucchini balls. Serve with Parmesan cheese, if desired.

Lentil Spaghetti Sauce

1 tbsp	vegetable oil	15 mL
2	cloves garlic, chopped	2
1	large onion, chopped	1
1	large stalk celery, chopped	1
2 cups	vegetable stock or water	500 mL
1 cup	red lentils, washed	250 mL
1	can (5½ oz/156 mL) tomato paste	1
1 tbsp	chopped fresh parsley	15 mL
½ tsp	dried oregano	2 mL
½ tsp	salt	2 mL
Pinch	cayenne pepper	Pinch
	Freshly grated Parmesan cheese	

1. In a large saucepan, heat oil over medium heat; cook garlic, onion and celery for about 5 minutes or until tender. Add vegetable stock and lentils; cover and cook over low heat for about 35 minutes or until lentils are tender.

2. Add tomato paste, ¾ cup (175 mL) water, parsley, oregano, salt and cayenne; cook, covered, for about 15 minutes or until lentils are soft and mushy. Serve over cooked spaghetti; sprinkle with cheese.

Excellent source of:
• Folate, iron and fiber

**MAKES
6 SERVINGS**

Lentils provide an abundance of carbohydrates, protein and fiber and can be the basis for an economical meal. Serve this sauce over the pasta of your choice or use it as sauce for lasagna. The combination of lentils and pasta in this recipe provides complete protein.

TIP

Lentils come in red, green and brown. Brown and green hold their shape better and are usually used in salads. Red, which break down during cooking, are used here because they dissolve in the sauce.

MAKES 6 TO 8 SERVINGS

This shepherd's pie rivals the beef version — creamy, thick and rich-tasting. Beans provide the meat-like texture.

TIPS

For a different twist, try sweet potatoes instead of potatoes.

Try other cheeses, such as mozzarella or Swiss.

Make ahead

Cover and store in the refrigerator for up to 1 day or transfer to an airtight container and store in the freezer for up to 3 weeks. Reheat gently.

Vegetarian Shepherd's Pie with Peppered Potato Topping

• Preheat oven to 350° F (180° C)
• 13- by 9-inch (3 L) baking dish

2 tsp	vegetable oil	10 mL
1 cup	chopped onions	250 mL
¾ cup	finely chopped carrots	175 mL
2 tsp	minced garlic	10 mL
1½ cups	prepared tomato pasta sauce	375 mL
1 cup	rinsed and drained canned red kidney beans	250 mL
1 cup	rinsed and drained canned chickpeas	250 mL
½ cup	vegetable stock or water	125 mL
1½ tsp	dried basil	7 mL
2	bay leaves	2
4 cups	diced potatoes	1 L
½ cup	2% milk	125 mL
⅓ cup	light sour cream	75 mL
¼ tsp	freshly ground black pepper	1 mL
¾ cup	shredded Cheddar cheese	175 mL
3 tbsp	freshly grated Parmesan cheese	45 mL

1. In a saucepan, heat oil over medium-high heat. Add onions, carrots and garlic; cook for 4 minutes or until onions are softened. Stir in tomato sauce, kidney beans, chickpeas, vegetable stock, basil and bay leaves. Reduce heat to medium-low and cook, covered, for 15 minutes or until vegetables are tender. Remove bay leaves. Transfer sauce to a food processor; pulse on and off just until chunky. Spread over bottom of baking dish.

2. Place potatoes in a saucepan and add cold water to cover; bring to a boil. Reduce heat and simmer for 10 to 12 minutes or until tender. Drain; mash with milk, sour cream and pepper. Spoon on top of sauce in baking dish. Sprinkle with Cheddar and Parmesan cheese. Bake, uncovered, for 20 minutes or until hot.

NUTRITIONAL ANALYSIS PER SERVING (1 OF 8)			
Energy: 237 kcal	Fat: 8 g	Fiber: 10.1 g	Iron: 2.4 mg
Protein: 10 g	Carbohydrate: 33 g	Calcium: 178 mg	Folate: 77 mcg

Zucchini, Mushroom and Bean Loaf with Tomato Sauce

- Preheat oven to 350° F (180° C)
- 9- by 5-inch (2 L) loaf pan sprayed with vegetable spray

1 tsp	vegetable oil	5 mL
1 cup	chopped onions	250 mL
½ cup	finely chopped carrots	125 mL
2 tsp	minced garlic	10 mL
2 cups	chopped zucchini	500 mL
1 cup	chopped mushrooms	250 mL
2	eggs	2
1½ cups	rinsed and drained canned chickpeas	375 mL
1½ cups	rinsed and drained canned white kidney beans	375 mL
⅓ cup	dry seasoned bread crumbs	75 mL
3 tbsp	chili sauce	45 mL
2 tbsp	freshly grated Parmesan cheese	25 mL
1 tsp	dried basil	5 mL
¾ cup	prepared tomato pasta sauce	175 mL

MAKES 6 TO 8 SERVINGS

This vegetarian loaf tastes a lot like chicken. The combination of puréed beans provides a meaty texture. This loaf is a good source of fiber.

TIP

Replace bottled chili sauce with barbecue sauce or ketchup.

Make ahead

Cover and store in the refrigerator for up to 1 day. Serve cold or reheated.

1. In a nonstick skillet, heat oil over medium-high heat. Add onions, carrots and garlic; cook for 4 minutes. Stir in zucchini and mushrooms; cook for 8 minutes or until softened.

2. In a food processor, combine zucchini mixture, eggs, chickpeas, kidney beans, bread crumbs, chili sauce, cheese and basil. Pulse on and off until finely chopped and well combined. Press into prepared loaf pan.

3. Bake, uncovered, for 40 minutes or until tester inserted in center comes out clean. Heat tomato sauce and serve with sliced loaf.

NUTRITIONAL ANALYSIS PER SERVING (1 OF 8)			
Energy: 188 kcal	Fat: 5 g	Fiber: 6.6 g	Iron: 2.5 mg
Protein: 9 g	Carbohydrate: 28 g	Calcium: 80 mg	Folate: 100 mcg

**MAKES
5 SERVINGS**

Yams, a popular ingredient in Southern dishes, take center stage in this fun-to-eat fajita recipe.

TIP

Although the true yam is different from the sweet potato, the terms tend to be used interchangeably in North America and refer to an elongated, brown-skinned tuber with an orange-colored flesh.

Roasted Yam Fajitas

- Preheat oven to 350°F (180°C)
- Baking sheet

Sauce

1/3 cup	orange juice	75 mL
1 tsp	grated lime zest	5 mL
2 tbsp	freshly squeezed lime juice	25 mL
1 tbsp	olive oil	15 mL
1 tbsp	minced garlic	15 mL
1 tsp	crushed dried oregano	5 mL
1 tsp	ground cumin	5 mL
1/4 tsp	hot pepper flakes	1 mL
1/4 tsp	freshly ground black pepper	1 mL

Filling

4	yams or sweet potatoes (1 1/2 lb/750 g)	4
2 tbsp	olive oil, divided	25 mL
	Salt and freshly ground black pepper	
1	red bell pepper, cut into strips	1
1	green bell pepper, cut into strips	1
1	onion, sliced	1
10	7- to 8-inch (18 to 20 cm) flour tortillas	10

Toppings

Chopped tomatoes
Shredded lettuce
Shredded cheese
Light sour cream

1. *Prepare the sauce:* In a bowl, combine orange juice, lime zest and juice, oil, garlic, oregano, cumin, hot pepper flakes and pepper; cover and let stand for at least 4 hours at room temperature. (Or refrigerate overnight.)

2. *Prepare the filling:* Peel yams and cut into 1/2-inch (1 cm) cubes; toss with 1 tbsp (15 mL) of the oil. Place on baking sheet; sprinkle with salt and pepper to taste. Bake in preheated oven for 20 to 25 minutes or until tender but not mushy. Cool completely.

3. In a large skillet, heat the remaining oil over medium-high heat; sauté red and green peppers and onion for about 5 minutes. Add yams and sauce; heat through (most of sauce will be absorbed).

4. Meanwhile, wrap tortillas in foil; bake in preheated oven for 5 to 10 minutes or until heated. (Or wrap in paper towels and microwave at High for 40 seconds.) Spoon yam filling into tortillas. Top with desired toppings.

NUTRITIONAL ANALYSIS PER SERVING

Energy: 668 kcal	Fat: 18 g	Fiber: 7.2 g	Iron: 4.3 mg
Protein: 12 g	Carbohydrate: 114 g	Calcium: 66 mg	Folate: 51 mcg

Health Tip

Sweet potatoes are nutritious. Like all orange-colored vegetables, they are a good source of vitamin A. They also contain potassium and vitamin C.

MAKES 4 SERVINGS

These tasty treats are a gift from the Middle East, where they are eaten the way hamburgers are in North America. Liberally garnished, they make a great lunch or light dinner.

Falafel in Pita

1	can (19 oz/540 mL) chickpeas, drained and rinsed	1
½ cup	sliced green onion	125 mL
2 tbsp	freshly squeezed lemon juice	25 mL
1 tbsp	minced garlic	15 mL
1 to 2 tsp	curry powder	5 to 10 mL
1	egg	1
2 tbsp	vegetable oil	25 mL
½ cup	all-purpose flour	125 mL
4	pita breads	4
	Chopped peeled cucumber	
	Chopped tomato	
	Shredded lettuce	
	Plain yogurt	

1. In a food processor, combine chickpeas, onion, lemon juice, garlic and curry powder. Process until blended but chickpeas retain their texture. Using your hands, shape into 4 large patties.

2. In a shallow bowl, lightly beat egg. In a skillet, heat oil over medium heat. Dip each patty into the egg, then into the flour, coating both sides well. Fry until golden and heated through, about 2 minutes per side.

3. Fill each pita bread with a falafel and garnish with cucumber, tomato, lettuce and yogurt, as desired.

NUTRITIONAL ANALYSIS PER SERVING			
Energy: 498 kcal	Fat: 10 g	Fiber: 7.6 g	Iron: 3.7 mg
Protein: 22 g	Carbohydrate: 86 g	Calcium: 65 mg	Folate: 166 mcg

Spinach Risotto

- Preheat oven to 400°F (200°C)
- Ovenproof saucepan with heatproof handle

2 tbsp	butter	25 mL
1 cup	diced onion	250 mL
1 cup	Arborio rice	250 mL
1 tbsp	minced garlic	15 mL
1	package (10 oz/300 g) frozen spinach, partially thawed (see tip, at right)	1
3 cups	vegetable stock	750 mL
3 tbsp	prepared sun-dried tomato pesto	45 mL
	Freshly grated Parmesan cheese	

1. In an ovenproof saucepan, melt butter over medium heat. Add onion and cook until softened, about 3 minutes. Add rice and cook, stirring, until the grains of rice are coated with butter, about 1 minute. Add spinach and cook, breaking up with a spoon, until thoroughly integrated into the rice, about 2 minutes. Stir in vegetable stock and pesto. Bring to a boil.

2. Transfer saucepan to preheated oven and bake, stirring partway through, until rice has absorbed the liquid, about 30 minutes. Remove from oven and sprinkle cheese over top. Serve immediately.

NUTRITIONAL ANALYSIS PER SERVING

Energy: 313 kcal	Fat: 7 g	Fiber: 3.2 g	Iron: 2.8 mg
Protein: 8 g	Carbohydrate: 55 g	Calcium: 139 mg	Folate: 114 mcg

Excellent source of:
- Folate

Good source of:
- Iron

Source of:
- Calcium and fiber

MAKES 4 SERVINGS

Although it needs to bake for 30 minutes, this method for cooking risotto eliminates the tedious task of stirring the liquid until it is absorbed. Add crusty rolls and a crisp green salad for a tasty meal.

TIPS

If you don't have a saucepan with an ovenproof handle, transfer the mixture to a deep 6-cup (1.5 L) baking dish after completing Step 1.

To partially thaw the spinach for this recipe, place the package in a microwave and heat on High for 3 minutes. It can easily be separated using a fork but will still have some ice crystals. Do not drain before adding to rice.

**MAKES
4 SERVINGS**

Enjoy this as a meal or snack — it's a great way to use up frozen leftover rice. You can easily divide the ingredients in half to serve 2.

TIP

Using a small amount of highly flavored sesame oil adds great taste without adding too much fat.

Egg and Mushroom Fried Rice

4	eggs	4
2 tsp	vegetable oil	10 mL
1 cup	sliced mushrooms	250 mL
1 tsp	minced garlic	5 mL
1 tsp	minced gingerroot (or ½ tsp/2 mL ground ginger)	5 mL
3 cups	cooked rice	750 mL
½ cup	frozen peas	125 mL
½ cup	chopped green onions	125 mL
⅓ cup	sodium-reduced soy sauce	75 mL
½ to 1 tsp	sesame oil	2 to 5 mL
Pinch	freshly ground black pepper	Pinch

1. In a small bowl, whisk eggs until well blended. Pour into a large nonstick skillet; cook, undisturbed, over low heat for 4 to 5 minutes or until bottom is lightly browned and mixture is almost set. Flip eggs over and cook for 1 to 2 minutes. Remove from pan; cool slightly. Cut into ¼-inch (5 mm) strips. Set aside.

2. In the same skillet, heat oil over medium-high heat. Add mushrooms; cook for 4 to 5 minutes or until lightly browned. Add garlic and ginger; cook for 1 minute. Stir in rice, peas and onions until combined. Stir in soy sauce, sesame oil and pepper; add cooked egg strips. Cook for 2 minutes or until piping hot.

NUTRITIONAL ANALYSIS PER SERVING			
Energy: 317 kcal	Fat: 9 g	Fiber: 2.2 g	Iron: 2.5 mg
Protein: 12 g	Carbohydrate: 46 g	Calcium: 60 mg	Folate: 63 mcg

Swiss Chard Frittata in a Pita

Excellent source of:
• Folate, iron and fiber

Good source of:
• Calcium

4	eggs	4
1 tsp	olive oil	5 mL
¼ cup	chopped onion	50 mL
½ tsp	minced garlic	2 mL
2 cups	packed chopped Swiss chard	500 mL
2 tbsp	chopped fresh basil (or ½ tsp/2 mL dried)	25 mL
¼ cup	freshly grated Parmesan cheese	50 mL
2	small (6-inch/15 cm) pita breads	2

MAKES 2 SERVINGS

This dish makes a delicious quick meal or snack. If you don't have any pita bread on hand, serve it with whole-grain toast.

1. In a small bowl, whisk together eggs and 1 tbsp (15 mL) water. Set aside.

2. In a small nonstick skillet, heat oil over medium-high heat. Add onion and garlic; cook for 1 to 2 minutes. Stir in chard and basil (it will cook down; if necessary, add it in 2 batches); cook for 3 to 4 minutes or until chard is wilted. Remove from pan; set aside.

3. Wipe skillet and place over medium heat. Add half of the chard mixture and half of the egg mixture. Cook for 3 to 5 minutes or until browned on the bottom but still not completely set on top; sprinkle with half of the cheese. Flip frittata over; cook for 1 to 2 minutes or until browned and completely set. Remove from pan and cut in half. Repeat with remaining ingredients to make second frittata.

4. Cut pitas in half; place frittata halves inside each half.

TIPS

Chopped fresh spinach can easily be substituted for the Swiss chard. Experiment with other greens, too, such as collard greens, kale, mustard greens, dandelion greens and rapini; they are all great substitutes for the chard in this recipe.

While this dish is already a good source of fiber, you can increase the fiber by using whole wheat pita bread instead of white pita bread.

NUTRITIONAL ANALYSIS PER SERVING

| Energy: 402 kcal | Fat: 18 g | Fiber: 9.0 g | Iron: 5.0 mg |
| Protein: 23 g | Carbohydrate: 40 g | Calcium: 213 mg | Folate: 126 mcg |

Spinach Frittata

MAKES 2 SERVINGS

A frittata is an Italian omelet in which the ingredients are cooked with the eggs rather than being folded into them, French style. There are several methods for making this versatile dish. This one — in which the eggs are partially cooked on top of the stove, then finished in the oven — is essentially foolproof.

TIP

If the handle of your skillet is not ovenproof, wrap it in aluminum foil.

• Preheat oven to 425°F (220°C)
• Ovenproof skillet with heatproof handle and lid

6	eggs, beaten	6
1 tbsp	vegetable oil	15 mL
½ cup	diced onion	125 mL
1 tsp	dried Italian seasoning	5 mL
½ tsp	salt	2 mL
	Freshly ground black pepper	
1	package (10 oz/300 g) frozen chopped spinach, thawed and squeezed dry, or 1 package (10 oz/300 g) spinach, washed, stems removed and chopped	1
¼ cup	freshly grated Parmesan cheese	50 mL
2 tbsp	prepared sun-dried tomato pesto	25 mL

1. In a bowl, lightly beat eggs. Set aside.
2. In an ovenproof skillet, heat oil over medium heat. Add onion and cook, stirring, until softened, about 3 minutes. Stir in Italian seasoning, salt and pepper to taste. Add spinach and stir well.
3. Reduce heat to low. Cover and cook until spinach is wilted, about 5 minutes. Slowly pour eggs over spinach. Increase heat to medium. Cover and cook until mixture begins to form a crust on the bottom, 2 to 3 minutes.
4. Sprinkle with cheese and transfer pan to preheated oven. Bake, uncovered, until eggs are set but frittata is still soft in the center, about 3 minutes. Cut into wedges and serve topped with a dollop of pesto.

NUTRITIONAL ANALYSIS PER SERVING

Energy: 416 kcal	Fat: 28 g	Fiber: 6.5 g	Iron: 7.7 mg
Protein: 27 g	Carbohydrate: 14 g	Calcium: 379 mg	Folate: 398 mcg

Sides

Couscous 266

Rapini with Balsamic Vinegar 267

Green Beans with Cashews 268

Green Beans and Tomato 269

Cauliflower Casserole 270

**MAKES
4 SERVINGS**

Couscous

¼ cup	freshly squeezed orange juice	50 mL
½ tsp	ground cinnamon	2 mL
¼ tsp	ground cloves	1 mL
¼ tsp	ground ginger	1 mL
¼ tsp	powdered turmeric	1 mL
1 cup	couscous	250 mL
½ cup	currants	125 mL

1. In a medium saucepan, bring 1 cup (250 mL) water, orange juice, cinnamon, cloves, ginger and turmeric to a boil. Stir in couscous. Remove from heat.

2. Let stand for 5 minutes, covered, until liquid is absorbed. Fluff with a fork. Stir in currants.

Variation

In place of water and orange juice, use chicken stock. Replace cinnamon, cloves, ginger and turmeric with 1 tsp (5 mL) dried thyme. Instead of currants, add ½ cup (125 mL) chopped green olives with pimientos. Season with freshly ground black pepper to taste.

NUTRITIONAL ANALYSIS PER SERVING			
Energy: 180 kcal	Fat: Trace	Fiber: 2.3 g	Iron: 0.9 mg
Protein: 6 g	Carbohydrate: 38 g	Calcium: 26 mg	Folate: 15 mcg

Health Tip

Pregnancy is a time when women are motivated to make positive dietary changes for the health of their unborn baby. These changes can be continued after the baby is born.

Rapini with Balsamic Vinegar

1	bunch rapini, washed, bottom 1½ inches (4 cm) of stalks trimmed	1
1 tsp	salt	5 mL
3 tbsp	balsamic vinegar	45 mL
2 tbsp	extra-virgin olive oil	25 mL
	Freshly ground black pepper	
	Few sprigs fresh basil or parsley, chopped	
¼ cup	thinly sliced red onion	50 mL
1 tsp	drained capers	5 mL
3 tbsp	shaved Parmesan or Pecorino cheese	45 mL

1. Prepare rapini. Cut off the top 2½ inches (6 cm) — the part that has the leaves and the flowers — and set aside. Cut the remaining stalks into 1-inch (2.5 cm) pieces.

2. In a large pot, bring 1½ inches (4 cm) of water to a boil. Add salt and chopped stalks and cook, uncovered, for 8 minutes, until tender. Add the reserved tops and cook, uncovered, for another 8 minutes. Drain, refresh with cold water and drain again.

3. Transfer drained rapini to a serving plate and spread out. In a small bowl, combine vinegar, olive oil, pepper to taste and chopped basil or parsley. Evenly dress the rapini with this sauce. Scatter slices of red onion and capers over the rapini and top with shaved cheese.

NUTRITIONAL ANALYSIS PER SERVING			
Energy: 97 kcal	Fat: 8 g	Fiber: 2.9 g	Iron: 0.8 mg
Protein: 3 g	Carbohydrate: 6 g	Calcium: 172 mg	Folate: 114 mcg

Excellent source of:
• Folate

Good source of:
• Calcium

Source of:
• Iron and fiber

MAKES 4 SERVINGS

The Italians use their unrivaled condiments and cheeses to create just the kind of culinary sorcery needed to make bitter greens pleasurable. These enhancements, which include olive oil, balsamic vinegar and Parmesan cheese, lend flavors and qualities that work with the bitterness and make it interesting.

Make ahead

Cover and keep at room temperature for up to 1 hour.

**MAKES
4 SERVINGS**

The simple addition of cashews and red onions to this dish transforms ordinary green beans into a formidable companion to any gourmet main course.

Green Beans with Cashews

1 lb	green beans, trimmed	500 g
2 tbsp	olive oil	25 mL
½ cup	slivered red onion	125 mL
⅓ cup	raw cashews	75 mL
¼ tsp	salt	1 mL
¼ tsp	freshly ground black pepper	1 mL
	Few sprigs fresh parsley, chopped	

1. Blanch green beans in a pot of boiling water for 5 minutes. Drain and immediately refresh in a bowl of ice-cold water. Drain and set aside.

2. In a large skillet, heat oil over medium-high heat for 30 seconds. Add onion, cashews, salt and pepper and stir-fry for 2 to 3 minutes, until the onions are softened. Add cooked green beans, increase heat to high and stir-fry actively for 2 to 3 minutes, until the beans feel hot to the touch. (Take care that you don't burn any cashews in the process.) Transfer to a serving plate and garnish with chopped parsley. Serve immediately.

NUTRITIONAL ANALYSIS PER SERVING			
Energy: 201 kcal	Fat: 14 g	Fiber: 4.6 g	Iron: 2.7 mg
Protein: 6 g	Carbohydrate: 16 g	Calcium: 60 mg	Folate: 56 mcg

Health Tip

Green beans are a good source of folate, which can help prevent neural tube defects.

Green Beans and Tomato

1 tbsp	tomato paste	15 mL
1 cup	warm water	250 mL
¼ cup	olive oil	50 mL
2	onions, sliced	2
¼ tsp	salt	1 mL
¼ tsp	freshly ground black pepper	1 mL
1	sweet or hot banana pepper	1
4	cloves garlic, thinly sliced	4
2	tomatoes, cut into thick wedges	2
1 tsp	granulated sugar	5 mL
	Few sprigs fresh parsley, roughly chopped	
1 lb	green beans, trimmed	500 g

1. In a small bowl, stir together tomato paste and water until dissolved. Set aside.

2. In a large, heavy-bottomed saucepan, heat oil over high heat for about 1 minute. Add onions, salt and pepper. Stir-fry for 2 minutes, until onions are softened. Add whole banana pepper and stir-fry for 1 minute. Add garlic and stir-fry for 30 seconds.

3. Add tomato wedges (skin and seeds are all right for this recipe) and stir-cook for 1 to 2 minutes, until softened. Add the dissolved tomato paste, sugar and most of the parsley (reserve some parsley for the final garnish). Stir-cook for 1 to 2 minutes, until contents are bubbling. Add green beans and stir, immersing the beans in the sauce until it has come back to a boil, about 30 seconds. Reduce heat to medium-low and simmer, uncovered, for 30 to 40 minutes, stirring occasionally, until the beans have lost 90% of their crunch.

4. Using tongs, transfer beans to a serving bowl, leaving behind as much of the sauce as possible. Increase heat to high and boil sauce until reduced to a syrupy consistency, about 5 to 7 minutes. If the sauce becomes too thick, add some water and bring back to boil. Pour sauce evenly over the beans. Garnish with the remaining parsley and serve.

NUTRITIONAL ANALYSIS PER SERVING (1 OF 6)			
Energy: 122 kcal	Fat: 8 g	Fiber: 3.8 g	Iron: 1.5 mg
Protein: 2 g	Carbohydrate: 12 g	Calcium: 48 mg	Folate: 43 mcg

Good source of:
- Folate

Source of:
- Iron and fiber

MAKES 4 TO 6 SERVINGS

These slow-simmered green beans belong to that group of oily, overcooked vegetables the Greeks call lathera (literally, "cooked in oil"). Given contemporary preferences for super-crunchy, sparsely sauced vegetables, they may seem seriously retro. But they offer their own reward.

Make ahead

Cover and keep at room temperature for up to 2 hours.

MAKES 4 TO 6 SERVINGS

For those who are not big vegetable fans, a casserole is a great way to change it up a little. This casserole makes a wonderful accompaniment to pork, beef or chicken dishes.

Cauliflower Casserole

- Preheat oven to 375°F (190°C)
- 6-cup (1.5 L) baking dish, lightly greased

1	cauliflower, cut in florets (about 6 cups/1.5 L)	1
2 tbsp	butter	25 mL
1	clove garlic, minced	1
3 tbsp	all-purpose flour	45 mL
1¼ cups	milk	300 mL
½ cup	shredded Cheddar cheese	125 mL
⅓ cup	freshly grated Parmesan cheese, divided	75 mL
¼ cup	chopped fresh parsley or dill	50 mL
½ tsp	salt	2 mL
¼ tsp	freshly ground black pepper	1 mL
½ cup	dry bread crumbs	125 mL

1. In a large pot of boiling water, cook cauliflower for 3 to 5 minutes, or until tender-crisp. Drain and transfer to prepared baking dish. Set aside.

2. In a medium saucepan, melt butter over medium heat. Add garlic and flour; reduce heat to low and cook, stirring, for 1 minute. Increase heat to medium and gradually stir in milk. Cook, stirring constantly, until mixture comes to a boil. Reduce heat and simmer, stirring constantly, for 2 to 3 minutes, or until thickened. Remove from heat and add Cheddar, ¼ cup (50 mL) of the Parmesan, parsley, salt and pepper; stir until cheese melts, about 2 minutes. Pour over cauliflower.

3. In a small bowl, combine bread crumbs and the remaining Parmesan. Sprinkle over cauliflower.

4. Bake, uncovered, in preheated oven for 30 minutes, or until bubbling.

NUTRITIONAL ANALYSIS PER SERVING			
Energy: 162 kcal	Fat: 9 g	Fiber: 2.7 g	Iron: 0.9 mg
Protein: 9 g	Carbohydrate: 13 g	Calcium: 224 mg	Folate: 67 mcg

Pasta

Pasta with Goat Cheese, Snow Peas
  and Tomato Coulis 272

Pasta Fagioli Capra 273

Hoisin Stir-fried Vegetables and Tofu
  over Rice Noodles 274

Spaghetti with Broccoli 275

Linguine with Tuna, White Beans and Dill . . . 276

Tuna Garden Pasta 277

Mushroom-Spinach Lasagna
  with Goat Cheese 278

Penne with Tuna and Peppers 280

**MAKES
4 SERVINGS**

Farfalle (bow tie pasta) and soft crumbled goat cheese, often called chèvre, are readily available in supermarkets and add a sophisticated note to this elegant recipe.

TIPS

For even better results, use finely chopped fresh basil instead of the dried — double or triple the quantity depending on your preference and add after the vegetables are cooked.

When tossing the pasta, add roasted garlic for an additional touch. To roast garlic, place 12 cloves of peeled garlic in foil with 1 tsp (5 mL) olive oil. Bake in 325°F (160°C) oven until soft, about 20 minutes.

Chèvre, soft or unripened goat cheese, is usually sold in a roll. It is lower in sodium than goat cheese that has been allowed to ripen.

Pasta with Goat Cheese, Snow Peas and Tomato Coulis

Tomato Coulis

½ cup	diced shallots	125 mL
¼ cup	diced celery	50 mL
2	cloves garlic, minced	2
1	can (28 oz/796 mL) tomatoes	1
2 tbsp	chopped fresh parsley	25 mL
1 tbsp	crushed dried basil	15 mL
2 tsp	packed brown sugar	10 mL
¼ tsp	salt	1 mL
¼ tsp	freshly ground black pepper	1 mL

Pasta

1 tbsp	olive oil	15 mL
8 oz	snow peas	250 g
1 tbsp	crushed dried basil	15 mL
4 cups	farfalle (bow tie pasta), cooked and drained	1 L
	Salt and freshly ground black pepper	
4 oz	soft crumbled goat cheese or shredded mozzarella	125 g

1. *Prepare the tomato coulis:* In a skillet, combine shallots, celery and ¼ cup (50 mL) water; cook over medium heat until soft. Add garlic, tomatoes, parsley, basil, sugar, salt and pepper; bring to a boil. Reduce heat and simmer for 10 minutes, stirring occasionally. Purée in a food processor. Keep warm.

2. *Prepare the pasta:* In a large skillet, heat oil over medium heat; cook snow peas and basil, stirring, for 3 to 5 minutes or until tender. Stir in pasta. Season with salt and pepper to taste.

3. To serve, place tomato coulis in a pasta bowl; top with pasta mixture. Sprinkle with goat cheese.

NUTRITIONAL ANALYSIS PER SERVING			
Energy: 385 kcal	Fat: 11 g	Fiber: 5.2 g	Iron: 5.0 mg
Protein: 15 g	Carbohydrate: 59 g	Calcium: 205 mg	Folate: 67 mcg

Pasta Fagioli Capra

3 tbsp	extra-virgin olive oil	45 mL
6	cloves garlic, finely chopped	6
2	bay leaves	2
1	stalk celery, finely chopped	1
1	small onion, finely chopped	1
1	small carrot, finely chopped	1
1	sprig thyme, leaves only, finely chopped	1
1 cup	chopped plum tomatoes, canned or fresh	250 mL
¼ cup	cooked romano beans	50 mL
¼ cup	cooked black-eyed peas	50 mL
¼ cup	cooked cannellini beans (white kidney beans) or navy beans	50 mL
¼ cup	cooked large lima beans	50 mL
¼ cup	cooked chickpeas	50 mL
6 cups	vegetable stock	1.5 L
	Salt and freshly ground black pepper	
	Freshly grated nutmeg	
1 cup	maccheroni (the straight, short variety), ditalini or tubetti	250 mL
½ cup	cooked peeled fava beans	125 mL
¼ cup	roughly chopped flat-leaf parsley	50 mL
	Olive oil	
6	slices of rustic country-style bread, brushed with olive oil and grilled or oven-toasted	6

1. In a large saucepan, heat oil over medium heat. Add garlic, bay leaves, celery, onion, carrot and thyme; cook for 5 minutes or until vegetables are softened. Stir in tomatoes; cook, stirring, for 3 minutes.

2. Stir in romano beans, black-eyed peas, kidney beans, lima beans and chickpeas. Add vegetable stock and bring to a boil. Reduce heat to simmer and cook for 15 minutes, skimming any foam that rises to the top. Season to taste with salt, pepper and nutmeg.

3. Stir in pasta and fava beans; return to a simmer and cook, stirring occasionally, for 10 minutes or just until pasta is tender.

4. Stir in parsley. Drizzle with olive oil and serve immediately with toasts.

MAKES 6 SERVINGS

Pasta fagioli combines beans, pasta and vegetables to make a delicious meal-in-a-bowl.

TIP

The combination of beans can be varied to suit your taste and may either be canned, dried, fresh or frozen. If using canned beans, rinse and drain well.

NUTRITIONAL ANALYSIS PER SERVING			
Energy: 328 kcal	Fat: 10 g	Fiber: 9.4 g	Iron: 3.8 mg
Protein: 11 g	Carbohydrate: 51 g	Calcium: 69 mg	Folate: 105 mcg

**MAKES
4 SERVINGS**

TIPS

Make sure to buy tofu that has been coagulated with calcium sulfate or calcium chloride. Read the ingredient list on the label for the coagulant. Otherwise, you won't get nearly as much calcium out of this recipe.

Be sure to use a firm or extra-firm variety of tofu or it will fall apart in the stir-fry.

Tofu can be replaced with 6 oz (175 g) cooked beans of your choice.

If rice noodles are not available, use regular pasta. Cook according to package directions.

Make ahead

Prepare sauce, cover and store in the refrigerator for up to 2 days.

Hoisin Stir-fried Vegetables and Tofu over Rice Noodles

Sauce

1/3 cup	hoisin sauce	75 mL
1/3 cup	soy sauce	75 mL
1/4 cup	rice wine vinegar	50 mL
1/4 cup	packed brown sugar	50 mL
1 tsp	minced garlic	5 mL
1 tsp	minced gingerroot	5 mL

Stir-fry

8 oz	thin rice vermicelli	250 g
2 tsp	vegetable oil	10 mL
2 1/4 cups	chopped red bell peppers	550 mL
2 1/4 cups	chopped leeks	550 mL
2 cups	sliced mushrooms	500 mL
1 1/4 cups	shredded carrots	300 mL
1 1/4 cups	chopped zucchini	300 mL
6 oz	firm tofu (see tip, at left), cubed	175 g

1. *Prepare the sauce:* In a small bowl, whisk together hoisin sauce, soy sauce, vinegar, brown sugar, garlic and ginger. Set aside.

2. *Prepare the stir-fry:* Pour boiling water over noodles to cover; soak for 10 minutes or until soft. Drain well.

3. In a nonstick wok or large saucepan sprayed with vegetable spray, heat oil over high heat. Add red peppers and leeks; stir-fry for 4 minutes. Add mushrooms and stir-fry for 2 minutes. Add carrots and zucchini; stir-fry for 2 minutes or until vegetables are tender-crisp. Add noodles, tofu and sauce; stir-fry for 2 minutes or until bubbly and hot. Serve immediately.

NUTRITIONAL ANALYSIS PER SERVING			
Energy: 379 kcal	Fat: 8 g	Fiber: 5.6 g	Iron: 8.8 mg
Protein: 13 g	Carbohydrate: 70 g	Calcium: 175 mg	Folate: 94 mcg

Spaghetti with Broccoli

12 oz	spaghetti	375 g
1 tbsp	olive oil	15 mL
1 cup	diced onion	250 mL
1 tbsp	minced garlic	15 mL
1 tsp	salt	5 mL
	Freshly ground black pepper	
1	can (28 oz/796 mL) tomatoes, coarsely chopped, including juice	1
4 cups	broccoli florets, thawed if frozen	1 L
	Freshly grated Parmesan cheese	

1. Cook spaghetti in a pot of boiling salted water until tender to the bite, about 7 minutes. Drain.

2. Meanwhile, in a skillet, heat oil over medium heat. Add onion and cook, stirring, until softened, about 3 minutes. Add garlic, salt and pepper to taste. Cook, stirring, for 1 minute.

3. Stir in tomatoes with juice and broccoli and bring to a boil. Reduce heat to low and simmer until broccoli is tender, about 15 minutes.

4. In a warm serving bowl, toss cooked spaghetti with sauce. Pass the Parmesan.

Variations

Spaghetti with Tuna: Omit the broccoli. After the sauce has finished simmering, stir in 1 can (6 oz/170 g) flaked tuna, drained. Serve immediately.

Spaghetti with Pancetta and Hot Pepper: Add 2 oz (60 g) diced pancetta and 1 whole hot dried chili pepper along with the onion. Cook, stirring, until the pancetta is lightly browned, about 4 minutes. Continue with recipe and remove chili before serving.

NUTRITIONAL ANALYSIS PER SERVING			
Energy: 477 kcal	Fat: 5 g	Fiber: 4.4 g	Iron: 3.5 mg
Protein: 17 g	Carbohydrate: 93 g	Calcium: 146 mg	Folate: 109 mcg

Health Tip

Broccoli should be included in the diet at least a few times every week. It is loaded with many nutrients, including protein, the B vitamins, calcium, iron, fiber and vitamin C.

Excellent source of:
• Folate

Good source of:
• Iron and fiber

Source of:
• Calcium

MAKES 4 SERVINGS

Spaghetti topped with this simple broccoli and tomato sauce is an ideal dish to serve to vegetarians. The variations, which use canned tuna or pancetta — an Italian cured bacon available at specialty food stores or well-stocked supermarkets — are equally tasty.

**MAKES
6 SERVINGS**

TIPS

For color variation, try red kidney beans or black beans instead of white beans.

For a more sophisticated meal, replace canned tuna with cooked tuna or swordfish.

Make ahead

Prepare sauce, cover and store in the refrigerator for up to 1 day. Reheat gently, adding more stock if too thick.

Linguine with Tuna, White Beans and Dill

12 oz	linguine	375 g
1 tbsp	olive oil	15 mL
1	can (19 oz/540 mL) white kidney beans, drained	1
¼ cup	freshly squeezed lemon juice	50 mL
2 tsp	crushed garlic	10 mL
1¾ cups	cold chicken stock	425 mL
4 tsp	all-purpose flour	20 mL
1	can (6.5 oz/185 g) flaked tuna packed in water, drained	1
½ cup	chopped fresh dill (or 1 tbsp/15 mL dried dillweed)	125 mL
⅓ cup	sliced black olives	75 mL
¼ cup	chopped green onions	50 mL

1. Cook pasta in boiling water according to package instructions or until firm to the bite. Drain and place in a serving bowl.

2. In a large nonstick skillet, heat oil; add beans, lemon juice and garlic. Cook for 2 minutes or until hot.

3. Meanwhile, in a small bowl combine chicken stock and flour until smooth. Add to bean mixture; simmer for 3 minutes or until sauce thickens slightly. Pour over pasta. Add tuna, dill, olives and green onions. Toss to combine.

NUTRITIONAL ANALYSIS PER SERVING			
Energy: 247 kcal	Fat: 5 g	Fiber: 5.8 g	Iron: 3.3 mg
Protein: 18 g	Carbohydrate: 32 g	Calcium: 52 mg	Folate: 93 mcg

Tuna Garden Pasta

2 tbsp	butter or margarine	25 mL
6	large mushrooms, sliced	6
1	small onion, sliced	1
2	cans (each 6.5 oz/185 g) water-packed chunk white tuna, drained	2
2 cups	chicken stock	500 mL
2 tbsp	all-purpose flour	25 mL
2 tbsp	chopped pimiento	25 mL
1 tsp	grated lemon zest	5 mL
2 tbsp	freshly squeezed lemon juice	25 mL
1 tsp	dried thyme	5 mL
¼ tsp	garlic powder	1 mL
Pinch	salt	Pinch
Pinch	freshly ground black pepper	Pinch
3	carrots, sliced	3
2	large bunches broccoli (florets only), chopped	2
8 oz	spaghettini	250 g
	Tomato slices	

1. In a large skillet, melt butter over medium heat. Cook mushrooms and onion for about 5 minutes or until tender. Stir in tuna. Combine chicken stock, flour, pimiento, lemon zest and juice, thyme, garlic powder, salt and pepper. Stir into tuna mixture; cook for about 5 minutes or until slightly thickened.

2. Steam carrots and broccoli over boiling water until tender-crisp. Drain well and add to tuna mixture.

3. In a large pot of boiling water, cook pasta according to package directions or until tender but firm; drain well. Stir tuna and vegetable sauce into pasta; garnish with tomato slices.

NUTRITIONAL ANALYSIS PER SERVING			
Energy: 314 kcal	Fat: 5 g	Fiber: 3.1 g	Iron: 3.0 mg
Protein: 25 g	Carbohydrate: 42 g	Calcium: 59 mg	Folate: 49 mcg

Good source of:
• Folate and iron

Source of:
• Calcium and fiber

MAKES 6 SERVINGS

The light sauce, prepared with chicken stock rather than milk or cream, highlights the flavors of the vegetables and tuna, which provide abundant protein, fiber, vitamins and iron.

TIPS

For variety, serve this with whole wheat spaghetti instead of spaghettini.

You may want to use minced garlic to taste instead of the garlic powder and 1 tbsp (15 mL) fresh thyme instead of the dried version. Add to the onion-mushroom mixture just before adding the tuna.

MAKES 4 TO 6 SERVINGS

Lasagna layered with meat, cheese and tomato sauce is so much a part of our gastronomic vocabulary that contemplating one with different ingredients requires a considerable stretch of the imagination. Still, there's a world of lasagnas out there. So if you're in the mood for a change, try this meatless variety — it's every bit as satisfying as the original.

TIPS

If expense or calories are a concern, you can substitute low-fat ricotta for the goat cheese in the filling, as well as 12 oz (375 g) low-fat mozzarella instead of the recommended mixture for the topping.

For noodles, either cook your own or use the "ready to bake" variety (preferably white ones, to contrast with the spinach).

Mushroom-Spinach Lasagna with Goat Cheese

• Preheat oven to 375°F (190°C)
• 13- by 9-inch (3 L) baking dish

12 oz	spinach, washed and trimmed	375 g
¼ cup	olive oil, divided	50 mL
¾ tsp	salt, divided	4 mL
½ tsp	freshly ground black pepper, divided	2 mL
12 oz	portobello mushrooms, trimmed and sliced ½-inch (1 cm) thick	375 g
2 tbsp	finely chopped garlic, divided	25 mL
½ tsp	hot pepper flakes	2 mL
2 cups	finely diced peeled tomatoes, with juices, or canned tomatoes	500 mL
1 tsp	balsamic vinegar	5 mL
½ tsp	dried rosemary, crumbled	2 mL
½ tsp	dried thyme	2 mL
9	cooked lasagna noodles (see tip, at left)	9
8 oz	goat cheese, divided (see tip, at left)	250 g
8 oz	shredded mozzarella (about 2 cups/500 mL)	250 g
4 oz	grated strong Italian cheese such as Crotonese, Asiago or aged provolone	125 g

1. In a large pot, bring about 1 inch (2.5 cm) salted water to boil. Add spinach, cover and cook for 1 minute. Uncover, turn the spinach, cover again and cook 1 minute more. Drain. Rinse under cold water; drain. Press lightly to extract more water and set aside in a colander to continue draining.

2. In a large nonstick skillet, heat 2 tbsp (25 mL) of the olive oil, ¼ tsp (1 mL) of the salt and ¼ tsp (1 mL) of the pepper over high heat for 1 minute. Add mushroom slices (they'll absorb all the oil immediately); stir-fry for 3 to 4 minutes or until browned and shiny. Add 1 tbsp (15 mL) of the garlic and stir-fry for 1 minute or until the garlic starts to brown. Transfer to a bowl and set aside.

3. In the same skillet, heat remaining olive oil, remaining salt, remaining pepper, hot pepper flakes and remaining garlic over high heat, stirring, for 1 minute. Add tomatoes, vinegar, rosemary and thyme; cook, stirring, until bubbling. Cook, stirring, for 2 more minutes or until the tomatoes are breaking up and a sauce forms. Remove from heat and set aside.

4. Spread the bottom of baking dish with 2 tbsp (25 mL) of the tomato sauce. Lay flat 3 of the lasagna noodles (they should cover the whole surface). Spread the spinach evenly over the surface. Dot half of the goat cheese evenly over the spinach. Cover with another layer of 3 noodles. Spread the mushrooms evenly over lasagna noodles. Dot remaining goat cheese over the mushrooms. Cover with the last layer of 3 noodles and spoon the rest of the tomato sauce evenly over the noodles. Mix the grated mozzarella and strong Italian cheeses; sprinkle evenly over the surface of the lasagna to create the topping.

5. Bake in preheated oven, uncovered, for 35 to 40 minutes or until the topping is rosy-browned and the inside is bubbling. Remove from oven and let rest, uncovered, for 10 minutes to temper. Lift portions carefully to retain the cheese on top and serve immediately.

NUTRITIONAL ANALYSIS PER SERVING (1 OF 6)			
Energy: 564 kcal	Fat: 34 g	Fiber: 5.3 g	Iron: 4.8 mg
Protein: 34 g	Carbohydrate: 34 g	Calcium: 669 mg	Folate: 154 mcg

**MAKES
4 SERVINGS**

*Canned tuna has
long been a great
convenience food,
and the substitution
of bottled roasted red
peppers for freshly
roasted dramatically
reduces the
preparation time.*

Penne with Tuna and Peppers

12 oz	penne	375 g
¼ cup	olive oil, preferably extra-virgin, divided, plus additional for drizzling	50 mL
1 tbsp	minced garlic	15 mL
2	roasted red bell peppers, cut into strips	2
2 tbsp	finely chopped parsley	25 mL
2 tbsp	drained capers	25 mL
1	can (6 oz/170 g) tuna, preferably Italian, packed in olive oil, drained	1
	Freshly ground black pepper	
¼ cup	toasted croutons or 2 tbsp (25 mL) coarse dry bread crumbs	50 mL

1. Cook penne in a pot of boiling salted water until tender to the bite, about 8 minutes. Drain.

2. In a warm serving bowl, combine hot penne with 2 tbsp (25 mL) of the olive oil. Keep warm.

3. Meanwhile, in a small saucepan over low heat, heat remaining olive oil. Add garlic and cook, stirring occasionally, until light golden, about 3 minutes. Add red pepper strips and stir until well coated with oil.

4. Add parsley and capers. Stir well and remove from heat. Stir in tuna and black pepper to taste. Spread sauce attractively over top of warm penne. Sprinkle with croutons. Drizzle with olive oil and serve.

NUTRITIONAL ANALYSIS PER SERVING			
Energy: 564 kcal	Fat: 19 g	Fiber: 4.2 g	Iron: 5.2 mg
Protein: 24 g	Carbohydrate: 74 g	Calcium: 31 mg	Folate: 277 mcg

Desserts

Cinnamon Baked Pears 282

Autumn Crumble 283

Buttermilk Oat-Banana Cake 284

Chocolate Cupcakes 285

Date Oatmeal Cake with Mocha Frosting 286

Sunflower Cookies. 287

Reverse Chocolate Chip Cookies. 288

Grandma's Rolled Oat Cookies 289

Lemony Biscotti 290

Almond Crescents 291

Berry Oatmeal Squares. 292

Vanilla Custard 293

Orange Crème Caramel 294

Strawberry Sorbet 295

**MAKES
4 SERVINGS**

**MAKES ABOUT
½ CUP (125 ML)
YOGURT SAUCE**

Here's another easy and delicious way to serve fruit. Try poaching peaches, nectarines, apples, fresh pineapple or oranges in this manner.

TIPS

Most pears are shipped before they are fully ripe in order to avoid damage. If your pears are overly firm, store them in a cool place to ripen before using in this recipe.

For added fiber, leave the skin on pears, apples, peaches and nectarines when serving.

Cinnamon Baked Pears

• Preheat oven to 350°F (180°C)
• Baking dish

4	pears	4
½ cup	blueberries	125 mL
2 tbsp	packed brown sugar	25 mL
1 tbsp	freshly squeezed lemon juice	15 mL
¼ tsp	ground cinnamon	1 mL

Yogurt Sauce

½ cup	low-fat plain yogurt	125 mL
1 tbsp	packed brown sugar	15 mL
½ tsp	ground cinnamon	2 mL
½ tsp	vanilla	2 mL

1. Peel pears and cut in half lengthwise; scoop out core. Place cut side down in shallow baking dish. Sprinkle blueberries around pears.

2. Combine ½ cup (125 mL) water, brown sugar, lemon juice and cinnamon; pour over pears. Bake, covered, in preheated oven for about 45 minutes or until pears are tender, basting occasionally with pan juices.

3. *Prepare the yogurt sauce:* In a small bowl, combine yogurt, brown sugar, cinnamon and vanilla. Serve pears with pan juices; spoon a dollop of yogurt sauce over cooked pear halves.

NUTRITIONAL ANALYSIS PER SERVING			
Energy: 160 kcal	Fat: 1 g	Fiber: 5.8 g	Iron: 0.8 mg
Protein: 3 g	Carbohydrate: 39 g	Calcium: 96 mg	Folate: 18 mcg

Autumn Crumble

- Preheat oven to 350°F (180°C)
- 8-inch (2 L) square baking pan, greased

1	egg	1
2 cups	mashed cooked acorn squash (1 large)	500 mL
1/3 cup	packed brown sugar	75 mL
1/4 cup	all-purpose or whole wheat flour	50 mL
1 tbsp	milk	15 mL
1 tsp	vanilla	5 mL
1 tsp	ground cinnamon	5 mL
1 tsp	ground nutmeg	5 mL
1/4 tsp	ground cloves	1 mL
2	large apples, peeled and chopped	2
1	large carrot, grated	1
1/2 cup	raisins	125 mL

Topping

1/2 cup	quick-cooking rolled oats	125 mL
1/4 cup	natural wheat bran	50 mL
1/4 cup	packed brown sugar	50 mL
2 tbsp	all-purpose or whole wheat flour	25 mL
2 tbsp	soft margarine	25 mL
1 tsp	ground cinnamon	5 mL

1. With electric mixer or in food processor, blend egg, squash, brown sugar, flour, milk, vanilla, cinnamon, nutmeg and cloves until smooth; stir in apples, carrot and raisins. Spread in prepared pan.

2. *Prepare the topping:* Combine oats, wheat bran, brown sugar, flour, margarine and cinnamon until crumbly; sprinkle over squash mixture. Bake in preheated oven for 30 to 35 minutes or until golden brown. Serve warm.

NUTRITIONAL ANALYSIS PER SERVING			
Energy: 214 kcal	Fat: 4 g	Fiber: 2.6 g	Iron: 2.1 mg
Protein: 3 g	Carbohydrate: 44 g	Calcium: 58 mg	Folate: 18 mcg

Good source of:
- Iron

Source of:
- Calcium, folate and fiber

MAKES 8 SERVINGS

Here's a crumble with a difference. Acorn squash and carrots, instead of fruit, provide the base for the crumble topping. The grains and fruit add dietary fiber, and the orange vegetables add vitamin A. Serve as a dessert with ice milk or frozen yogurt, or as a side dish with pork chops.

TIP

Try using cooked pumpkin or canned pumpkin purée instead of squash in this recipe.

**MAKES
12 SERVINGS**

The glaze poured over this fabulous cake makes it extra moist and delicious.

TIPS

This recipe is a great way to use over-ripe bananas. If you can't use bananas that are becoming ripe, pop them into a resealable plastic bag and freeze them. They will turn black, but once they are thawed and the skins are removed, they will be perfect for this recipe.

This recipe makes about 2 cups (500 mL) of glaze.

Buttermilk Oat-Banana Cake

- Preheat oven to 350°F (180°C)
- 8-inch (2 L) square baking pan, lightly greased and floured

1 cup	buttermilk	250 mL
⅔ cup	rolled oats	150 mL
⅓ cup	oat bran or wheat bran	75 mL
1 cup	granulated sugar	250 mL
¼ cup	butter or margarine	50 mL
1	egg	1
1 tsp	vanilla	5 mL
2	ripe bananas, mashed	2
1½ cups	all-purpose flour	375 mL
1 tsp	baking soda	5 mL
1 tsp	baking powder	5 mL

Glaze

½ cup	granulated sugar	125 mL
½ cup	buttermilk	125 mL
¼ cup	butter or margarine	50 mL
½ tsp	baking soda	2 mL

1. In a small bowl, pour buttermilk over oats and oat bran. Let stand for 10 minutes.

2. In a medium bowl, cream sugar and butter. Beat in egg and vanilla. Combine bananas and buttermilk mixture with creamed ingredients. Sift together flour, baking soda and baking powder. Stir dry ingredients into banana mixture; blend well.

3. Pour batter into prepared pan. Bake in preheated oven for 45 minutes or until tester inserted in center comes out clean. Let stand for 5 minutes.

4. *Prepare the glaze:* In a small saucepan over medium heat, combine sugar, buttermilk, butter and baking soda; bring just to a boil. (Watch closely; mixture will foam.)

5. Poke holes with tester (a metal skewer or a wooden toothpick) all over cake surface; pour glaze over cake while still warm. Cool cake before cutting.

NUTRITIONAL ANALYSIS PER SERVING			
Energy: 277 kcal	Fat: 8 g	Fiber: 2.0 g	Iron: 1.1 mg
Protein: 4 g	Carbohydrate: 49 g	Calcium: 52 mg	Folate: 14 mcg

Chocolate Cupcakes

- Preheat oven to 325°F (160°C)
- 12-cup muffin tin, lined with paper cups

1 cup	all-purpose flour	250 mL
½ cup	unsweetened cocoa powder	125 mL
1½ tsp	baking powder	7 mL
¾ cup	granulated sugar	175 mL
¼ cup	packed brown sugar	50 mL
⅔ cup	butter, softened	150 mL
4	eggs	4
½ cup	white chocolate chips	125 mL
¼ cup	semi-sweet chocolate chips	50 mL

1. In a small bowl, combine flour, cocoa and baking powder.

2. In a large bowl, using an electric mixer, cream sugar, brown sugar and butter until smooth. Add eggs, one at a time, beating well after each. Stir in flour mixture until well combined. Fold in white and semi-sweet chocolate chips. Spoon evenly into prepared muffin cups.

3. Bake in preheated oven for 15 to 20 minutes, or until a tester inserted in the center of a cupcake comes out clean. Let cool to room temperature on a wire rack.

NUTRITIONAL ANALYSIS PER SERVING (1 CUPCAKE)			
Energy: 273 kcal	Fat: 16 g	Fiber: 1.0 g	Iron: 1.5 mg
Protein: 4 g	Carbohydrate: 32 g	Calcium: 41 mg	Folate: 16 mcg

Health Tip

Desserts do not need to be avoided completely in a healthy diet. Try to choose sweets and other less nutritious foods less often, but remember that all foods can be part of a well-balanced diet.

Source of:
- Folate and iron

MAKES 12 CUPCAKES

A great treat for yourself, with or without company! These freeze well, so try making double the batch, freeze and have as a treat any time!

Make ahead

Place in an airtight container and store at room temperature for up to 1 day, or wrap in plastic, then place in a freezer bag and store in the freezer for up to 2 months.

**MAKES
16 SERVINGS**

**MAKES ¾ CUP
(175 ML) FROSTING**

*Here's a delicious
old-fashioned cake
that combines dates,
walnuts and oats
with a yummy mocha
frosting.*

TIPS

Most of the dates sold in
North America are dried
and high in concentrated
sugar. As a result, they are
a great source of energy.
Take some along on hikes
or whenever you think you
may need a power snack.

If desired, use butter
instead of margarine in
this recipe.

Date Oatmeal Cake with Mocha Frosting

- Preheat oven to 350°F (180°C)
- 9-inch (2.5 L) square baking pan, greased

Cake

1 cup	rolled oats	250 mL
1½ cups	boiling water	375 mL
1 cup	all-purpose flour	250 mL
1 tsp	baking soda	5 mL
¼ tsp	salt	1 mL
1 cup	packed brown sugar	250 mL
½ cup	margarine	125 mL
1 tsp	vanilla	5 mL
1 cup	chopped dates	250 mL
½ cup	chopped walnuts	125 mL

Mocha Frosting

1½ cups	sifted confectioner's (icing) sugar	300 mL
2 tbsp	margarine	25 mL
2 tsp	unsweetened cocoa powder	10 mL
1 tbsp	strong coffee, cooled	15 mL
1 tsp	vanilla	5 mL

1. *Prepare the cake:* In a small bowl, combine oats and boiling water; let stand until cool.

2. In a separate bowl, combine flour, baking soda and salt. Set aside.

3. In a large bowl, cream brown sugar and margarine until fluffy. Beat in vanilla, rolled oats mixture and flour mixture. Stir in dates and walnuts. Pour mixture into prepared pan and bake in preheated oven for 30 to 35 minutes or until cake tester inserted in center comes out clean. Set aside to cool.

4. *Prepare the Mocha Frosting:* In a bowl, blend together sugar, margarine, cocoa, coffee and vanilla until fluffy. If necessary, thin icing with extra coffee to reach desired consistency. Spread over cooled cake.

NUTRITIONAL ANALYSIS PER SERVING			
Energy: 273 kcal	Fat: 11 g	Fiber: 2.3 g	Iron: 1.3 mg
Protein: 3 g	Carbohydrate: 43 g	Calcium: 26 mg	Folate: 8 mcg

Sunflower Cookies

- Preheat oven to 350°F (180°C)
- Cookie sheets, lightly greased

¾ cup	lightly packed brown sugar	175 mL
¾ cup	granulated sugar	175 mL
½ cup	butter or margarine	125 mL
1	egg, beaten	1
½ tsp	vanilla	2 mL
½ tsp	baking soda, dissolved in 2 tsp (10 mL) hot water	2 mL
1 cup	unsalted shelled sunflower seeds	250 mL
½ cup	all-purpose flour	125 mL
½ cup	whole wheat flour	125 mL
½ cup	large-flake rolled oats	125 mL
½ cup	chocolate chips	125 mL
½ cup	raisins	125 mL
⅓ cup	natural wheat bran	75 mL
⅓ cup	wheat germ	75 mL
1 tsp	salt	5 mL

1. In a large bowl, cream brown sugar, granulated sugar and butter until fluffy. Stir in egg, vanilla and baking soda dissolved in hot water. Add sunflower seeds, all-purpose flour, whole wheat flour, oats, chocolate chips, raisins, wheat bran, wheat germ and salt; combine thoroughly.

2. Drop batter a spoonful at a time onto lightly greased or nonstick cookie sheets. Bake in preheated oven for about 10 minutes.

NUTRITIONAL ANALYSIS PER SERVING (2 COOKIES)

Energy: 134 kcal	Fat: 6 g	Fiber: 1.6 g	Iron: 0.8 mg
Protein: 2 g	Carbohydrate: 18 g	Calcium: 14 mg	Folate: 14 mcg

MAKES 5 DOZEN COOKIES

The crunchiness of nuts and seeds and the sweetness of raisins and chocolate chips make this healthy cookie one that everyone will enjoy.

TIP

Since sunflower seeds are high in fat, check them for freshness before using to ensure that they haven't become rancid.

**MAKES ABOUT
30 COOKIES**

*A favorite for young
and old alike.*

TIP

For additional chocolate
flavor, add ¼ cup (50 mL)
semi-sweet chocolate chips
with the white chocolate
chips.

Make ahead

Place in an airtight
container and store at
room temperature for
up to 5 days or in the
freezer for up to 3 months.

Reverse Chocolate Chip Cookies

• Preheat oven to 375°F (190°C)
• Baking sheets, greased

1 cup	quick-cooking rolled oats	250 mL
1 cup	all-purpose flour	250 mL
¼ cup	unsweetened cocoa powder	50 mL
½ tsp	baking powder	2 mL
½ tsp	baking soda	2 mL
¼ tsp	salt	1 mL
1	egg	1
1 cup	packed brown sugar	250 mL
½ cup	butter, softened	125 mL
½ tsp	vanilla	2 mL
1½ cups	white chocolate chips	375 mL

1. In a medium bowl, combine oats, flour, cocoa, baking powder, baking soda and salt.

2. In a large bowl, using an electric mixer, beat egg, brown sugar, butter and vanilla until smooth. Stir in flour mixture until well combined. Fold in chocolate chips.

3. Form dough into 1-inch (2.5 cm) round balls and place 2 inches (5 cm) apart on prepared baking sheets. Bake in preheated oven for 8 to 10 minutes or until cookies are set. Let cool to room temperature on a wire rack.

NUTRITIONAL ANALYSIS PER SERVING (1 COOKIE)			
Energy: 135 kcal	Fat: 6 g	Fiber: 0.1 g	Iron: 0.7 mg
Protein: 2 g	Carbohydrate: 18 g	Calcium: 30 mg	Folate: 4 mcg

Grandma's Rolled Oat Cookies

- Preheat oven to 325°F (160°C)
- Cookie sheets, lightly greased

Cookie Dough

1½ cups	all-purpose flour	375 mL
1½ cups	rolled oats	375 mL
1 tsp	baking soda	5 mL
½ cup	shortening	125 mL
½ cup	hot water	125 mL

Filling

2 cups	chopped dates	500 mL
¼ cup	granulated sugar	50 mL
1 tsp	vanilla	5 mL

1. *Prepare the cookie dough:* Combine flour, oats and baking soda. Cut in shortening until mixture resembles coarse crumbs. Add sufficient water to shape dough into a roll. Wrap in waxed paper; refrigerate overnight.

2. Cut cookie dough into thin wafers (⅛ inch/3 mm). Place on lightly greased or nonstick cookie sheet. Bake in preheated oven for about 10 minutes.

3. *Prepare the filling:* Cook dates, ½ cup (125 mL) water and sugar on low heat for about 30 minutes, stirring occasionally. Stir in vanilla.

4. When cookies and filling are cool, spread about 1 tbsp (15 mL) date filling between 2 cookies.

NUTRITIONAL ANALYSIS PER SERVING (2 COOKIES)			
Energy: 188 kcal	Fat: 7 g	Fiber: 3.0 g	Iron: 1.0 mg
Protein: 2 g	Carbohydrate: 30 g	Calcium: 12 mg	Folate: 8 mcg

Source of:
- Iron and fiber

MAKES 3 DOZEN COOKIES

These unsweetened cookies taste like a Scottish oatcake; the sweet date filling complements the oatmeal. They are every bit as warm and comforting as when Grandma made them.

TIPS

In this recipe, refrigerating the cookie dough overnight makes it easier to slice. Remove dough from the refrigerator about 15 minutes before using.

Although dates are high in naturally-occurring sugar, they contribute vitamins, minerals and fiber.

Lemony Biscotti

MAKES ABOUT
34 BISCOTTI

So refreshing, and wonderful with a cup of tea or milk.

TIP

After Step 2, you can place dough in the refrigerator for up to 2 hours to harden, if desired, for easier management.

Make ahead

Place in an airtight container and store at room temperature for up to 2 weeks.

- Preheat oven to 325°F (160°C)
- Baking sheets, greased

1½ cups	all-purpose flour	375 mL
½ cup	cornmeal	125 mL
1 tsp	baking powder	5 mL
Pinch	salt	Pinch
1 cup	granulated sugar	250 mL
½ cup	butter, softened	125 mL
1 tbsp	grated lemon zest	15 mL
½ tsp	vanilla	2 mL
2	eggs	2

1. In a medium bowl, combine flour, cornmeal, baking powder and salt.

2. In a large bowl, using an electric mixer, beat sugar, butter, lemon zest and vanilla until smooth. Add eggs, one at a time, beating well after each. Stir in flour mixture until a soft dough forms.

3. Divide dough in half and form into two 10-inch (25 cm) logs. Place at least 2 inches (5 cm) apart on prepared baking sheet.

4. Bake in preheated oven for 30 minutes, until lightly browned. Let cool to room temperature on baking sheet. Reduce oven temperature to 275°F (140°C).

5. Transfer logs to a cutting board. Using a serrated knife, slice into ½-inch (1 cm) pieces. Place flat on sheet and bake for 35 minutes, until dry. Turn over and bake for 20 minutes, until dry. Let cool to room temperature on a wire rack.

NUTRITIONAL ANALYSIS PER SERVING (3 BISCOTTI)			
Energy: 246 kcal	Fat: 9 g	Fiber: 0.9 g	Iron: 0.9 mg
Protein: 3 g	Carbohydrate: 36 g	Calcium: 15 mg	Folate: 12 mcg

Almond Crescents

Source of:
- Folate and iron

- Preheat oven to 325°F (160°C)
- Baking sheets, ungreased

1¼ cups	all-purpose flour	300 mL
1 cup	ground almonds	250 mL
⅓ cup	confectioner's (icing) sugar, divided	75 mL
¾ cup	butter, softened	175 mL
1 tsp	vanilla	5 mL

1. In a medium bowl, combine flour and almonds. Add ¼ cup (50 mL) of the confectioner's sugar and mix well. Add butter and vanilla and mix until smooth.

2. Using about 2 tsp (10 mL) dough for each cookie, form into crescent shapes and place 2 inches (5 cm) apart on baking sheet. Bake in preheated oven for 10 to 12 minutes, or until edges are barely brown. Remove from oven and sprinkle with the remaining confectioner's sugar. Let cool to room temperature on a wire rack.

NUTRITIONAL ANALYSIS PER SERVING (2 CRESCENTS)

Energy: 218 kcal	Fat: 18 g	Fiber: 0.4 g	Iron: 0.8 mg
Protein: 4 g	Carbohydrate: 14 g	Calcium: 38 mg	Folate: 12 mcg

Health Tip

Almonds are a great source of monounsaturated fats, which have been associated with a reduced risk of heart disease.

MAKES 30 COOKIES

This dessert is mildly sweet, with the addition of healthy almonds.

TIP

Freeze to have ready for visitors or for an afternoon snack.

Make ahead

Place in an airtight container and store at room temperature for up to 5 days or in the freezer for up to 3 months.

MAKES 12 SQUARES

Delicious as a snack on its own, or heated slightly and served with vanilla ice cream on top!

TIP

If you prefer, use a combination of blueberries and raspberries, keeping the total amount at 3 cups (750 mL).

Make ahead

Place in an airtight container and store at room temperature for up to 2 days, or individually wrap, then place in an airtight container and store in the freezer for up to 2 months.

Berry Oatmeal Squares

• Preheat oven to 350°F (180°C)
• 8-inch (2 L) square metal baking pan, greased

1½ cups	all-purpose flour	375 mL
1½ cups	quick-cooking rolled oats	375 mL
½ cup	packed brown sugar	125 mL
¾ cup	butter, softened	175 mL
3 cups	fresh or frozen blueberries or raspberries	750 mL
2 tbsp	granulated sugar	25 mL
1 tbsp	cornstarch	15 mL
2 tsp	freshly squeezed lemon juice	10 mL

1. In a medium bowl, combine flour, oats and brown sugar. Add butter and, using a spoon, mix to form a crumbly mixture.

2. Spoon about two-thirds of the oat mixture into baking pan and press down to form a firm layer. Bake in preheated oven for about 10 minutes, until lightly browned on edges.

3. In another medium bowl, combine berries, sugar, cornstarch and lemon juice. Sprinkle over oat crust in baking pan. Cover with the remaining oat mixture and pat down firmly. Bake for 50 minutes, or until berries are bubbly. Let cool in pan on a wire rack. Cut into 12 squares.

NUTRITIONAL ANALYSIS PER SERVING (1 SQUARE)			
Energy: 260 kcal	Fat: 12 g	Fiber: 3.0 g	Iron: 1.5 mg
Protein: 4 g	Carbohydrate: 34 g	Calcium: 23 mg	Folate: 13 mcg

Vanilla Custard

Source of:
- Calcium, folate and iron

- Preheat toaster oven to 350°F (180°C)
- 8-inch (2 L) square baking dish

2	eggs	2
2	egg yolks	2
1½ cups	milk or light (5%) cream	375 mL
¼ cup	granulated sugar	50 mL
1 tsp	vanilla	5 mL
Pinch	salt	Pinch
Pinch	ground nutmeg	Pinch

MAKES 4 SERVINGS

A satisfying and soothing dessert. Top with fresh raspberries or blueberries.

1. In a large bowl, beat together eggs, egg yolks, milk, sugar, vanilla, salt and nutmeg. Pour into four 4-oz (125 mL) ramekins.

2. Place ramekins in baking dish. Do not crowd dishes. Pour boiling water into baking dish until it comes halfway up sides of ramekins.

3. Bake in preheated toaster oven for 35 minutes, or until custard is just set and knife inserted in center comes out clean.

4. Remove ramekins from water bath and cool on wire racks. Cover and refrigerate for 4 hours or until completely chilled.

NUTRITIONAL ANALYSIS PER SERVING			
Energy: 175 kcal	Fat: 9 g	Fiber: 0.0 g	Iron: 1.0 mg
Protein: 8 g	Carbohydrate: 16 g	Calcium: 143 mg	Folate: 34 mcg

**MAKES
8 SERVINGS**

This recipe is a lighter, but even tastier, variation of traditional crème caramel. It makes a nice balance to a heavier main course.

Make ahead

Cover with foil or plastic wrap and store in the refrigerator for up to 2 days.

Orange Crème Caramel

• Preheat oven to 350°F (180°C)
• 8-inch (2 L) round baking pan

1 cup	granulated sugar, divided	250 mL
5	eggs	5
2½ cups	hot milk	625 mL
1 tbsp	grated orange zest	15 mL
1 tsp	vanilla	5 mL

1. In a small heavy saucepan, combine ½ cup (125 mL) of the sugar and ¼ cup (50 mL) water. Cook over medium heat, stirring constantly, until sugar is dissolved. (Be careful not to let the mixture boil at this stage.) Increase heat to medium-high and boil, without stirring, for 6 to 8 minutes or until mixture caramelizes and is golden in color. Pour immediately into baking pan, tilting pan to cover bottom.

2. In a medium bowl, stir together eggs and the remaining sugar until blended. Stir in hot milk, orange zest and vanilla; avoid overmixing. Pour into pan over caramel mixture. Place baking pan in a larger pan of boiling water. Bake in preheated oven for 40 to 45 minutes or until mixture is set. Remove from hot water. Cool on a rack. Refrigerate until ready to serve.

3. To remove from pan, run a spatula carefully around custard. Invert a rimmed serving plate over custard and turn over. Serve in wedges with caramel sauce from the pan.

NUTRITIONAL ANALYSIS PER SERVING			
Energy: 194 kcal	Fat: 5 g	Fiber: 0.1 g	Iron: 0.7 mg
Protein: 6 g	Carbohydrate: 31 g	Calcium: 117 mg	Folate: 24 mcg

Strawberry Sorbet

- **8-inch (2 L) square pan**

1½ cups	fresh or frozen unsweetened strawberries	375 mL
2 cups	unsweetened apple juice	500 mL
¼ cup	granulated sugar	50 mL
¼ tsp	ground cinnamon	1 mL
2 tbsp	cold water	25 mL
4 tsp	cornstarch	20 mL

1. Wash and hull fresh strawberries or thaw frozen strawberries. In a blender or food processor, blend strawberries and apple juice until almost smooth.

2. In a medium saucepan, over medium heat, cook strawberry mixture, sugar and cinnamon, stirring frequently, for about 5 minutes or until sugar is dissolved. Combine water and cornstarch; stir into hot mixture. Cook for about 3 minutes or until thickened and clear. Chill for 1 hour. Pour into pan; cover and freeze for about 3 hours or until firm.

3. Break frozen mixture into chunks; beat with electric mixer at medium speed until fluffy. Transfer to an airtight container and freeze until firm. Transfer from freezer to refrigerator about 15 minutes before serving.

NUTRITIONAL ANALYSIS PER SERVING			
Energy: 87 kcal	Fat: Trace	Fiber: 0.8 mg	Iron: 0.5 mg
Protein: Trace	Carbohydrate: 22 g	Calcium: 13 mg	Folate: 7 mcg

Health Tip

When you're craving sweets, this recipe is an excellent lower-fat alternative to ice cream. While it is not a source of any of the key nutrients highlighted in this book, it is a source of vitamin C, a powerful antioxidant.

The perfect low-fat ending to any meal, this sorbet can be made with virtually any fruit. Try raspberries, peaches, blueberries, kiwi fruit, cantaloupe or any other seasonal fruit.

TIP

Beating the sorbet during the freezing process helps to keep it from becoming too solid and helps to reduce the formation of ice crystals.

Nutritional Analysis

The nutrient analyses for all the recipes were prepared using Vision Software Technologies Inc., version 5.2. The nutrient databases used are the Canadian Nutrient File 1998 and the USDA National Nutrient Database for Standard Reference. This also includes the evaluation of recipe servings as sources of nutrients.

The nutrient analyses were based on:

- imperial measures and weights (except for food typically packaged and used in metric);
- the larger number of servings where there is a range;
- the smaller amount where there is a range;
- the first ingredient listed where there is a choice;
- the exclusion of "optional" ingredients; and
- the exclusion of ingredients with non-specified or "to taste" amounts.

The evaluation of recipe servings as sources of nutrients combine U.S. and Canadian regulations. Bearing in mind that the two countries have different reporting standards, the highest standard was always used. As a result, some recipes that would have been identified as an excellent source of a particular nutrient in one country may be listed only as a source or a good source because the standard is higher in the other country.

Contributing Authors

Julia Aitkin
Easy Entertaining Cookbook
A recipe from this book is found on page 189.

Byron Ayanoglu
The New Vegetarian Gourmet
A recipe from this book is found on page 170.
125 Best Vegetarian Recipes
Recipes from this book are found on pages 157, 159 (top), 161, 178, 184, 192, 251, 267–69 and 278.

Johanna Burkhard
Fast & Easy Cooking
A recipe from this book is found on page 235.

Pat Crocker
The Healing Herbs Cookbook
A recipe from this book is found on page 253.

Dietitians of Canada
Dietitians of Canada Cook Great Food
Recipes from this book are found on pages 142–48, 150, 152, 156 (top), 159 (bottom), 163, 164, 166, 167, 175, 176, 179 (top), 180, 181, 185, 193 (bottom), 194, 197, 201, 202, 207, 213, 216, 218, 219, 227, 232, 239, 242, 244, 248, 249, 254, 255, 258, 262, 263, 272, 277, 282–84, 286, 287, 289, 294 and 295.

Judith Finlayson
The Convenience Cook
Recipes from this book are found on pages 168, 169, 173, 174, 179 (bottom), 186, 190, 193 (top), 195, 196, 198, 200, 211, 217, 223, 226, 229, 230, 233, 243, 246, 260, 261, 264, 275 and 280.

Tracy Kett
The Organic Gourmet
A recipe from this book is found on page 172.

Ilana Simon
125 Best Indoor Grill Recipes
Recipes from this book are found on pages 203, 204, 208, 209, 212, 220, 234, 245, 250 (top) and 266.

Kathleen Sloan
Rustic Italian Cooking
Recipes from this book can be found on pages 171 and 273.

Linda Stephen
125 Best Toaster Oven Recipes
Recipes from this book are found on pages 154, 221, 222, 236, 238 and 293.

Editors of Robert Rose
The Beans, Lentils and Tofu Gourmet
Recipes from this book are found on pages 158, 160, 256, 257, 274 and 276.

Resources

This list of resources is sorted by topic, beginning with pregnancy and nutrition, then proceeding alphabetically through more specific topics.

Pregnancy & Nutrition

American College of Obstetricians
  and Gynecologists
409 12th St, S.W., PO Box 96920
Washington, DC 20090-6920
Tel: 202-638-5577 or 1-800-762-2264
www.acog.org

American Dietetic Association
120 South Riverside Plaza, Suite 2000
Chicago, IL 60606-6995
Tel: 1-800-877-1600
www.eatright.org

American Pregnancy Association
1425 Greenway Dr, Suite 440
Irving, TX 75038
Tel: 1-800-672-2296
www.americanpregnancy.org

Dietitians of Canada
480 University Ave, Suite 604
Toronto, ON M5G 1V2
Tel: 416-596-0857
Fax: 416-596-0603
www.dietitians.ca

Health Canada
Office of Nutrition Policy and Promotion
Tower A, Qualicum Towers
2936 Baseline Rd, 3rd Floor A.L. 3303D
Ottawa, ON K1A 0K9
Tel: 613-957-8329
E-mail: healthy_eating@hc-sc.gc.ca
www.hc-sc.gc.ca/fn-an/nutrition/prenatal/
  national_guidelines_tc-lignes_directrices
  _nationales_tm_e.html

March of Dimes
Pregnancy and Newborn Health Education
  Center
1275 Mamaroneck Ave
White Plains, NY 10605
www.marchofdimes.com

Motherisk
The Hospital for Sick Children
555 University Ave
Toronto, ON M5G 1X8
Tel: 416-813-6780
www.motherisk.org

Other Motherisk Services
Nausea and Vomiting in Pregnancy:
  1-800-436-8477
Motherisk HIV Healthline and Network:
  1-888-246-5840
Motherisk Alcohol and Substance Use
  Line: 1-877-FAS-INFO (327-4636)

The Society of Obstetricians and
  Gynaecologists of Canada
780 Echo Dr
Ottawa, ON K1S 5R7
Tel: 613-730-4192 or 1-800-561-2416
Fax: 613-730-4314
E-mail: helpdesk@sogc.com
www.sogc.medical.org

U.S. Department of Health and Human
  Services
The National Women's Health Information
  Center
Pregnancy and a Healthy Diet
Tel: 1-800-994-9662
www.womenshealth.gov

Allergy & Pregnancy

American Academy of Allergy, Asthma
  and Immunology
555 East Wells Street, Suite 1100
Milwaukee, WI 53202-3823
Tel: 414-272-6071 or 1-800-822-2762
E-mail: info@aaaai.org
www.aaaai.org

Food Allergy and Anaphylaxis Network
11781 Lee Jackson Hwy, Suite 160
Fairfax, VA 22033-3309
Tel: 800-929-4040
Fax: 703-691-2713
E-mail:faan@foodallergy.org
www.foodallergy.org

Breastfeeding

Canadian Lactation Consultants Association
www.clca-accl.ca

International Lactation Consultants Association
1500 Sunday Drive, Suite 102
Raleigh, NC 27607
Tel: 919-861-5577 Fax: 919-787-4916
E-mail: info@ilca.org
www.ilca.org

La Leche League International
1400 N. Meacham Rd
Schaumburg, IL 60173-4808
Tel: 847-519-7730
www.lalecheleague.org

Pregnancy & Dental Health

American Dental Association
211 East Chicago Ave
Chicago, IL 60611-2678
Tel: 312-440-2500
www.ada.org

Canadian Dental Association
1815 Alta Vista Dr
Ottawa, ON K1G 3Y6
Tel: 613-523-1770
www.cda-adc.ca

Food Safety & Pregnancy

Canadian Diabetes Association
National Office
1400-522 University Ave
Toronto, ON M5G 2R5
Tel: 1-800 BANTING (226-8464)
E-mail: info@diabetes.ca
www.diabetes.ca

Center for Science in the Public Interest (United States)
1875 Connecticut Ave, N.W., Suite 300
Washington, DC 20009
Tel: 202-332-9110 Fax: 202-265-4954
E-mail: cspi@cspinet.org
www.cspinet.org

Centre for Science in the Public Interest (Canada)
CTTC Bldg, Suite 4550
1125 Colonel By Drive
Ottawa, ON K1S 5R1
Tel: 613-244-7337 Fax: 613-244-1559
E-mail: jefferyb@istar.ca
www.cspinet.org/canada

Environmental Protection Agency
Ariel Rios Building
1200 Pennsylvania Ave, N.W.
Washington, DC 20460
Tel: 202-272-0167
www.epa.gov

United States Department of Agriculture
Food Safety and Inspection Service
www.fsis.usda.gov

USDA Meat & Poultry Hotline
Tel: 1-888-MPHotline (1-888-674-6854)
  or 1-800-256-7072 (TTY)
E-mail: mphotline.fsis@usda.gov

FSIS Technical Service Center
Tel: 402-221-7400 Fax: 402-221-7438
Hotline 1-800-233-3935
E-mail: TechCenter@fsis.usda.gov

USDA Animal and Plant Health Inspection Service (APHIS)
4700 River Road
Riverdale, MD 20737
Tel: 1-866-536-7593 or 202-720-7943
www.aphis.usda.gov

United States Food and Drug Administration
Center for Food Safety and Applied Nutrition
5600 Fishers Lane
Rockville, MD 20857
Tel: 1-888-INFO-FDA (1-888-463-6332)
  or 1-888-SAFEFOOD
www.cfsan.fda.gov

References

This list of references is sorted by topic, beginning with general pregnancy, then proceeding alphabetically through more specific topics related to pregnancy and nutrition.

General Pregnancy

American Dietetic Association. Position of the American Dietetic Association: Nutrition and lifestyle for a healthy pregnancy outcome. JADA 2002;102(10):1479–90.

Butte NF. Carbohydrate and lipid metabolism in pregnancy: Normal compared with gestational diabetes mellitus. Am J Clin Nutr 2000;71(5 Suppl):1256S–61S.

Butte NF, Wong WW, Treuth MS, Ellis KJ, O'Brian Smith E. Energy requirements during pregnancy based on total energy expenditure and energy deposition. Am J Clin Nutr 2004;79(6):1078–87.

Curtis GB, Schuler J. Your Pregnancy Week by Week. 4th ed. New York: Fisher Books, 2000.

Douglas A. The Mother of All Pregnancy Books. Toronto, ON: Macmillan Canada, 2000.

Gale CR, O'Callaghan FJ, Godfrey KM, Law CM, Martyn CN. Critical periods of brain growth and cognitive function in children. Brain 2004;127(Pt 2):321–29.

George GC, Hanss-Nuss H, Milani TJ, Freeland-Graves JH. Food choices of low-income women during pregnancy and postpartum. J Am Diet Assoc 2005;105(6):899–907.

Godfrey KM, Barker DJ. Fetal nutrition and adult disease. Am J Clin Nutr 2000;71 (5 Suppl):1344S–52S.

Grischke EM. [Nutrition during pregnancy—current aspects]. MMW Fortschr Med 2004;146(11):29–30,2.

Hacker NS, Moor JG. Essentials of Obstetrics and Gynecology. 3rd ed. St. Louis, MO: WB Saunders, 1998.

Health Canada. Nutrition for a Healthy Pregnancy: National Guidelines for the Childbearing Years. Minister of Public Works and Government Services, 1999.

Hurley KM, Caulfield LE, Sacco LM, Costigan KA, Dipietro JA. Psychosocial influences in dietary patterns during pregnancy. J Am Diet Assoc 2005;105(6):963–66.

Jovanovic L. Nutrition and pregnancy: The link between dietary intake and diabetes. Curr Diab Rep 2004;4(4):266–72.

Kaiser LL, Allen L. Position of the American Dietetic Association: Nutrition and lifestyle for a healthy pregnancy outcome. J Am Diet Assoc 2002;102(10):1479–90.

Kalhan SC. Protein metabolism in pregnancy. Am J Clin Nutr 2000;71(5 Suppl):1249S–55S.

King JC. Physiology of pregnancy and nutrient metabolism. Am J Clin Nutr 2000;71(5 Suppl):1218S–25S.

Kramer MS, Kakuma R. Energy and protein intake in pregnancy. Cochrane Database Syst Rev 2003(4):CD000032.

Lof M, Olausson H, Bostrom K, Janerot-Sjoberg B, Sohlstrom A, Forsum E. Changes in basal metabolic rate during pregnancy in relation to changes in body weight and composition, cardiac output, insulin-like growth factor I, and thyroid hormones and in relation to fetal growth. Am J Clin Nutr 2005;81(3):678–85.

Moore VM, Davies MJ, Willson KJ, Worsley A, Robinson JS. Dietary composition of pregnant women is related to size of the baby at birth. J Nutr 2004;134(7):1820–26.

Mennella JA, Jagnow CP, Beauchamp GK. Prenatal and postnatal flavor learning by human infants. Pediatrics 2001;107(6):E88.

Picciano MF. Pregnancy and lactation: Physiological adjustments, nutritional requirements and the role of dietary supplements. J Nutr 2003;133: 1997S–2002S.

Society of Obstetricians and Gynaecologists of Canada. Healthy Beginnings: Your Handbook for Pregnancy and Birth. 2nd ed. Ottawa, ON: Society of Obstetricians and Gynaecologists of Canada, 2000.

Udipi SA, Ghugre P, Antony U. Nutrition in pregnancy and lactation. J Indian Med Assoc 2000;98(9):548–57.

Vobecky JS. Nutritional aspects of preconceptional period as related to pregnancy and early infancy. Prog Food Nutr Sci 1986;10(1-2):205–36.

Worthington-Roberts BS, Rodwell Williams S. Nutrition Throughout the Lifecycle. 3rd ed. St. Louis, MO: Mosby-Year Book, 1996.

Wu G, Bazer FW, Cudd TA, Meininger CJ, Spencer TE. Maternal nutrition and fetal development. J Nutr 2004;134(9): 2169–72.

Young GL, Jewell D. Interventions for leg cramps in pregnancy. Cochrane Database Syst Rev 2002;(1):CD000121.

Young GL, Jewell D. Interventions for varicosities and leg oedema in pregnancy. Cochrane Database Syst Rev 2000;(2): CD001066.

Alcohol & Pregnancy

Gabriel K, Hofmann C, Glavas M, Weinberg J. The hormonal effects of alcohol use on the mother and fetus. Alcohol Health Res World 1998;22(3):170–77.

Passaro KT, Little RE, Savitz DA, Noss J. The effect of maternal drinking before conception and in early pregnancy on infant birthweight. The ALSPAC Study Team. Avon Longitudinal Study of Pregnancy and Childhood. Epidemiology 1996;7(4):377–83.

Walpole I, Zubrick S, Pontre J. Is there a fetal effect with low to moderate alcohol use before or during pregnancy? J Epidemiol Community Health 1990;44(4):297–301.

Allergy & Pregnancy/Lactation

Arshad SH. Primary prevention of asthma and allergy. J Allergy Clin Immunol 2005;226(1):4–13.

Friedman NJ, Zeiger RS. Prevention and natural history of food allergy. In Pediatric Allergy: Principles and Practice. Yeung Dym (ed). St. Louis, MO: Mosby, 2003.

Breastfeeding

Ahluwalia IB, Morrow B, Hsia J. Why do women stop breastfeeding? Findings from the pregnancy risk assessment and monitoring system. Pediatrics 2005;116:1408–12.

American Academy of Pediatrics. Breastfeeding and the use of human milk. Work Group on Breastfeeding. Pediatrics 1997;100(6):1035–39.

American Dietetic Association. Position of the American Dietetic Association: Breaking the barriers to breastfeeding. JADA 2001;101(10):1213–20.

Bachrach VR, Schwarz E, Bachrach LR. Breastfeeding and the risk of hospitalization for respiratrory disease in infancy: A meta-analysis. Arch Pediatr Adolesc Med 2003;157(3)237–43.

Della-Giustina K, Chow G. Medications in pregnancy and lactation. Emerg Med Clin North Am 2003;21(3):585–613.

Dewey KG. Impact of breastfeeding on maternal nutritional status. Adv Exp Med Biol 2004;554:91–100.

Health Canada. Exclusive Breastfeeding Duration. 2004 Health Canada Recommendation. Fact Sheet, 2004.

Health Canada. Vitamin D Supplementation for Breastfed Infants. 2004 Health Canada Recommendation. Fact Sheet, 2004.

Kronborg H, Vaeth M. The influence of psychosocial factors on the duration of breastfeeding. Scand J Pub Health 2004;32(3):210–16.

Newman J, Pitman T. Dr. Jack Newman's Guide to Breastfeeding. New York: HarperCollins, 2000.

Oddy WH, Sly PD, de Klerk NH, Landau LI, Kendall GE, Holt PG, Stanley FJ. Breastfeeding and respiratory morbidity in infancy: A birth cohort study. Arch Dis Child 2003;88(3):224–28.

Riordan J. Breastfeeding and Human Lactation. 3rd ed. Sudbury, UK: Jones and Bartlett, 2005.

Wosje KS, Kalkwarf HJ. Lactation, weaning and calcium supplementation: Effects on body composition in postpartum women. Am J Clin Nutr 2004;80(2):423–29.

Calcium and Vitamin D & Pregnancy

Ala-Houhala M. 25-Hydroxyvitamin D levels during breast-feeding with or without maternal or infantile supplementation of vitamin D. J Pediatr Gastroenterol Nutr 1985;4(2):220–26.

Ala-Houhala M, Koskinen T, Terho A, Koivula T, Visakorpi J. Maternal compared with infant vitamin D supplementation. Arch Dis Child 1986;61(12):1159–63.

Arab L, Carriquiry A, Steck-Scott S, Gaudet MM. Ethnic differences in the nutrient intake adequacy of premenopausal US women: Results from the Third National Health Examination Survey. J Am Diet Assoc 2003;103(8):1008–14.

Harkness LS, Cromer BA. Vitamin D deficiency in adolescent females. J Adolesc Health 2005;37(1):75.

Hashim N, Norliza ZA. Calcium status among pregnant women. Asia Pac J Clin Nutr 2004;13(Suppl):S97.

Pawley N, Bishop NJ. Prenatal and infant predictors of bone health: The influence of vitamin D. Am J Clin Nutr 2004;80 (6 Suppl):1748S–51S.

Reichrath J, Querings K. Vitamin D deficiency during pregnancy: A risk factor not only for fetal growth and bone metabolism but also for correct development of the fetal immune system? Am J Clin Nutr 2005;81(5):1177; author reply 1178.

Ritchie LD, King JC. Dietary calcium and pregnancy-induced hypertension: Is there a relation? Am J Clin Nutr 2000;71 (5 Suppl):1371S–74S.

Salle BL, Delvin EE, Lapillonne A, Bishop NJ, Glorieux FH. Perinatal metabolism of vitamin D. Am J Clin Nutr 2000;71(5 Suppl):1317S–24S.

Shenoy SD, Swift P, Cody D, Iqbal J. Maternal vitamin D deficiency, refractory neonatal hypocalcaemia, and nutritional rickets. Arch Dis Child 2005;90(4): 437–38.

Specker B. Vitamin D requirements during pregnancy. Am J Clin Nutr 2004;80 (6 Suppl):1740S–47S.

Villar J, Belizan JM. Same nutrient, different hypotheses: Disparities in trials of calcium supplementation during pregnancy. Am J Clin Nutr 2000;71(5 Suppl):1375S–79S.

Caffeine & Pregnancy

Dews PB, O'Brien CP, Bergman J. Caffeine: Behavioral effects of withdrawal and related issues. Food Chem Toxicol 2002;40(9):1257–61.

Fernandes O, Sabharwal M, Smiley T, Pastuszak A, Koren G, Einarson T. Moderate to heavy caffeine consumption during pregnancy and relationship to spontaneous abortion and abnormal fetal growth: A meta-analysis. Reprod Toxicol 1998;12(4):435–44.

Frary CD, Johnson RK, Wang MQ. Food sources and intakes of caffeine in the diets of persons in the United States. J Am Diet Assoc 2005;105(1):110–13.

Giannelli M, Doyle P, Roman E, Pelerin M, Hermon C. The effect of caffeine consumption and nausea on the risk of miscarriage. Paediatr Perinat Epidemiol 2003;17(4):316–23.

James JE. Critical review of dietary caffeine and blood pressure: A relationship that should be taken more seriously. Psychosom Med 2004;66(1):63–71.

Jensen TK, Henriksen TB, Hjollund NH, Scheike T, Kolstad H, Giwercman A, et al. Caffeine intake and fecundability: A follow-up study among 430 Danish couples planning their first pregnancy. Reprod Toxicol 1998;12(3):289–95.

Rogers PJ, Heatherley SV, Hayward RC, Seers HE, Hill J, Kane M. Effects of caffeine and caffeine withdrawal on mood and cognitive performance degraded by sleep restriction. Psychopharmacology (Berl) 2005;179(4):742–52.

Sata F, Yamada H, Suzuki K, Saijo Y, Kato EH, Morikawa M, et al. Caffeine intake, CYP1A2 polymorphism and the risk of recurrent pregnancy loss. Mol Hum Reprod 2005;11(5):357–60.

Signorello LB, McLaughlin JK. Maternal caffeine consumption and spontaneous abortion: A review of the epidemiologic evidence. Epidemiology 2004;15(2):229–39.

Tolstrup JS, Kjaer SK, Munk C, Madsen LB, Ottesen B, Bergholt T, et al. Does caffeine and alcohol intake before pregnancy predict the occurrence of spontaneous abortion? Hum Reprod 2003;18(12):2704–10.

Constipation and Hemorrhoids & Pregnancy

American Dietetic Association. Position of the American Dietetic Association: Health implications of dietary fiber. JADA 2002;102(7):993–1000.

American Gastroenterological Association. American Gastroenterological Association medical position statement: Diagnosis and treatment of hemorrhoids. Gastroenterology 2004;126:1461–62.

American Gastroenterological Association. American Gastroenterological Association medical position statement: Guidelines on constipation. Gatroenterology 2000; 119:1761–78.

Cravings & Pregnancy

Hook EB. Dietary cravings and aversions during pregnancy. Am J Clin Nutr 1978;31(8):1355–62.

Eating Disorders & Pregnancy

Abraham S. Obstetricians and maternal body weight and eating disorders during pregnancy. J Psychosom Obstet Gynaecol 2001;22(3):159–63.

Davies K, Wardle J. Body image and dieting in pregnancy. J Psychosom Res 1994; 38(8):787–99.

Franko DL, Spurrell EB. Detection and management of eating disorders during pregnancy. Obstet Gynecol 2000;95 (6 Pt 1):942–46.

Kouba S, Hallstrom T, Lindholm C, Hirschberg AL. Pregnancy and neonatal outcomes in women with eating disorders. Obstet Gynecol 2005;105(2):255–60.

Morrill ES, Nickols-Richardson HM. Bulimia nervosa during pregnancy: A review. J Am Diet Assoc 2001;101(4):448–54.

Siega-Riz AM, Herrmann TS, Savitz DA, Thorp JM. Frequency of eating during pregnancy and its effect on preterm delivery. Am J Epidemiol 2001;153(7): 647–52.

Essential Fatty Acids & Pregnancy

Denomme J, Stark KD, Holub BJ. Directly quantitated dietary (n-3) fatty acid intakes of pregnant Canadian women are lower than current dietary recommendations. J Nutr 2005;135(2):206–11.

Freeman MP, Hibbeln JR, Wisner KL, Brumbach BH, Watchman M, Gelenberg AJ. Randomized dose-ranging pilot trial of omega-3 fatty acids for postpartum depression. Acta Psychiatr Scand 2006; 113(1):31–35.

Haggarty P. Effect of placental function on fatty acid requirements during pregnancy. Eur J Clin Nutr 2004;58(12):1559–70.

Hornstra G. Essential fatty acids in mothers and their neonates. Am J Clin Nutr 2000;71(5 Suppl):1262S–69S.

Larque E, Zamora S, Gil A. Dietary trans fatty acids in early life: A review. Early Hum Dev 2001;65 (Suppl):S31–41.

Mojska H. Influence of trans fatty acids on infant and fetus development. Acta Microbiol Pol 2003;52 (Suppl):67–74.

Sakamoto M, Kubota M, Liu XJ, Murata K, Nakai K, Satoh H. Maternal and fetal mercury and n-3 polyunsaturated fatty acids as a risk and benefit of fish consumption to fetus. Environ Sci Technol 2004;38(14):3860–63.

Saldeen P, Saldeen T. Women and omega-3 fatty acids. Obstet Gynecol Surv 2004; 59(10):722–30.

Exercise & Pregnancy

Artal R. Exercise and pregnancy. Clin Sports Med 1992;11(2):363–77.

Artal R, O'Toole M. Guidelines of the American College of Obstetricians and Gynecologists for exercise during pregnancy and the postpartum period. Br J Sports Med 2003;37(1):6–12; discussion.

Clapp JF, 3rd. The effects of maternal exercise on fetal oxygenation and feto-placental growth. Eur J Obstet Gynecol Reprod Biol 2003;110 (1 Suppl):S80–85.

Clapp JF, 3rd. Exercise during pregnancy. A clinical update. Clin Sports Med 2000; 19(2):273–86.

Clapp JF, 3rd, Kim H, Burciu B, Lopez B. Beginning regular exercise in early pregnancy: Effect on fetoplacental growth. Am J Obstet Gynecol 2000;183(6):1484–88.

Clapp JF, 3rd, Kim H, Burciu B, Schmidt S, Petry K, Lopez B. Continuing regular exercise during pregnancy: Effect of exercise volume on fetoplacental growth. Am J Obstet Gynecol 2002;186(1):142–47.

Davies GA, Wolfe LA, Mottola MF, MacKinnon C. Joint SOGC/CSEP clinical practice guideline: Exercise in pregnancy and the postpartum period. Can J Appl Physiol 2003;28(3):330–41.

Davies GA, Wolfe LA, Mottola MF, MacKinnon C, Arsenault MY, Bartellas E, et al. Exercise in pregnancy and the postpartum period. J Obstet Gynaecol Can 2003;25(6):516–29.

Downs DS, Hausenblas HA. Exercising for two: Examining pregnant women's second trimester exercise intention and behavior using the framework of the theory of planned behavior. Women's Health Issues 2003;13(6):222–28.

Larson-Meyer DE. Effect of postpartum exercise on mothers and their offspring: A review of the literature. Obes Res 2002;10(8):841–53.

Mottola MF. Exercise in the postpartum period: Practical applications. Curr Sports Med Rep 2002;1(6):362–68.

Mottola MF, Campbell MK. Activity patterns during pregnancy. Can J Appl Physiol 2003;28(4):642–53.

Ning Y, Williams MA, Dempsey JC, Sorensen TK, Frederick IO, Luthy DA. Correlates of recreational physical activity in early pregnancy. J Matern Fetal Neonatal Med 2003;13(6):385–93.

O'Toole ML, Sawicki MA, Artal R. Structured diet and physical activity prevent postpartum weight retention. J Women's Health (Larchmt) 2003;12(10):991–98.

Paisley TS, Joy EA, Price RJ, Jr. Exercise during pregnancy: A practical approach. Curr Sports Med Rep 2003;2(6):325-30.

Santos IA, Stein R, Fuchs SC, Duncan BB, Ribeiro JP, Kroeff LR, Carballo MT, Schmidt MI. Aerobic exercise and submaximal functional capacity in overweight pregnant women: A randomized trial. Obstet Gynecol 2005;106(2):216–18.

Stevenson L. Exercise in pregnancy. Part 1: Update on pathophysiology. Can Fam Physician 1997;43:97–104.

Stevenson L. Exercise in pregnancy. Part 2: Recommendations for individuals. Can Fam Physician 1997;43:107-11.

Symons Downs D, Hausenblas HA. Women's exercise beliefs and behaviors during their pregnancy and postpartum. J Midwifery Women's Health 2004;49(2):138–44.

Treuth MS, Butte NF, Puyau M. Pregnancy-related changes in physical activity, fitness, and strength. Med Sci Sports Exerc 2005;37(5):832–37.

Wolfe LA, Davies GA. Canadian guidelines for exercise in pregnancy. Clin Obstet Gynecol 2003;46(2):488–95.

Wolfe LA, Mottola MF. Aerobic exercise in pregnancy: An update. Can J Appl Physiol 1993;18(2):119–47.

Folate & Pregnancy

Daltveit AK, et al. Changes in knowledge and attitudes of folate, and use of dietary supplements among women of reproductive age in Norway 1998 to 2000. Scand J Public Health 2004;32(4):264–71.

Guthrie H, Picciano MF. Human Nutrition. St. Louis, MO: Mosby-Year Book, 1995.

Health Canada. Folic Acid and Birth Defects. Fact Sheet.

House JD, et al. Folate and vitamin B12 status of women in Newfoundland at their first prenatal visit. CMAJ 2000;162(11):1557–59.

Liu S, et al. A comprehensive evaluation of food fortification with folic acid for the primary prevention of neural tube defects. BMC Pregnancy and Childbirth 2004;4:20.

Ray JG, Vermeulen MJ, Boss SC, Cole DE. Declining rate of folate insufficiency among adults following increased folic acid food fortification in Canada. Can J Public Health 2002;93(4):249–53.

Tam LE, et al. A survey of preconceptional folic acid use in a group of Canadian women. J Obstet Gynaecol Can 2005;27(3):232–36.

Food Safety & Pregnancy

American Academy of Pediatrics Committee on Drugs. The transfer of drugs and other chemicals into human milk. Pediatrics 1994;93:137–50.

American Pregnancy Association. Foods to Avoid During Pregnancy. Fact Sheet.

Center for Science in the Public Interest. Unexpected Consequences: Miscarriage and Birth Defects from Tainted Foods, 2000.

Corrion ML, Ostrea EM, Jr., Bielawski DM, Posecion NC, Jr., Seagraves JJ. Detection of prenatal exposure to several classes of environmental toxicants and their metabolites by gas chromatography-mass spectrometry in maternal and umbilical cord blood. J Chromatogr B Analyt Technol Biomed Life Sci 2005;822(1-2):221–29.

Daniels JL, et al. Fish intake during pregnancy and early cognitive development of offspring. Epidemiology 2004;15(4):394–402.

Koren G. Exposure to electromagnetic fields during pregnancy. Can Fam Physician 2003;49:151, 153.

Longnecker MP, Klebanoff MA, Dunson DB, Guo X, Chen Z, Zhou H, et al. Maternal serum level of the DDT metabolite DDE in relation to fetal loss in previous pregnancies. Environ Res 2005;97(2):127–33.

Nielsen SS, Mueller BA, De Roos AJ, Viernes HM, Farin FM, Checkoway H. Risk of brain tumors in children and susceptibility to organophosphorus insecticides: The potential role of paraoxonase (PON1). Environ Health Perspect 2005;113(7): 909–13.

Organization of Teratology Information Services. Listeriosis and Pregnancy. Fact Sheet, 2004.

Pitkin RM, Reynolds WA, Stegink LD et al. Glutamate metabolism and placental transfer in pregnancy. In LJ Filer, Garattini S, Kare MR et al (eds), Glutamic Acid: Advances in Biochemistry and Physiology. New York: Raven Press, 1999:103–10.

Robert E. Intrauterine effects of electromagnetic files (low frequency, mid-frequency RD, and microwave): Review of epidemiologic studies. Teratology 1999; 59:292–98.

US Food and Drug Administration: Center for Food Safety and Applied Nutrition. Keep Your Baby Safe: Eat Hard Cheeses Instead of Soft Cheeses During Pregnancy. Fact Sheet, 1997.

Yagev Y, Koren G. Eating fish during pregnancy. Risk of exposure to toxic levels of methylmercury. Can Fam Physician 2002;48:1619–21.

Gestational Diabetes & Pregnancy

Lauenborg J, Hansen T, Jensen DM, Vestergaard H, Molsted-Pedersen L, Hornnes P, et al. Increasing incidence of diabetes after gestational diabetes: A long-term follow-up in a Danish population. Diabetes Care 2004;27(5):1194–99.

Linne Y, Barkeling B, Rossner S. Natural course of gestational diabetes mellitus: Long term follow up of women in the SPAWN study. Bjog 2002;109(11):1227–31.

Iron & Pregnancy

Allen LH. Anemia and iron deficiency: Effects on pregnancy outcome. Am J Clin Nutr 2000;71(5 Suppl):1280S–84S.

Ball MJ, Bartlett MA. Dietary intake and iron status of Australian vegetarian women. Am J Clin Nutr 1999;70(3):353–58.

Deegan H, Bates HM, McCargar LJ. Assessment of iron status in adolescents: Dietary, biochemical and lifestyle determinants. J Adolesc Health 2005; 37(1):75.

Hallberg L, Hulthen L. Prediction of dietary iron absorption: An algorithm for calculating absorption and bioavailability of dietary iron. Am J Clin Nutr 2000;71(5):1147–60.

Scholl TO. Iron status during pregnancy: Setting the stage for mother and infant. Am J Clin Nutr 2005;81(5):1218S–22S.

Scholl TO, Hediger ML, Fischer RL, Shearer JW. Anemia vs iron deficiency: Increased risk of preterm delivery in a prospective study. Am J Clin Nutr 1992;55(5):985–88.

Zhou SJ, Makrides M, Gibson RA, Baghurst P. Effect of iron supplementation in pregnancy on IQ of children at 4 years of age. Asia Pac J Clin Nutr 2004;13(Suppl):S39.

Multiple Pregnancy

Brown JE, Carlson M. Nutrition and multifetal pregnancy. JADA 2000;100(3):343–48.

Kaiser LL, Allen L. Position of the American Dietetic Association: Nutrition and lifestyle for a healthy pregnancy outcome. J Am Diet Assoc 2002;102(10):1479–90.

Klein L. Nutritional recommendations for multiple pregnancy. JADA 2005;105(7): 1050–52.

Nausea and Vomiting & Pregnancy

Arsenault MY, Lane CA, MacKinnon CJ, Bartellas E, Cargill YM, Klein MC, et al. The management of nausea and vomiting of pregnancy. J Obstet Gynaecol Can 2002;24(10):817-31; quiz 832–33.

Betz O, Kranke P, Geldner G, Wulf H, Eberhart LH. [Is ginger a clinically relevant antiemetic? A systematic review of randomized controlled trials]. Forsch Komplementarmed Klass Naturheilkd 2005;12(1):14–23.

Borrelli F, Capasso R, Aviello G, Pittler MH, Izzo AA. Effectiveness and safety of ginger in the treatment of pregnancy-induced nausea and vomiting. Obstet Gynecol 2005;105(4):849–56.

Bsat FA, Hoffman DE, Seubert DE. Comparison of three outpatient regimens in the management of nausea and vomiting in pregnancy. J Perinatol 2003;23(7):531–35.

Chandra K, Einarson A, Koren G. Taking ginger for nausea and vomiting during pregnancy. Can Fam Physician 2002; 48:1441–42.

Chandra K, Magee L, Einarson A, Koren G. Nausea and vomiting in pregnancy: Results of a survey that identified interventions used by women to alleviate their symptoms. J Psychosom Obstet Gynaecol 2003;24(2):71–75.

Jednak MA, Shadigian EM, Kim MS, Woods ML, Hooper FG, Owyang C, et al. Protein meals reduce nausea and gastric slow wave dysrhythmic activity in first trimester pregnancy. Am J Physiol 1999;277 (4 Pt 1):G855–61.

Jewell D, Young G. Interventions for nausea and vomiting in early pregnancy. Cochrane Database Syst Rev 2003(4):CD000145.

Meltzer DI. Selections from current literature. Complementary therapies for nausea and vomiting in early pregnancy. Fam Pract 2000;17(6):570–73.

Niebyl JR, Goodwin TM. Overview of nausea and vomiting of pregnancy with an emphasis on vitamins and ginger. Am J Obstet Gynecol 2002;186(5 Suppl Understanding):S253–55.

Philip B. Hyperemesis gravidarum: Literature review. Wmj 2003;102(3):46–51.

Portnoi G, Chng LA, Karimi-Tabesh L, Koren G, Tan MP, Einarson A. Prospective comparative study of the safety and effectiveness of ginger for the treatment of nausea and vomiting in pregnancy. Am J Obstet Gynecol 2003;189(5):1374–77.

Quinla JD, Hill DA. Nausea and vomiting of pregnancy. Am Fam Physician 2003;68(1): 121–28.

Sahakian V, Rouse D, Sipes S, Rose N, Niebyl J. Vitamin B6 is effective therapy for nausea and vomiting of pregnancy: A randomized, double-blind placebo-controlled study. Obstet Gynecol 1991; 78(1):33–36.

Smith C, Crowther C, Willson K, Hotham N, McMillian V. A randomized controlled trial of ginger to treat nausea and vomiting in pregnancy. Obstet Gynecol 2004;103(4): 639–45.

Sripramote M, Lekhyananda N. A randomized comparison of ginger and vitamin B6 in the treatment of nausea and vomiting of pregnancy. J Med Assoc Thai 2003;86(9): 846–53.

Swallow BL, Lindow SW, Masson EA, Hay DM. Psychological health in early pregnancy: Relationship with nausea and vomiting. J Obstet Gynaecol 2004;24(1):28–32.

Verberg MF, Gillott DJ, Al-Fardan N, Grudzinskas JG. Hyperemesis gravidarum, a literature review. Hum Reprod Update 2005.

Weigel RM, Weigel MM. Nausea and vomiting of early pregnancy and pregnancy outcome. A meta-analytical review. Br J Obstet Gynaecol 1989;96(11):1312–18.

Willetts KE, Ekangaki A, Eden JA. Effect of a ginger extract on pregnancy-induced nausea: A randomised controlled trial. Aust N Z J Obstet Gynaecol 2003;43(2):139–44.

Pica & Pregnancy

Corbett RW, Ryan C, Weinrich SP. Pica in pregnancy: Does it affect pregnancy outcomes? MCN Am J Matern Child Nurs 2003;28(3):183-89; quiz 190–91.

Lopez LB, Ortega Soler CR, de Portela ML. [Pica during pregnancy: A frequently underestimated problem]. Arch Latinoam Nutr 2004;54(1):17–24.

Postpartum Depression

Carter AS, Wood Baker C, Brownell KD. Body mass index, eating attitudes, and symptoms of depression and anxiety in pregnancy and the postpartum period. Psychosomatic Med 2000; 62:264–70.

Chen TH, Lan TH, Yang CY, Juang KD. Postpartum mood disorders may be related to a decreased insulin level after delivery. Med Hypotheses 2005;Nov. 28.

Corwin EJ, Murray-Kolb LE, Beard JL. Low hemoglobin level is a risk factor for postpartum depression. J Nutr 2003; 133:4139–42.

De Vriese SR, Christophe AB, Maes M. Lowered serum n-3 polyunsaturated fatty acid (PUFA) levels predict the occurrence of postpartum depression: Further evidence that lowered n-PUFAs are related to major depression. Life Sci 2003; 73:3181–87.

Hibbeln, JR. Seafood consumption, the DHA content of mothers' milk and prevalence rates of postpartum depression: A cross-national, ecological analysis. Journal of Affective Disorders 2002;69:15–29.

Recreational Drug Use & Pregnancy

Fried PA, Barnes MV, Drake ER. Soft drug use after pregnancy compared to use before and during pregnancy. Am J Obstet Gynecol 1985;151(6):787–92.

Fried PA, Watkinson B, Willan A. Marijuana use during pregnancy and decreased length of gestation. Am J Obstet Gynecol 1984;150(1):23–27.

Smoking & Pregnancy

Biederman J. Attention-deficit/hyperactivity disorder: A selective overview. Biol Psychiatry 2005;57(11):1215–20.

Ernst M, Moolchan ET, Robinson ML. Behavioral and neural consequences of prenatal exposure to nicotine. J Am Acad Child Adolesc Psychiatry 2001;40(6): 630–41.

Fried PA, O'Connell CM. A comparison of the effects of prenatal exposure to tobacco, alcohol, cannabis and caffeine on birth size and subsequent growth. Neurotoxicol Teratol 1987;9(2):79–85.

Grange G, Vayssiere C, Borgne A, Ouazana A, L'Huillier JP, Valensi P, et al. Description of tobacco addiction in pregnant women. Eur J Obstet Gynecol Reprod Biol 2005; 120(2):146–51.

Hofhuis W, Merkus PJ, de Jongste JC. [Negative effects of passive smoking on the (unborn) child]. Ned Tijdschr Geneeskd 2002;146(8):356–59.

Jensen MS, Mabeck LM, Toft G, Thulstrup AM, Bonde JP. Lower sperm counts following prenatal tobacco exposure. Hum Reprod 2005.

Jurado D, Munoz C, Luna Jde D, Munoz-Hoyos A. Is maternal smoking more determinant than paternal smoking on the respiratory symptoms of young children? Respir Med 2005;99(9):1138–44.

Kyrklund-Blomberg NB, Granath F, Cnattingius S. Maternal smoking and causes of very preterm birth. Acta Obstet Gynecol Scand 2005;84(6):572–77.

Linnet KM, Wisborg K, Obel C, Secher NJ, Thomsen PH, Agerbo E, et al. Smoking during pregnancy and the risk for hyperkinetic disorder in offspring. Pediatrics 2005;116(2):462–67.

Linnet KM, Dalsgaard S, Obel C, Wisborg K, Henriksen TB, Rodriguez A, et al. Maternal lifestyle factors in pregnancy risk of attention deficit hyperactivity disorder and associated behaviors: Review of the current evidence. Am J Psychiatry 2003; 160(6):1028.

Stocks J, Dezateux C. The effect of parental smoking on lung function and development during infancy. Respirology 2003;8(3): 266–85.

Wisborg K, Henriksen TB, Hedegaard M, Secher NJ. Smoking during pregnancy and preterm birth. Br J Obstet Gynaecol 1996;103(8):800–5.

Supplements and Herbs & Pregnancy

Azais-Braesco V, Pascal G. Vitamin A in pregnancy: Requirements and safety limits. Am J Clin Nutr 2000;71(5 Suppl):1325S–33S.

Chan TY. The prevalence, use and harmful potential of some Chinese herbal medicines in babies and children. Vet Hum Toxicol 1994;36(3):238–40.

Favier M, Faure P. [Supplements during pregnancy: Fad or necessity?]. Rev Fr Gynecol Obstet 1994;89(4):210–15.

King JC. Determinants of maternal zinc status during pregnancy. Am J Clin Nutr 2000;71(5 Suppl):1334S–43S.

Lee BE, Hong YC, Lee KH, Kim YJ, Kim WK, Chang NS, et al. Influence of maternal serum levels of vitamins C and E during the second trimester on birth weight and length. Eur J Clin Nutr 2004;58(10):1365–71.

Merialdi M, Caulfield LE, Zavaleta N, Figueroa A, Costigan KA, Dominici F, et al. Randomized controlled trial of prenatal zinc supplementation and fetal bone growth. Am J Clin Nutr 2004;79(5):826–30.

Pinn G. Herbs used in obstetrics and gynaecology. Aust Fam Physician 2001; 30(4):351–54, 356.

Stapleton H. The use of herbal medicine in pregnancy and labour. Part I: An overview of current practice. Complement Ther Nurs Midwifery 1995;1(5):148–53.

Vahratian A, Siega-Riz AM, Savitz DA, Thorp JM, Jr. Multivitamin use and the risk of preterm birth. Am J Epidemiol 2004; 160(9):886–92.

Weiss R, Fogelman Y, Bennett M. Severe vitamin B12 deficiency in an infant associated with a maternal deficiency and a strict vegetarian diet. J Pediatr Hematol Oncol 2004;26(4):270–71.

Wilkinson JM. What do we know about herbal morning sickness treatments? A literature survey. Midwifery 2000;16(3):224–28.

Wong HB. Effects of herbs and drugs during pregnancy and lactation. J Singapore Paediatr Soc 1979;21(3-4):169–78.

Teenage Pregnancy

Gutierrez Y, King JC. Nutrition during teenage pregnancy. Pediatr Ann 1993;22(2):99–108.

Story M, Stang J. Nutrition and the Pregnant Adolescent: A Practical Reference Guide. Minneapolis, MN: Center for Leadership, Education and Training in Maternal and Child Nutrition, University of Minnesota, 2000.

Water Contamination & Pregnancy

Zender R, Bachand AM, Reif JS. Exposure to tap water during pregnancy. J Expo Anal Environ Epidemiol 2001;11(3):224–30.

Weight & Pregnancy

Abrams B, Altman SL, Pickett KE. Pregnancy weight gain: Still controversial. Am J Clin Nutr 2000;71(5 Suppl):1233S–41S.

Carmichael SL, Shaw GM, Schaffer DM, Laurent C, Selvin S. Dieting behaviors and risk of neural tube defects. Am J Epidemiol 2003;158(12):1127–31.

Devine CM, Bove CF, Olson CM. Continuity and change in women's weight orientations and lifestyle practices through pregnancy and the postpartum period: The influence of life course trajectories and transitional events. Soc Sci Med 2000;50(4):567–82.

Dewey KG, McCrory MA. Effects of dieting and physical activity on pregnancy and lactation. Am J Clin Nutr 1994;59(2 Suppl):446S-52S; discussion 452S–53S.

Galtier-Dereure F, Boegner C, Bringer J. Obesity and pregnancy: Complications and cost. Am J Clin Nutr 2000;71(5 Suppl):1242S–48S.

Hickey CA. Sociocultural and behavioral influences on weight gain during pregnancy. Am J Clin Nutr 2000;71(5 Suppl):1364S–70S.

Keppel KG, Taffel SM. Pregnancy-related weight gain and retention: Implications of the 1990 Institute of Medicine guidelines. Am J Public Health 1993;83(8):1100–3.

Lederman SA. The effect of pregnancy weight gain on later obesity. Obstet Gynecol 1993;82(1):148–55.

Linne Y, Barkeling B, Rossner S. Long-term weight development after pregnancy. Obes Rev 2002;3(2):75–83.

McCrory MA. Does dieting during lactation put infant growth at risk? Nutr Rev 2001;59(1 Pt 1):18–21.

Muscati SK, Gray-Donald K, Koski KG. Timing of weight gain during pregnancy: Promoting fetal growth and minimizing maternal weight retention. Int J Obes Relat Metab Disord 1996;20(6):526–32.

Olson CM, Strawderman MS, Hinton PS, Pearson TA. Gestational weight gain and postpartum behaviors associated with weight change from early pregnancy to 1 y postpartum. Int J Obes Relat Metab Disord 2003;27(1):117–27.

Polley BA, Wing RR, Sims CJ. Randomized controlled trial to prevent excessive weight gain in pregnant women. Int J Obes Relat Metab Disord 2002;26(11):1494–502.

Rooney BL, Schauberger CW. Excess pregnancy weight gain and long-term obesity: One decade later. Obstet Gynecol 2002;100(2):245–52.

Shaw GM, Todoroff K, Carmichael SL, Schaffer DM, Selvin S. Lowered weight gain during pregnancy and risk of neural tube defects among offspring. Int J Epidemiol 2001;30(1):60–65.

Stotland NE, Haas JS, Brawarsky P, Jackson RA, Fuentes-Afflick E, Escobar GJ. Body mass index, provider advice, and target gestational weight gain. Obstet Gynecol 2005;105(3):633–38.

Thorsdottir I, Birgisdottir BE. Different weight gain in women of normal weight before pregnancy: Postpartum weight and birth weight. Obstet Gynecol 1998;92(3):377–83.

Vegetarianism & Pregnancy

American Dietetic Association, Dietitians of Canada. Position of the American Dietetic Association and Dietitians of Canada: Vegetarian diets. JADA 2003;103:748–65.

Koebnick C, et al. Long-term ovo-lacto vegetarian diet impairs vitamin B12 status in pregnant women. J Nutr 2004;134:3319–26.

Acknowledgments

THIS BOOK IS A VERY LARGE UNDERTAKING and could not have been done without the support of so many people.

We are very grateful for the valuable contributions and reviews provided by the following colleagues: Debbie O'Connor, Kirsten Smith, Erin Love, Gloria Green, Diana Mager, Suzanne Simpson, Kellie Welch, Jennifer Buccino, Vanita Pais, Esther Assor, Louise Bannister, Jaimie Kennedy, Kellie Sherwood, Joan Brennan, Susan Dello, Debbie Stone, Joyce Touw, Charlotte Miller, Sandy Fraser, Suhail Al-Saleh and Myla Moretti (Motherisk program). Thanks to Naomi Shuman and Linda Chow for data entry, recipe analysis and countless hours of meticulous attention to detail. A special, heartfelt thank you to Debbie O'Connor for her ongoing support and encouragement.

We would like to thank Heidi Falckh at The Hospital for Sick Children for all of her dedication, as well as Bob Dees and Marian Jarkovich at Robert Rose Publishing for their guidance throughout this project. A special thanks to Bob Hilderley and Sue Sumeraj for taking our words and producing this wonderful work.

Thank you to those who offered to share your tasty recipes, including Leya Aronson, Inta Huns, Mabel Rosaroso, Denise Robichaud, Rosa Lasky, Connie Saab and Kristen Lasky. And, of course, a big thanks to the ever-indulgent recipe testers, Natali, Matt, Katelyn, Avery, Blair and David.

From Daina to Blair, Natali and Matis (our Matty). You are everything and more to me. *Mīlu jūs*. Blair, my thanks and appreciation for all these years of encouragement and devotion. How lucky I am. To my mom, Ilze Kalnins. You have taught me so much. *Paldies, Paldies*. And to Joanne, my genuine sincere thanks. Once again, you made the preparation of this book a truly wonderful experience. I am indebted to your patience, understanding and support throughout the project. And, of course, to your great insights and knowledge. We have a special personal and professional friendship, and I am so very proud of that.

Joanne would like to thank David, Katelyn and Avery for all that they are. You are my heart and soul. I could not have done any of this without your constant support. Thank you to my mom and to Lynn O'Connor for taking care of Katelyn and Avery so I could finish writing. To Daina I would like to say that I truly admire you. I am continually amazed at your dedication, knowledge and experience. Three books later and I am so proud of all we've learned together. I couldn't ask for a better partner to write with. You help to motivate me and keep me focused. I value your friendship and wish you great things always.

Index

Entries in bold indicate recipe titles.

A

ace K (acesulfame potassium), 42

alcohol

and breastfeeding, 120–21, 124, 125

and pregnancy, 41, 76

allergies (food), 9, 77–78

breastfeeding and, 122–23

almonds

Almond Crescents, 291

Chicken Salad Amandine, 196

Chickpea-Herb Burgers, 253

Crunchy Broccoli Salad, 182

Mandarin Orange Salad with Almonds, 181

No-Bake Trail Mix, 164

Sonoma Chicken Salad, 183

American Dietetic Association, 49

amino acids, 20, 21

anemia, 29, 30, 48, 67, 81, 83–84. *See also* iron

appetizers, 155–64

apples and apple juice

Autumn Crumble, 283

Strawberry Sorbet, 295

Apricot Bran Bread, 147

Asian Cucumber Salad, 179

Asian Turkey and Noodle Soup, 176

aspartame, 42

Autumn Crumble, 283

B

babies. *See also* breastfeeding

and iron, 103

nutrition for, 130

sleeping habits, 115

and vitamin D, 100, 124

weight of, 55, 107, 113

Baked Chicken and Potato Dinner, 201

Baked Fish with Tomatoes and Roasted Red Pepper, 217

Baked Lemon Salmon with Mango Salsa, 221

bananas

Banana Berry Wake-Up Shake, 142

Banana Bread, 145

Banana Oat Bran Muffins, 153

Banana Oatmeal Muffins, 154

Breakfast Muesli to Go, 143

Buttermilk Oat-Banana Cake, 284

Barbecue Sauce, 239

beans, dried. *See also* beans, fresh

Bean Salad, Tasty, 188

Black and White Bean Salsa, 160

Black Bean Salsa, 159

Chicken Tacos, 211

Fassolada, 170

Linguine with Tuna, White Beans and Dill, 276

Mixed Winter Beans, 248

Pasta Fagioli Capra, 273

Rice and Bean Salad, 187

Turkey Chili, 214

Tuscan Bean Salad, 190

20-Minute Chili, 235

Vegetarian Chili, 252

Vegetarian Shepherd's Pie with Peppered Potato Topping, 256

White Bean Salad with Lemon-Dill Vinaigrette, 189

White Bean Soup with Swiss Chard, 171

Zucchini, Mushroom and Bean Loaf with Tomato Sauce, 257

beans, fresh

Bean Salad, Tasty, 188

Green Beans and Tomato, 269

Green Beans with Cashews, 268

Pasta Fagioli Capra, 273

beef

Beef Fajitas, 232

Beef Lettuce Wraps, 240

Beef Souvlaki, 234

Beef Stroganoff, 233

Cabbage Rolls, Quick and Easy, 241

Meatball Pasta Sauce, 237

Meatballs with Teriyaki Sauce, 236

Meatloaf, Homestyle, 238

Meatloaf "Muffins" with Barbecue Sauce, 239

Thai-Style Beef Salad, 198

20-Minute Chili, 235

beets

Beet and Feta Salad, 186

Borscht, 174

bell peppers. *See also green and red varieties (below)*

Baked Chicken and Potato Dinner, 201

Beef Fajitas, 232

Lentil Salad, 191

Orange Ginger Pork and Vegetables, 244

Roasted Yam Fajitas, 258

Turkey Chili, 214

Vegetarian Chili, 252

bell peppers, green

Just Peachy Pork, 243

Spiced Veal Stir-fry, 242

20-Minute Chili, 235

Vietnamese Chicken and Rice Noodle Salad, 197

bell peppers, red

Baked Fish with Tomatoes and Roasted Red Pepper, 217

Chicken Tacos, 211

Ginger Chili Sweet Potato Soup, 168

bell peppers, red (*continued*)
    Hoisin Stir-fried Vegetables and Tofu over Rice Noodles, 274
    Penne with Tuna and Peppers, 280
    Rice and Bean Salad, 187
    Salmon with Roasted Vegetables, 219
    Southwestern Sweet Potato Soup, 167
    Turkiaki Fiesta, 213
berries. *See also* blueberries; cranberries; strawberries
    Banana Berry Wake-Up Shake, 142
    Berry Oatmeal Squares, 292
    Breakfast Muesli to Go, 143
Best-Ever Baked Chicken, 200
Big-Batch Bran Muffins, 150
birth control pills, 114
Black and White Bean Salsa, 160
Black Bean Salsa, 159
blood pressure, 94–96
blood sugar, 20, 85
blueberries
    Berry Oatmeal Squares, 292
    Cinnamon Baked Pears, 282
    Cranberry Oat Muffins (tip), 152
BMI (body mass index), 54, 70
BMR (basal metabolic rate), 14
body image, 54–55
bok choy. *See* cabbage
Borscht, 174
bran cereal
    Apricot Bran Bread, 147
    Big-Batch Bran Muffins, 150
    Carrot Bran Muffins, 151
    Fiber-Full Bran Pancakes, 144
breakfast dishes, 141–54, 163
Breakfast Muesli to Go, 143
breastfeeding, 98–125. *See also* breast milk; breasts
    benefits, 104–5
    biting during, 117
    duration, 124–25

    exercise and, 128
    guidelines, 102–3
    issues, 113–21
    latching, 102, 117
    and nutrition, 107–8
    positions, 110–11
    prescription drugs and, 114, 120
    questions and answers, 124–25
    sufficiency, 106–7, 108
breast milk. *See also* breastfeeding
    expressing, 109
    nutrients in, 99–103, 106–7
    oversupply, 114–15
    poor supply, 113–14
    preterm, 99
    protective factors in, 106–7
    storing, 109, 112
breasts
    blocked ducts, 118
    engorgement, 117, 119
    problems with, 116–17
    surgically altered, 115
broccoli
    Crunchy Broccoli Salad, 182
    Spaghetti with Broccoli, 275
    Sweet and Spicy Shrimp with Broccoli, 228
    Tuna Garden Pasta, 277
Bruschetta with Beans, 190
bulgur wheat
    Bulgur Salad, 194
    Tabbouleh, 192
    Vegetarian Chili, 252
buttermilk
    Banana Oatmeal Muffins, 154
    Big-Batch Bran Muffins, 150
    Buttermilk Oat-Banana Cake, 284
    Carrot Bran Muffins, 151
    Chicken Nuggets (tip), 212
    Healthy Cheese 'n' Herb Bread, 146

C

cabbage
    as breast engorgement remedy, 119
    Cabbage Rolls, Quick and Easy, 241
    Mixed Winter Beans, 248
    Orange Ginger Pork and Vegetables, 244
    Stir-fried Vegetables with Tofu, 249
caffeine
    and breastfeeding, 121, 125
    and pregnancy, 39–40
calcium, 27–28
    before pregnancy, 57–58
    recommended intake, 28, 58
    sources, 28, 57, 135–36
    in teeth, 91
    vegetarians and, 68
calorie intake, 14–16
    before pregnancy, 49–56
    breastfeeding and, 101
    of fetus, 15
    in first trimester, 72
    in second trimester, 82–83
    in vegetarians, 67
Canada's Food Guide, 52–53
carbohydrates, 16–19
    in breast milk, 100
    recommended intake, 18
    sources, 19
carrots
    Carrot Bran Muffins, 151
    Carrot Orange Soup, 166
    Chickpea-Herb Burgers, 253
    Hoisin Stir-fried Vegetables and Tofu over Rice Noodles, 274
    Mixed Winter Beans, 248
    Orange Ginger Pork and Vegetables, 244
    Spiced Veal Stir-fry, 242
    Stir-fried Vegetables with Tofu, 249
    Tuna Garden Pasta, 277
    Vietnamese Chicken and Rice Noodle Salad, 197

Cauliflower Casserole, 270
Cauliflower Popcorn Snack, 162
celery
  Beet and Feta Salad, 186
  Fassolada, 170
  Mandarin Orange Salad
    with Almonds, 181
  Orange Ginger Pork and
    Vegetables, 244
  Spiced Veal Stir-fry, 242
  Stir-fried Vegetables with
    Tofu, 249
  Turkiaki Fiesta, 213
cesarean section, 128
cheese. *See also specific types of*
  cheese (below)
  Beef Fajitas, 232
  Cauliflower Casserole, 270
  Chicken Tacos, 211
  concerns about, 9, 33, 36
  Cottage Cheese Herb Dip,
    156
  Healthy Cheese 'n' Herb
    Bread, 146
  Vegetarian Shepherd's Pie
    with Peppered Potato
    Topping, 256
  White Bean Soup with Swiss
    Chard, 171
cheese, feta
  Beet and Feta Salad, 186
  Bulgur Salad, 194
  Greek Summer Salad, 184
  Lentil Salad, 191
  Sonoma Chicken Salad, 183
cheese, goat
  Mushroom-Spinach Lasagna
    with Goat Cheese, 278
  Pasta with Goat Cheese,
    Snow Peas and Tomato
    Coulis, 272
  Portobello Mushrooms with
    Goat Cheese, 161
cheese, Parmesan
  Baked Chicken, Best-Ever,
    200
  Baked Chicken and Potato
    Dinner, 201

Chicken Nuggets, 212
Crispy Chicken, 205
Meatballs with Teriyaki
  Sauce (variation), 236
Parmesan-Crusted Snapper
  with Tomato Olive Sauce,
  226
Parmesan Herb-Baked Fish
  Fillets, 216
Pesto Chicken Thighs, 204
Sole and Spinach Casserole,
  224
Spinach Frittata, 264
Swiss Chard Frittata in a
  Pita, 263
chicken
  Baked Chicken, Best-Ever,
    200
  Baked Chicken and Potato
    Dinner, 201
  Chicken Nuggets, 212
  Chicken Salad Amandine, 196
  Chicken Tacos, 211
  Crispy Chicken, 205
  Curried Chicken, 210
  Ginger, Soy and Lime
    Chicken, 203
  Greek Lemon Chicken, 208
  Grilled Honey-Ginger
    Chicken Breasts, 206
  Honey Dijon Chicken, 207
  Hot and Sour Chicken Soup,
    175
  Meatballs with Teriyaki
    Sauce, 236
  Pesto Chicken Thighs, 204
  Sonoma Chicken Salad, 183
  Sticky Sesame Chicken, 209
  Teriyaki Pork Chops
    (variation), 245
  Turkiaki Fiesta, 213
  Vietnamese Chicken and
    Rice Noodle Salad, 197
  Yogurt-Marinated Chicken,
    202
chickpeas
  Bean Salad, Tasty, 188
  Chickpea-Herb Burgers, 253

  Chickpea Tofu Stew, 251
  Falafel in Pita, 260
  Hummus, 158
  Mixed Winter Beans, 248
  Pasta Fagioli Capra, 273
  Spaghetti with Zucchini
    Balls and Tomato Sauce,
    254
  Tofu and Chickpea Garlic
    Dip, 158
  Vegetarian Shepherd's Pie
    with Peppered Potato
    Topping, 256
  Warm Chickpea Salad, 193
  Zucchini, Mushroom and
    Bean Loaf with Tomato
    Sauce, 257
chocolate chips
  Banana Oatmeal Muffins
    (variation), 154
  Chocolate Cupcakes, 285
  Reverse Chocolate Chip
    Cookies, 288
  Sunflower Cookies, 287
cholesterol, 19, 22, 24–25
  in breast milk, 100
cilantro
  Black and White Bean Salsa,
    160
  Rice and Bean Salad, 187
  Sweet and Tasty Tofu, 250
Cinnamon Baked Pears, 282
cocoa powder
  Chocolate Cupcakes, 285
  Date Oatmeal Cake with
    Mocha Frosting, 286
  Reverse Chocolate Chip
    Cookies, 288
coconut
  Granola, 163
  No-Bake Trail Mix, 164
coconut milk
  Coconut Shrimp Curry, 230
  Curried Chicken, 210
coffee, 12, 125. *See also* caffeine
Coffee Cake, 149
colostrum, 99
constipation, 10, 19, 20, 88

corn
    Bean Salad, Tasty, 188
    Black and White Bean Salsa, 160
    Black Bean Salsa, 159
    Bulgur Salad, 194
    Chicken Tacos, 211
    Ginger Chili Sweet Potato Soup, 168
    Southwestern Sweet Potato Soup, 167
    Turkey Chili, 214
corn flakes cereal
    Chicken Nuggets, 212
    Crispy Chicken, 205
cornmeal
    Lemony Biscotti, 290
    Spaghetti with Zucchini Balls and Tomato Sauce, 254
Cottage Cheese Herb Dip, 156
Couscous, 266
Crab Cakes, The Narrows, 227
cramps (in legs), 92
cranberries
    Cranberry Oat Muffins, 152
    Muesli Mix, 143
Creamy Microwave Oatmeal, 144
Crispy Chicken, 205
Crunchy Broccoli Salad, 182
cucumber
    Asian Cucumber Salad, 179
    Greek Summer Salad, 184
    Mango, Strawberry and Cucumber Salad, 179
    Mango-Cucumber Salad, 178
    Sonoma Chicken Salad, 183
    Thai-Style Beef Salad, 198
    Tzatziki Sauce, 159
    Vietnamese Chicken and Rice Noodle Salad, 197
Curried Chicken, 210
Curried Lentil and Spinach Soup, 173
cyclamate, 43

D

dairy products, 39. *See also* cheese; milk
dates
    Big-Batch Bran Muffins, 150
    Date Oatmeal Cake with Mocha Frosting, 286
    Grandma's Rolled Oat Cookies, 289
dental health, 9, 90–91
depression, post-partum, 129
desserts, 281–95
DHA (docosahexaenoic acid), 69
diabetes, gestational, 84–86
Dietitians of Canada, 49
diets. *See also* weight management
    and breastfeeding, 126
    low-carbohydrate, 19, 55
    vegetarian, 65–69
diet soda, 9
dips, 156–60
DRI (dietary recommended intake), 18
drugs, 64
    and breastfeeding, 114, 120

E

E. coli, 35
eating disorders, 55
eclampsia, 94
Eggplant Dip, 157
eggs, 39
    Egg and Mushroom Fried Rice, 262
    The Narrows Crab Cakes, 227
    Orange Crème Caramel, 294
    Spinach Frittata, 264
    Swiss Chard Frittata in a Pita, 263
    Vanilla Custard, 293
electromagnetic fields (EMFs), 39
energy. *See* calorie intake
enzymes, 106
Equal®, 42

estrogen, 114
exercise, 12, 63, 96
    and breastfeeding, 128
    in first trimester, 75, 81
    post-partum, 127–28
    in second trimester, 86, 88, 89–90

F

Falafel in Pita, 260
Fassolada, 170
fatigue, 80–81, 96
fats, 21–25
    in breast milk, 100
    recommended intake, 25
    saturated *vs.* unsaturated, 21–22
    sources, 22
fatty acids
    monounsaturated, 21
    omega 3, 23–24, 37, 62, 129
    omega 6, 23–24, 62
    polyunsaturated, 21–22
    recommended intake, 23, 62
    sources, 24
    trans fatty acids, 22–23
fetal alcohol syndrome (FAS), 76
fiber, 19–20, 88
    recommended intake, 19, 20
    sources, 20, 139–40
Fiber-Full Bran Pancakes, 144
fish, 36–38, 124. *See also* salmon; tuna
    Baked Fish with Tomatoes and Roasted Red Pepper, 217
    Parmesan-Crusted Snapper with Tomato Olive Sauce, 226
    Parmesan Herb-Baked Fish Fillets, 216
    Sole and Spinach Casserole, 224
    South Side Halibut, 218
flatulence (gas), 20
fluid intake, 88, 125. *See also* water (drinking)

fluoride, 47

folate (folic acid), 8, 25–27
  recommended intake, 26, 64
  sources, 27, 59, 136–38
  vegetarians and, 69

food guides, 48
  Canada's Food Guide, 52–53
  MyPyramid (USDA), 50

foods. *See also* food guides; food safety
  aversion to, 78
  to avoid, 36–41
  calorie content, 73
  contaminants in, 36
  cravings for, 7, 78
  illnesses from, 32–35
  organic, 45

food safety, 32–47
  cooking temperatures, 35
  handling practices, 34
  quick guide, 44

foremilk, 101

fruit and fruit juices, 39. *See also specific types of fruit*
  Cinnamon Baked Pears, 282
  Granola, 163
  Just Peachy Pork, 243
  Meatballs with Teriyaki Sauce (variation), 236
  No-Bake Trail Mix, 164
  Roasted Yam Fajitas, 258

G

garlic
  Chickpea Tofu Stew, 251
  Eggplant Dip, 157
  Garlic Chili Shrimp, 229
  Green Beans and Tomato, 269
  Homestyle Meatloaf, 238
  Pasta Fagioli Capra, 273
  Pesto Chicken Thighs, 204
  Spaghetti with Zucchini Balls and Tomato Sauce, 254
  Tasty Bean Salad, 188
  Tzatziki Sauce, 159
  White Bean Soup with Swiss Chard, 171

Yogurt-Marinated Chicken, 202

gas (flatulence), 20

gastric reflux, 87

ginger, 81

Ginger, Soy and Lime Chicken, 203

Ginger Chili Sweet Potato Soup, 168

gingivitis, 90

glucose tolerance, 85, 86

glycemic index, 18–19

Grandma's Rolled Oat Cookies, 289

Granola, 163

Greek Lemon Chicken, 208

Greek Summer Salad, 184

Green Beans and Tomato, 269

Green Beans with Cashews, 268

greens. *See also* spinach
  Beef Lettuce Wraps, 240
  Beet and Feta Salad, 186
  Chicken Salad Amandine, 196
  Greens with Strawberries, 180
  Mandarin Orange Salad with Almonds, 181
  Mango, Strawberry and Cucumber Salad, 179
  Mediterranean Potato Salad, 195
  Portobello Mushrooms with Goat Cheese, 161
  Rapini with Balsamic Vinegar, 267
  Sonoma Chicken Salad, 183
  Sweet Green Pea Soup, 169
  Swiss Chard Frittata in a Pita, 263
  Thai-Style Beef Salad, 198
  White Bean Soup with Swiss Chard, 171

Grilled Honey-Ginger Chicken Breasts, 206

Grilled Tofu, 250

gums. *See* dental health

H

Healthy Cheese 'n' Herb Bread, 146

heartburn, 87

hemorrhoids, 10, 89

herbal products, 8, 11, 41
  and breastfeeding, 114

Herb-Flavored Vinaigrette, 195

herbs, fresh
  Linguine with Tuna, White Beans and Dill, 276
  Pesto Chicken Thighs, 204
  Sweet Green Pea Soup (variation), 169
  Tabbouleh, 192
  Warm Chickpea Salad, 193

Hermesetas®, 43

hindmilk, 101

Hoisin Stir-fried Vegetables and Tofu over Rice Noodles, 274

Homestyle Meatloaf, 238

Honey Dijon Chicken, 207

Honey Dill Salmon with Dijon, 220

Honey Mustard Salmon, 222

hormones, 80, 90, 98–99, 114
  in breast milk, 106

Hot and Sour Chicken Soup, 175

hot dogs, 38

Hummus, 158

hypertension, gestational, 94–96

I

implants (breast), 115

iron, 29–30, 59–60. *See also* anemia
  for babies, 103
  deficiency of, 60, 67, 83–84
  in first trimester, 76, 81
  in second trimester, 83–84
  sources, 30, 61, 138–39
  in vegetarian diet, 67

J

Just Peachy Pork, 243

K

ketosis, 86

L

lactation, 98–99. *See also* breastfeeding
lactation consultants, 125
lactose, 17
leg problems, 92, 93–94
lemon
   Baked Lemon Salmon with Mango Salsa, 221
   Greens with Strawberries, 180
   Lemony Biscotti, 290
   Lemony Lentil Soup with Spinach, 173
lentils
   Lemony Lentil Soup with Spinach, 173
   Lentil Dip, 156
   Lentil Salad, 191
   Lentil Spaghetti Sauce, 255
   Savory Red Lentil Soup, 172
   Vegetarian Chili (tip), 252
lettuce. *See* greens
lifestyle choices, 63–64, 76–77
Linguine with Tuna, White Beans and Dill, 276
linoleic acid, 24
linolenic acid, 23–24, 69
listeriosis, 32–33, 36

M

macronutrients, 16–25, 51
maltose, 17
Mandarin Orange Salad with Almonds, 181
mangoes
   Baked Lemon Salmon with Mango Salsa, 221
   Mango, Strawberry and Cucumber Salad, 179
   Mango-Cucumber Salad, 178
mastitis, 116
meal plans, 132–34. *See also* recipes

meat, 38. *See also* beef; pork
   Savory Lamb Chops, 246
   Spiced Veal Stir-fry, 242
Meatball Pasta Sauce, 237
Meatballs with Teriyaki Sauce, 236
Meatloaf "Muffins" with Barbecue Sauce, 239
meconium, 107
medications, 64
Mediterranean Potato Salad, 195
mercury contamination, 36, 38
metabolism, 14
micronutrients, 25–31
microwave ovens, 11, 39
milk
   Banana Berry Wake-Up Shake, 142
   Meatloaf "Muffins" with Barbecue Sauce, 239
   Orange Crème Caramel, 294
   Vanilla Custard, 293
Mixed Winter Beans, 248
Mocha Frosting, 286
monosaccharides, 17
morning sickness. *See* nausea and vomiting
MSG (monosodium glutamate), 11, 121
Muesli Mix, 143
muffins, 145, 150–54
multiples, 15
   breastfeeding, 111
   and weight gain, 71, 74, 75
multivitamins, 8, 74, 77, 124
mushrooms
   Asian Turkey and Noodle Soup, 176
   Beef Stroganoff, 233
   Crunchy Broccoli Salad, 182
   Egg and Mushroom Fried Rice, 262
   Hoisin Stir-fried Vegetables and Tofu over Rice Noodles, 274
   Hot and Sour Chicken Soup, 175

   Mushroom-Spinach Lasagna with Goat Cheese, 278
   Portobello Mushrooms with Goat Cheese, 161
   Sole and Spinach Casserole, 224
   Spiced Veal Stir-fry, 242
   Stir-fried Vegetables with Tofu, 249
   Tuna Garden Pasta, 277
   White Bean Soup with Swiss Chard, 171
   Zucchini, Mushroom and Bean Loaf with Tomato Sauce, 257
MyPyramid food guide (USDA), 50

N

The Narrows Crab Cakes, 227
nausea and vomiting, 7, 79–80
neotame, 43
neural tube defects, 26
nipples, 117, 118. *See also* breasts
nitrates, 45
No-Bake Trail Mix, 164
noodles
   Asian Turkey and Noodle Soup, 176
   Beef Stroganoff, 233
   Crunchy Broccoli Salad, 182
   Hoisin Stir-fried Vegetables and Tofu over Rice Noodles, 274
   Vietnamese Chicken and Rice Noodle Salad, 197
NutraSweet®, 42
nutrition
   before pregnancy, 48–69
   breastfeeding and, 107–8
   for children, 130
   in first trimester, 72–75, 81
   in multiple pregnancy, 74
   post-partum, 98–129
   in second trimester, 86
nuts, 9. *See also specific types of nuts*; peanuts

Granola, 163
Green Beans with Cashews, 268

O
oat bran
Banana Oat Bran Muffins, 153
Buttermilk Oat-Banana Cake, 284
Muesli Mix, 143
oatmeal
Autumn Crumble, 283
Banana Oat Bran Muffins, 153
Banana Oatmeal Muffins, 154
Berry Oatmeal Squares, 292
Breakfast Muesli to Go, 143
Buttermilk Oat-Banana Cake, 284
Cranberry Oat Muffins, 152
Creamy Microwave Oatmeal, 144
Date Oatmeal Cake with Mocha Frosting, 286
Granola, 163
Healthy Cheese 'n' Herb Bread, 146
Meatloaf "Muffins" with Barbecue Sauce, 239
Muesli Mix, 143
Reverse Chocolate Chip Cookies, 288
Rolled Oat Cookies, Grandma's, 289
Spaghetti with Zucchini Balls and Tomato Sauce, 254
Sunflower Cookies, 287
obesity. *See* overweight
olives
Couscous (variation), 266
Eggplant Dip, 157
Greek Summer Salad, 184

Linguine with Tuna, White Beans and Dill, 276
Tofu and Chickpea Garlic Dip, 158
Warm Chickpea Salad, 193
omega 3 fatty acids, 23–24, 37, 62, 129
omega 6 fatty acids, 23–24, 62
onions
Beef Fajitas, 232
Beef Souvlaki, 234
Chickpea Tofu Stew, 251
Curried Chicken, 210
Green Beans and Tomato, 269
Mango-Cucumber Salad, 178
Thai-Style Beef Salad, 198
Turkiaki Fiesta, 213
Tuscan Bean Salad, 190
oranges and orange juice
Carrot Orange Soup, 166
Couscous, 266
Greens with Strawberries, 180
Mandarin Orange Salad with Almonds, 181
Orange Crème Caramel, 294
Orange Ginger Pork and Vegetables, 244
Roasted Yam Fajitas, 258
Sunny Orange Shake, 142
organic foods, 45
overweight, 48, 49–51. *See also* weight gain; weight management

P
Parmesan-Crusted Snapper with Tomato Olive Sauce, 226
Parmesan Herb-Baked Fish Fillets, 216
pasta
Linguine with Tuna, White Beans and Dill, 276
Mushroom-Spinach Lasagna with Goat Cheese, 278
Pasta Fagioli Capra, 273

Pasta with Goat Cheese, Snow Peas and Tomato Coulis, 272
Penne with Tuna and Peppers, 280
Spaghetti with Broccoli, 275
Spaghetti with Zucchini Balls and Tomato Sauce, 254
Tuna Garden Pasta, 277
peanuts, 9, 78, 122, 125
Pears, Cinnamon Baked, 282
peas. *See also* snow peas
Egg and Mushroom Fried Rice, 262
Pasta Fagioli Capra, 273
Sweet Green Pea Soup, 169
pecans
Coffee Cake, 149
Sonoma Chicken Salad, 183
Zucchini Nut Loaf, 148
Penne with Tuna and Peppers, 280
peppers, chili. *See also* bell peppers
Green Beans and Tomato, 269
Hot and Sour Chicken Soup, 175
Mango-Cucumber Salad, 178
Southwestern Sweet Potato Soup, 167
Spaghetti with Broccoli (variation), 275
Pesto Chicken Thighs, 204
pets, 34
phytate, 31
phytoestrogens, 38
pica, 84
pine nuts
Pesto Chicken Thighs, 204
Portobello Mushrooms with Goat Cheese, 161
pita breads
Beef Souvlaki, 234
Falafel in Pita, 260
Swiss Chard Frittata in a Pita, 263

PKU (phenylketonuria), 42
pollution, 36, 38, 121
polysaccharides, 17
pork
    Cabbage Rolls, Quick and Easy, 241
    Just Peachy Pork, 243
    Orange Ginger Pork and Vegetables, 244
    Teriyaki Pork Chops, 245
    Portobello Mushrooms with Goat Cheese, 161
post-partum depression, 129
potatoes. *See also* sweet potatoes
    Baked Chicken and Potato Dinner, 201
    Mediterranean Potato Salad, 195
    Salmon with Roasted Vegetables, 219
    Southwestern Sweet Potato Soup, 167
    Vegetarian Shepherd's Pie with Peppered Potato Topping, 256
poultry. *See* chicken; turkey
pre-eclampsia, 93, 94–96
pregnancy
    first trimester, 70–81
    foods to avoid, 36–41
    multiple, 15, 71, 74–75
    nutrient needs before, 56–62
    in older women, 56
    second trimester, 16, 82–91
    teenage, 56
    third trimester, 16, 92–97
    weight gain during, 12, 14, 70–72, 74, 95
progesterone, 80, 90
protein, 21
    in breast milk, 100
    in first trimester, 72–74
    recommended intake, 21, 74
    in vegetarian diet, 67
protein shakes/bars, 10
pumpkin seeds
    Autumn Crumble (tip), 283
    Granola, 163

Q

Quick and Easy Cabbage Rolls, 241
quick breads, 145–48

R

raisins and currants
    Autumn Crumble, 283
    Big-Batch Bran Muffins, 150
    Carrot Bran Muffins, 151
    Couscous, 266
    Creamy Microwave Oatmeal, 144
    Sonoma Chicken Salad, 183
    Sunflower Cookies, 287
    Zucchini Nut Loaf (tip), 148
Rapini with Balsamic Vinegar, 267
Raspberry Basil Vinaigrette, 193
recipes. *See also* meal plans
    for calcium, 135–36
    for fiber, 139–40
    for first trimester, 73
    for folate, 136–38
    for iron, 138–39
    for vegetarians, 247–64
Reverse Chocolate Chip Cookies, 288
rice
    Beef Lettuce Wraps, 240
    Cabbage Rolls, Quick and Easy, 241
    Egg and Mushroom Fried Rice, 262
    Rice and Bean Salad, 187
    Spinach and Rice Salad, 185
    Spinach Risotto, 261
Roasted Yam Fajitas, 258
Rolled Oat Cookies, Grandma's, 289

S

saccharin, 43
salads, 177–98
Salami and White Bean Salad, 190

salmon
    Baked Lemon Salmon with Mango Salsa, 221
    Honey Dill Salmon with Dijon, 220
    Salmon Burgers, 223
    Salmon with Roasted Vegetables, 219
    Soy-Glazed Salmon, 222
salmonellosis, 34–35
Savory Lamb Chops, 246
Savory Red Lentil Soup, 172
seafood, 227–30
sesame seeds
    Beef Lettuce Wraps, 240
    Crunchy Broccoli Salad, 182
    Granola, 163
    Healthy Cheese 'n' Herb Bread, 146
    Sticky Sesame Chicken, 209
    Turkiaki Fiesta, 213
shakes, 142
shrimp
    Coconut Shrimp Curry, 230
    Garlic Chili Shrimp, 229
    Sweet and Spicy Shrimp with Broccoli, 228
side dishes, 265–70
sleep, 81
    babies and, 115
smoking, 63–64
snacks, 91, 155–64
snow peas
    Asian Turkey and Noodle Soup, 176
    Pasta with Goat Cheese, Snow Peas and Tomato Coulis, 272
    Stir-fried Vegetables with Tofu, 249
    Turkiaki Fiesta, 213
sodium, 11
Sole and Spinach Casserole, 224
Sonoma Chicken Salad, 183
soups, 165–76
South Side Halibut, 218

Southwestern Sweet Potato Soup, 167
soy, 38, 123
Soy-Glazed Salmon, 222
Spaghetti with Broccoli, 275
Spaghetti with Zucchini Balls and Tomato Sauce, 254
Spiced Veal Stir-fry, 242
spinach
  Borscht, 174
  Lemony Lentil Soup with Spinach, 173
  Mushroom-Spinach Lasagna with Goat Cheese, 278
  Sole and Spinach Casserole, 224
  Spinach and Rice Salad, 185
  Spinach Frittata, 264
  Spinach Risotto, 261
  Swiss Chard Frittata in a Pita (tip), 263
Splenda®, 43
starches, 17
Sticky Sesame Chicken, 209
Stir-fried Vegetables with Tofu, 249
strawberries
  Greens with Strawberries, 180
  Mandarin Orange Salad with Almonds (tip), 181
  Mango, Strawberry and Cucumber Salad, 179
  Strawberry Sorbet, 295
stress, 80
stretch marks, 10, 97
Sucaryl®, 43
sucralose, 43
sucrose, 17
sugars, 16–17
Sugar Twin®, 43
Sunett®, 42
sunflower seeds
  Chickpea-Herb Burgers, 253
  Crunchy Broccoli Salad, 182
  Granola, 163
  Sonoma Chicken Salad, 183

Sunflower Cookies, 287
Sunny Orange Shake, 142
supplements. See also multivitamins
  iron, 84
  omega 3, 24
  vitamin and mineral, 27, 64, 76–77, 100
Sweet and Spicy Shrimp with Broccoli, 228
Sweet and Tasty Tofu, 250
sweeteners, artificial, 9, 42–43
Sweet Green Pea Soup, 169
sweet potatoes
  Ginger Chili Sweet Potato Soup, 168
  Roasted Yam Fajitas, 258
  Salmon with Roasted Vegetables, 219
  Southwestern Sweet Potato Soup, 167
  Vegetarian Shepherd's Pie with Peppered Potato Topping (tip), 256
Swiss chard. See greens

T

Tabbouleh, 192
Tacos, Chicken, 211
Tasty Bean Salad, 188
teeth, 9, 90–91
Teriyaki Pork Chops, 245
Teriyaki Sauce, 236
Thai-Style Beef Salad, 198
thrush, 116, 117
tofu
  Chickpea Tofu Stew, 251
  Grilled Tofu, 250
  Hoisin Stir-fried Vegetables and Tofu over Rice Noodles, 274
  Hot and Sour Chicken Soup, 175
  Stir-fried Vegetables with Tofu, 249
  Sweet and Tasty Tofu, 250
  Tofu and Chickpea Garlic Dip, 158

tomatoes
  Baked Fish with Tomatoes and Roasted Red Pepper, 217
  Beef Fajitas, 232
  Beef Souvlaki, 234
  Black and White Bean Salsa, 160
  Black Bean Salsa, 159
  Bulgur Salad, 194
  Chickpea Tofu Stew, 251
  Curried Chicken, 210
  Fassolada, 170
  Greek Summer Salad, 184
  Green Beans and Tomato, 269
  Lentil Salad, 191
  Mixed Winter Beans, 248
  Mushroom-Spinach Lasagna with Goat Cheese, 278
  Pasta Fagioli Capra, 273
  Pasta with Goat Cheese, Snow Peas and Tomato Coulis, 272
  Savory Red Lentil Soup, 172
  Spaghetti with Broccoli, 275
  Spaghetti with Zucchini Balls and Tomato Sauce, 254
  Tabbouleh, 192
  Thai-Style Beef Salad, 198
  Turkey Chili, 214
  Vegetarian Chili, 252
  White Bean Salad with Lemon-Dill Vinaigrette, 189
tortillas
  Beef Fajitas, 232
  Roasted Yam Fajitas, 258
toxemia, 94–96
toxoplasmosis, 33–34
trans fatty acids, 22–23
trihalomethanes (THMs), 46
tumors, pregnancy, 90–91
tuna
  Linguine with Tuna, White Beans and Dill, 276

tuna (*continued*)

Mediterranean Potato Salad, 195

Penne with Tuna and Peppers, 280

Spaghetti with Broccoli (variation), 275

Tuna Garden Pasta, 277

Tuscan Bean Salad, 190

turkey

Asian Turkey and Noodle Soup, 176

Meatballs with Teriyaki Sauce, 236

Turkey Chili, 214

Turkiaki Fiesta, 213

20-Minute Chili, 235

Tuscan Bean Salad, 190

20-Minute Chili, 235

Tzatziki Sauce, 159

V

Vanilla Custard, 293

vegetables, 39. *See also specific types of vegetables*

Autumn Crumble, 283

Hoisin Stir-fried Vegetables and Tofu over Rice Noodles, 274

Lentil Salad, 191

Mixed Winter Beans, 248

Salmon with Roasted Vegetables, 219

Vegetarian Chili, 252

vegetarians, 30, 65–69

recipes for, 247–64

Vegetarian Shepherd's Pie with Peppered Potato Topping, 256

Vietnamese Chicken and Rice Noodle Salad, 197

vitamin A, 77

vitamin B-12, 30–31

recommended intake, 30, 68

vegetarians and, 68

vitamin B-6 (pyridoxine), 81

vitamin D, 28–29, 58

babies and, 100, 124

in breast milk, 101

vegetarians and, 68

vitamin K, 101

vitamin supplements, 27, 64, 76–77. *See also specific vitamins*; multivitamins

W

walnuts

Date Oatmeal Cake with Mocha Frosting, 286

Healthy Cheese 'n' Herb Bread (tip), 146

Zucchini Nut Loaf, 148

Warm Chickpea Salad, 193

water (drinking), 12, 45–47. *See also* fluid intake

for baby, 124

bottled, 46–47

weight gain, 12, 14, 70–72. *See also* overweight

in babies, 107, 113

in multiple pregnancies, 71, 74, 75

and pre-eclampsia, 95

weight management, 15, 51, 54–55. *See also* overweight

after pregnancy, 126–27

Weight Watchers® sweetener, 43

wheat bran

Autumn Crumble, 283

Banana Oat Bran Muffins, 153

Buttermilk Oat-Banana Cake, 284

Meatloaf "Muffins" with Barbecue Sauce, 239

Muesli Mix, 143

Sunflower Cookies, 287

wheat germ

Fiber-Full Bran Pancakes, 144

Granola, 163

Muesli Mix, 143

Sunflower Cookies, 287

White Bean Salad with Lemon-Dill Vinaigrette, 189

White Bean Soup with Swiss Chard, 171

Y

yams. *See* sweet potatoes

yogurt

Banana Berry Wake-Up Shake, 142

Breakfast Muesli to Go, 143

Cinnamon Baked Pears, 282

Coffee Cake, 149

Cottage Cheese Herb Dip, 156

Crispy Chicken, 205

Sunny Orange Shake, 142

Tzatziki Sauce, 159

Yogurt-Marinated Chicken, 202

Z

zinc, 31, 60–62

recommended intake, 31, 62

vegetarians and, 68

zucchini

Bulgur Salad, 194

Hoisin Stir-fried Vegetables and Tofu over Rice Noodles, 274

Salmon with Roasted Vegetables, 219

Spaghetti with Zucchini Balls and Tomato Sauce, 254

Zucchini, Mushroom and Bean Loaf with Tomato Sauce, 257

Zucchini Nut Loaf, 148